The City & Guilds textbook

Level 2

Diploma in Care
FOR THE ADULT CARE WORKER APPRENTICESHIP

❚ Maria Ferreiro Peteiro

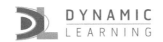

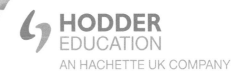

Hachette UK's policy is to use papers that are natural, renewable and recyclable products and made from wood grown in well-managed forests and other controlled sources. The logging and manufacturing processes are expected to conform to the environmental regulations of the country of origin.

Orders: please contact Hachette UK Distribution, Hely Hutchinson Centre, Milton Road, Didcot, Oxfordshire, OX11 7HH. Telephone: +44 (0)1235 827827. Email education@hachette.co.uk
Lines are open from 9 a.m. to 5 p.m., Monday to Friday. You can also order through our website: www.hoddereducation.co.uk

ISBN: 978 1 5104 2911 6

© Maria Ferreiro Peteiro 2018

First published in 2018 by
Hodder Education,
An Hachette UK Company
Carmelite House
50 Victoria Embankment
London EC4Y 0DZ
www.hoddereducation.co.uk

Impression number 10 9 8 7 6 5

Year   2023

Cover photo © kolinko_tanya - stock.adobe.com
Illustrations by Aptara Inc.
Typeset in India by Aptara Inc.
Printed and bound by CPI Group (UK) Ltd, Croydon, CR0 4YY

A catalogue record for this title is available from the British Library.

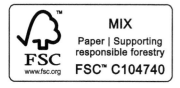

Contents

Optional units:

Popular optional units are available online at:
www.hoddereducation.co.uk/cityandguilds/adultcareextras

Acknowledgements and About the Author

About the Author

Maria Ferreiro Peteiro commenced her career in Health and Social Care in 1990 living and working in a lay community in France alongside individuals with a range of disabilities and health conditions. Maria's journey continued through a range of services and settings in the UK that included working within and leading provision for young and older adults who have learning disabilities, physical disabilities, dementia, mental health needs, challenging needs and sensory impairments. Having achieved her BA (Hons) in Health and Social Care, Maria embarked on delivering a range of Health and Social Care programmes and qualifications in both college and work-based settings. The experience she gained in work and academic settings led Maria to become a qualified assessor, internal and external quality assurer. Maria continues to practise in the Social Care field with adults, children and young people, and continues to externally quality assure vocational-based qualifications in Health and Social Care and Children and Young People's Services at Levels 2, 3 and 5.

Author's acknowledgements

I wish to thank Stephen, Imogen and the Hodder team for all their hard work and a very special thank you must go to my very supportive and encouraging editor Sundus.

To my husband Chris, your support and understanding were fantastic! And to my dog Simba, my extra-long walks with you couldn't have come at a better time!

Picture credits

Every effort has been made to trace and acknowledge ownership of copyright. The publishers will be glad to make suitable arrangements with any copyright holders whom it has not been possible to contact. The author and publishers would like to thank the following for permission to reproduce copyright material.

p.1 © Jacob Lund/stock.adobe.com; p.9 © dglimages/stock.adobe.com; p.10 © Cultura Creative (RF)/Alamy Stock Photo; p.16 © John Birdsall/REX/Shutterstock; p.17 © belahoche/stock.adobe.com; p.27 left © godfer/stock.adobe.com, right © jovannig/stock.adobe.com; p.28 © Sandor Kacso/stock.adobe.com; p.43 © Jules Selmes/Hodder Education; p.46 © Jacob Lund/stock.adobe.com; p.56 © Dan Race/Fotolia; p.66 © BSIP SA/Alamy Stock Photo; p.83 © Monkey Business Images/Shutterstock.com; p.87 © digitalskillet1/stock.adobe.com; p.96 © Adam Wasilewski/stock.adobe.com; p.104 © Andrey Popov/stock.adobe.com; p.106 © Photographee.eu/Fotolia; p.111 © Catchlight Visual Services/Alamy Stock Photo; p.118 © Rido/stock.adobe.com; p.120 © dglimages/stock.adobe.com; p.122 © Monkey Business Images/Shutterstock.com; p.130 M.Dörr & M.Frommherz/stock.adobe.com; p.135 © Monkey Business/stock.adobe.com; p.139 © JackF/stock.adobe.com; p.149 © Kacso Sandor/123RF.com; p.152 © Robert Kneschke/stock.adobe.com; p.182 © Alexander Raths/stock.adobe.com; p.186 © ACP prod/stock.adobe.com; p.207 © Monkey Business/stock.adobe.com; p.217 © Alamy Stock Photo; p.230 © JackF /stock.adobe.com; p.233 © Jules Selmes/Hodder Education; p.239 © mnirat/stock.adobe.com; p.248 © jdwfoto/stock.adobe.com; p.254 © Jules Selmes/Hodder Education; p.259 © Monkey Business/Fotolia; p. 261 © M.Dörr & M.Frommherz/stock.adobe.com; p.273 © Alexander Raths/Fotolia; p.280 © Peter Maszlen/stock.adobe.com; p.289 © deanm1974/Fotolia; p.298 © belahoche/stock.adobe.com; p.300 © Photographee.eu/stock.adobe.com; p.309 © Photographee.eu/Fotolia; p.323 © Monkey Business/stock.adobe.com; p.346 © Alamy Stock Photo; p.355 © Crown Copyright; p.377 © bilderzwerg/stock.adobe.com

This book contains public sector information licensed under the Open Government Licence v3.0.

How to use this book

This textbook covers all nine mandatory units for the City & Guilds Level 2 Diploma in Care.

Key features of the book

Learning outcomes

LO1: Understand why communication is important in the work setting

LO2: Be able to meet the communication and language needs, wishes and preferences of individuals

Learn about what you are going to cover in each unit.

AC 1.1 **Identify different reasons why people communicate**
What is communication?
When you communicate, you are:

Learning outcomes and assessment criteria are clearly stated and fully mapped to the specification.

Getting started

Think about a time when you have been outside your care setting, perhaps at a party or in a noisy environment when you were with a friend? How did the environment affect your communication?

Short activity or discussion to introduce you to the topic.

Key terms

RNIB stands for the Royal National Institute of Blind People. This is a UK charity that provides information, advice, practical and emotional support to people affected by sight loss.

Understand important terms and concepts.

Reflect on it

3.1 Barriers
Reflect on the different people you communicate with in your work setting. What barriers are there to communicating effectively with each person?

Learn to reflect on your own experiences, skills and practice, and develop the skills necessary to become a reflective practitioner.

Research it

3.2 Reducing barriers

Research ways of reducing communication barriers in the environment. You might like to look at the following website for useful tips

Royal College of Nursing, First Steps, Barriers to communication:

http://rcnhca.org.uk/top-page-001/barriers-to-communication

Enhance your understanding of topics with research-led activities encouraging you to explore an area in more detail.

Evidence opportunity

4.4 When to seek advice and why

Discuss with your manager when it may be necessary to seek advice about confidentiality in your work setting and the reasons why.

Test your understanding of the assessment criteria, apply your knowledge and generate evidence.

Dos and don'ts when dealing with others	
Do	Explain the reasons why you are unable to give out information to family members.
Don't	Feel pressured to give family members information just because they are related to the individual and even if they have the individual's interests at heart.

Useful advice and tips for best practice.

6Cs

C

Courage

Courage is required when speaking up for an individual. Not doing so may put the individual at risk and may mean that their communication and language needs,

Understand how each of the 6Cs (care, compassion, competence, communication, courage and commitment) can be applied in each unit.

Case study

2.3 Seeking advice about communication

Riya is new to care and has recently begun working as a domiciliary care worker providing care and support to older adults living in their own homes. Her main tasks and responsibilities

Learn about real-life scenarios and think about issues you may face in the workplace.

Knowledge: do you know how to identify barriers to communication?
Do you know the reasons why you may be having difficulties communicating with an individual? Do you know how to reduce any barriers?
Why is it important to check that communication has been understood by an individual?
Do you know what sources of information are available if you are finding it difficult to communicate with an individual in the care setting where you work?
Did you know that you have just answered questions about how to identify barriers and where to find support available in relation to communication?

Test your understanding of some of the knowledge, skills and behaviours you need at the end of each learning outcome.

Reflective exemplar	
Introduction	I work as a personal assistant with Jo, a young man who has learning disabilities and lives on his own in a flat. My duties involve supporting Jo to use public transport to travel to and from his workplace and go shopping every week for food and household goods.
What happened?	Last week when I was supporting Jo with food shopping in the supermarket, one of the cashiers

Explore examples of reflective accounts tailored to the content of the unit and understand how you can write your own accounts.

Suggestions for using the activities	
LO4 Be able to apply principles and practices relating to confidentiality at work	
4.1 Evidence opportunity (page 31)	Tell your assessor about your understanding of the term 'confidentiality'. You could also write a personal statement or reflective account about your experience of the meaning of the term 'confidentiality' in relation to your work role and setting.

Summaries of all the activities in the unit that can be used to show your knowledge and skills for the assessment criteria. This also includes other suggestions for using the activities and presenting your knowledge and skills. These are suggestions and your assessor will be able to provide more guidance on how you can evidence your knowledge and skills.

Legislation	
Relevant Act	**It states that:**
Data Protection Act 1998	information and data must be: processed fairly and lawfully; used only for the purpose it was intended to be used for; be adequate, relevant, accurate and up to date; held for no longer than is necessary; used in line with the rights of individuals; kept secure; and not transferred to other countries without the individual's permission.
General Data Protection Regulation (GDPR) 2018	In May 2018 the General Data Protection Regulation came into force. It provides detailed guidance to organisations on how to govern and manage people's personal information.

Summaries of legislation relevant to the study of each unit.

Resources for further reading and research

Books

Butler, S.J. (2004) *Hearing and Sight Loss – A Handbook for Professional Carers*, Age Concern

Weblinks

www.alzheimers.org.uk Alzheimer's Society – information on communication methods and strategies to use with individuals who have Alzheimer's disease

Includes references to books, websites and other sources for further reading and research.

Introduction

The qualification

Becoming a care worker is a choice that people make at different points in their life. Perhaps you decided you wanted to become a care worker when you were at school, or perhaps you have had a role in another profession and made the decision later in life. Whenever you made the decision to enter the care profession, for whatever reason, or whether you decided to work in a residential care home or assist someone to live independently in their own home, it is certain that the profession you are entering is a rewarding one; one where you provide a valuable service to those you care for.

In order to achieve the Level 2 Diploma in Care, you need to be in a job role where you provide care and support; for example you may be an adult care worker, support worker or personal assistant.

This book contains all nine mandatory units that you will need to complete for the City & Guilds Level 2 Diploma in Care. The mandatory units cover safeguarding and protection, your responsibilities as a care worker, communication, the duty of care you have to those you support, how you must handle information, your personal development, equality and inclusion, health, safety and well-being and person-centred approaches which are so key to ensuring the individual is at the centre of the support you provide.

You will also need to complete a number of optional units to achieve the diploma. Some popular optional units are available online at: www.hoddereducation.co.uk/cityandguilds/adultcareextras

The qualification will allow you to learn, develop and demonstrate the skills and knowledge required for employment and/or career progression in healthcare and adult care settings. The qualification is also linked to the following Trailblazer Apprenticeships:

- Adult Care Worker (mandatory in the standard)
- Healthcare Support Worker (optional for on programme).

Study skills

To complete the diploma to the best of your ability, you will need to ensure you develop the skills that are essential not only in providing high-quality care in the setting, but also when preparing assignments and documentation for your portfolio and other assessments. Here, we briefly discuss some of the skills that you will need to learn and develop for study as you progress through the diploma.

Spelling, punctuation, grammar

Being able to clearly express what you want to say is essential for good communication and ensuring others understand you. In your role, it is likely that you will write letters, reports and add notes to care or support plans and documents that will be seen by others. Ensuring that the information in these documents can be easily understood is important so that others are able to understand what is written and to ensure efficient practice. It also means that those you work with will view you as someone who is competent with good command of vocabulary, spelling, punctuation and grammar; this will reflect positively on you as a professional. Writing in full sentences, placing words in sentences in the correct order and using the correct punctuation shows that you take pride in your work. You will also need to apply these skills when you provide evidence and assignments for your portfolio so that you are able to demonstrate your knowledge and convey this in a grammatically correct, clear and accessible way.

Skills of reflection

Reflection is one of the key skills you will need to develop as a care worker. It encourages you to think back on your practice and consolidate what you have learned so that you can make changes and improvements. It involves thinking back over a situation or event that happened and understanding what you gained from the experience and the improvements or changes you will make, or have already made. For example, you may have attended a training update on safeguarding and, as a result, gained a greater insight into your role and the responsibilities for safeguarding individuals from abuse. This in turn means that your awareness on how to do this in your day-to-day work activities has been raised.

It is important to remember that reflecting involves thinking about what did not go well but also what did go well. It can be very tempting to just think about the negatives, and what went badly in a situation. This, of course, will help you to improve. However, it is important to think positively, and also focus on what went well so that you are able to repeat your behaviour and skills in other situations and also pass on good practice. In this way, you are always developing in your role and providing the best possible care which is why it is so important that you take time to reflect.

In each of the units, you will find an example of a reflective account. These will guide you with the different steps involved in writing your own reflective accounts, including:

- an introduction that sets the scene
- an account of the occasion, details of what happened
- a reflection of what worked well
- a reflection of what did not go as well
- a reflection of what you could do to improve
- all the assessment criteria it is directly linked to.

Research

Research involves exploring and finding out information about a topic to further develop your knowledge and understanding of it. Depending on the topic, research can be carried out in different ways such as by using the internet, books and/or journals. You are likely to use research skills not only for studying for this qualification but also in your personal life and at work. For example, you may have carried out research in relation to the best restaurant to go to in your local area or you may have been asked to explore different activities that an individual you care for can participate in at work. In health and/or social care, there are many examples of how and why research is used. For example, to find a cure for Alzheimer's, to gain a better understanding of diabetes or to find out how to improve work practices when supporting individuals with care or support needs.

If you think about an occasion when you successfully carried out research, you will have used a range of different skills and have gone through a process to be able to carry it out effectively. You would have begun by thinking about the purpose of carrying out the research, what you wanted to find out and why. You would then have set out a plan for how to do this, including deciding on the methods of collating the information, the sources of information to use and a timescale for doing this. You would then have moved on to collating the information, interpreting the information you collated before finally reviewing your research against the original purpose of your research and presenting your findings. In this way, you are able to develop your knowledge and skills beyond the setting and discover new, up-to-date background information which will help you to keep on top of what is happening in your profession and related stories.

Reading

In your role, you will read various documents; it might be this textbook, news articles as part of research or care plans, for example. You will therefore need to know when you need to read documents in depth, and when you can 'skim' read. Skim reading refers to reading to gain an overview or insight into the context of a topic. For example, you may 'skim' through a unit by reading the introduction or titles of each section to gain an insight into what the unit is about. However, in order to fully understand the unit and content of any document, you will need to carefully read the content in detail and not just the key points like when you skim read. It is important that you understand when you should read documents in detail and when you can skim read.

Time management

Managing your time effectively involves being able to achieve timescales set for the completion of, for example, assignments. This means being able to complete them on time whilst not compromising on the quality of your work, and allowing yourself enough time. To be able to manage your time effectively you need to be realistic about what you can and cannot do. There is no point in setting yourself an unrealistic target; not only will you not achieve this but not doing so will make you feel negative about yourself. Planning how to best manage your time is key! Perhaps you have children so you plan to study in the evenings or night when they have gone to bed and you have no distractions, or perhaps you care for a family member and find mornings a better time to study. Make a plan and stick to it by ensuring you review it from time to time to check that you are on track.

Referencing

Referencing the work and ideas of others means that you will not be plagiarising (a topic you will learn more about below). Referencing shows that you have carried out research in detail, and that you have read widely. It also shows that you have thought about and connected the ideas of others such as theorists and authors. It means you can show that you have a valid and credible basis for your work and ideas. Referencing also enables those reading your work to explore in more detail the topic you have referenced and to find out more about it.

Plagiarism

Plagiarism occurs when you do not acknowledge the work or ideas of others and claim that it is your own. This is unethical and illegal and has serious consequences including not being allowed to continue to study for your qualification. Therefore, referencing the work and ideas of others when submitting your work and assignments is a must.

Command words

The knowledge-based command words that you will find across this book and the specification will include 'describe', 'explain' and 'identify' for example, and will set out what you are expected to know or understand. The skills-based command words will include 'demonstrate' and 'use', for example, and these will set out what you will be expected to do or show through your work practice. Your assessor will be able to provide more guidance on the definitions of command words.

Assignments and work products

Work products

Work products can include plans and records of what you have produced during your everyday work activities. For example, you may have evidence of a social activity you carried out with an individual in the form of a short video film, or an entry you made in the daily report book about the assistance you provided to an individual with care or support needs with regard to eating and drinking.

Work products may also include other records that you and others may contribute to such as your supervision record (you and your manager would discuss this) or an individual's risk assessment (you and your colleagues would contribute to this). Sometimes work products can be included in your portfolio, but you should speak to your assessor who will be able to provide more guidance on this.

You will also need to ensure **confidentiality** when you include any work products in your portfolio that relate to an individual you care for or others including the individual's family, friends, or those you work with.

Assignments

Assignments are opportunities for you to show how you apply the knowledge and skills you have gained during your studies. An assignment could include a scenario or a brief that sets out the tasks that you are required to complete. For example, you may be given a scenario of an individual with care needs who discloses that they are being abused; you may be tasked with showing your knowledge and understanding of what actions to take when an individual makes a disclosure of abuse and how to report it. Or you may be given a brief that requires you to plan and deliver a recreational activity with an individual. You will also be asked to demonstrate skills as part of other tasks.

Assessment

How will I be assessed?

In order to achieve the Level 2 Diploma in Care, you will need to have a completed

portfolio of evidence covering the assessment criteria for each unit that you study, including the mandatory and optional units required. City & Guilds advise that the majority of assessment for this competence-based qualification will take place in the workplace under real work conditions.

The portfolio will contain evidence of your knowledge, skills and behaviours. The portfolio can be a physical paper-based file or a digital e-portfolio, and can include personal statements, reflective accounts, records of discussions, witness testimonies, assignments and work products, some of which we discuss below.

Observations

These are real-life observations of your practices in the setting where you work and will more often than not be carried out by your assessor.

Your assessor

Your assessor will be the main person who will plan and discuss the observations of your work practices with you and will be responsible for recording your observations. Expert witnesses may also on occasions be used but you will agree this with your assessor, this is discussed in more detail below. Observations of your work practices must reflect your everyday work activities and will therefore be carried out in the adult care setting where you work. You will be responsible for obtaining permission from those in your care setting for your observations to take place. This may, for example, involve seeking permission before the observation takes place and you may need to gain this permission from your employer, the individuals with care or support needs, individuals' families, friends and other professionals.

It may not be possible to plan all of your observations as some of them may be 'unexpected events' that occur in your work setting such as a fire drill or an individual having difficulties communicating. Your assessor will be responsible for collating this unplanned evidence if they deem it suitable to do so.

Witness testimonies

Witness testimonies can be used as evidence of your work practices that have been witnessed.

Your manager, for example, will be able to provide witness testimonies of your practice in the setting.

Witness testimonies can be provided orally or in writing and must be recorded. They must include your name, the date, time, venue and details of the work activity observed as well as the details of the witness including their name, designation/role and contact details (for example, telephone number or email address). Again, it will be a good idea to ensure it is okay to include this information.

Expert witnesses

Expert witnesses may be able to observe your working practices if they have current expertise in a specialist area such as diabetes care or when the observation is of a sensitive area such as end of life care. However, expert witnesses can be used only in specific circumstances and when agreed with your assessor.

Professional discussions

Professional discussions are planned and structured and are carried out between you and your assessor; it is an in-depth discussion that is led by you. It is a good way of presenting evidence through discussion, clearly showing the knowledge you have gained, the skills you have developed and the behaviours you have. It is a way of showing how you have met the requirements of the qualification. Your portfolio can form the basis of the discussion and so can other pieces of evidence that you may have collated such as work products and witness testimonies can also be discussed.

Personal statements and reflective accounts

Written accounts detailing knowledge and skills related to the assessment criteria can also be included in your portfolio.

Recognition of prior learning

Relevant prior credited learning that you have undertaken will also be recognised. This can take the form of not only certificated courses but may also include work placements or volunteering opportunities you have undertaken.

End-point assessment

The Level 2 Diploma in Care is linked to the Adult Care Worker Apprenticeship. If you are completing this qualification as part of an apprenticeship, you will need to complete the end-point assessment. You can find out more about this at: www.hoddereducation.co.uk/cityandguilds/adultcareextras

6Cs

The 6Cs are values which underpin Compassion in Practice, the national strategy that was developed for nurses, midwives and care staff, and was launched in December 2012. They are values which should underpin your practice; you are expected not just to know what these are, but also be able to demonstrate them in your practice. You can find out more here: www.skillsforcare.org.uk/Documents/Standards-legislation/6Cs/6Cs-in-social-care-guide.pdf

- **Care** is at the heart of the work we do, helping to improve the lives of individuals we support, and something we should always be striving to improve.
- **Communication** is key to forming and maintaining strong successful relationships with those we support and work with.
- **Compassion** and treating those we support with kindness and empathy are essential for upholding bonds and ensuring individuals trust us to care for them with respect and dignity.
- **Courage** allows us to speak up for those we care for especially when we have concerns, and doing the right thing for them in order to ensure that their rights are upheld. It also means having the courage to try and test new practice.
- **Competence** means fulfilling our roles to the best of our ability, understanding the needs of those we provide support for, and having the expertise and knowledge to effectively carry out our roles.
- **Commitment** means to be dedicated to providing high-quality care and helping to improve the lives of those we provide support for.

You can find out more about the Skills for Care definitions of the 6Cs here: www.skillsforcare.org.uk/Documents/Standards-legislation/6Cs/6Cs-in-social-care-guide.pdf

The 6Cs are also addressed in each unit in this textbook with clear links to how they are relevant to the content of the unit or assessment criteria.

Knowledge, Skills, Behaviours

Knowledge: This includes your understanding of the units you study and reasons for why you practise the way you do at work. It will also include understanding of a range of topics and areas such as legislation, different cultures, how to build good relationships, how to communicate and interact with others, and expectations that others, such as your employer, individuals and individuals' families, have of you. Knowledge will also cover more than just your knowledge and understanding of health and/or social care; it will include wider knowledge of cultures and the people you will work with, for example.

Skills: There are a wide range of skills that you will learn, practise and develop in your role and as you complete this diploma. This will include skills in communicating, safeguarding individuals, reporting and recording and also the skills that make you unique and bring out your qualities such as showing compassion, warmth, kindness and empathy. You will also develop and be required to show the skills you have when studying for this qualification such as your ability to interpret information, describe an event or analyse a task so that you can make improvements.

Behaviours: These include how you put into practice the personal qualities you have. For example, how do you use verbal and non-verbal communication to show your empathy towards an individual? How do you convey your happiness when an individual tells you that they have achieved the goal that they have been working towards? Your behaviours reflect the kind of person you are, for example, professional, kind and considerate.

You can access more information about this City & Guilds qualification and specification by searching for 'Adult Care' or '3095' on their website: www.cityandguilds.com

Communication in care settings (203)

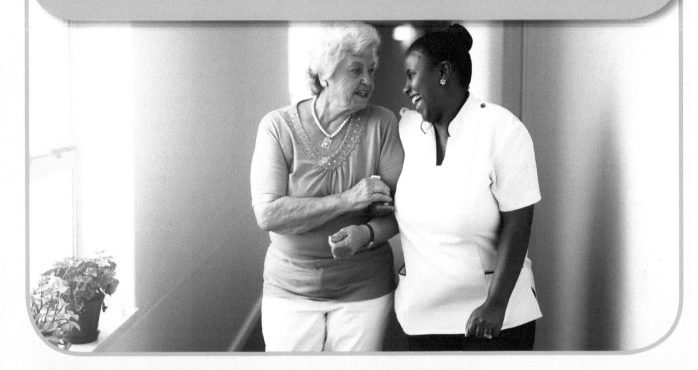

About this unit

Credit value: 3
Guided learning hours: 20

Working in care involves making a positive impact on the lives of young people, adults, their families and carers. Good communication is essential for developing caring relationships and working successfully as part of a team.

In this unit you will learn about why it is important to communicate effectively, and the different **methods** and technological aids you can use to do so. You will learn how to adapt the way you communicate so that you meet individuals' communication and language needs, their wishes and **preferences**. You will understand how to overcome and reduce **barriers** that may

get in the way of communicating effectively, for example cultural differences, to ensure that your communication is understood. You will be able to show how to communicate clearly and responsibly with people of different backgrounds, in ways that respect equality and diversity, and use a range of techniques while keeping information safe and confidential.

You will also have an opportunity to explore the personal qualities, values and behaviours that are expected of **adult care workers** and **personal assistants** when communicating with **individuals** and **others** at work.

Learning outcomes

LO1: Understand why communication is important in the work setting

LO2: Be able to meet the communication and language needs, wishes and preferences of individuals

LO3: Be able to reduce barriers to communication

LO4: Be able to apply principles and practices relating to confidentiality at work

Key terms

Communication methods are ways of interacting with others using non-verbal and verbal techniques, and technological aids. See AC 2.2 for a breakdown of these different methods of communication.

Preferences are wishes based on beliefs, values and culture.

Barriers can be anything that prevent or stop you or others from communicating and understanding the communication. See AC 3.1 for examples of different barriers to communication.

Services, in this unit, refer to organisations that provide translation, interpreting, speech and language and advocacy. See AC 3.4 for a breakdown of the different services available.

Adult care workers enable individuals with care and support needs to live independently and safely.

Personal assistants work directly for one individual with care and support needs, usually within the individual's own home.

Individuals are those requiring care or support.

Others refers to individuals' families, carers, advocates (see page 14 for definition), team members and other professionals.

Care settings can include adult, children and young people's health settings and adult care settings. However, this qualification focuses on adult care settings in particular.

Work settings can include one specific location or a range of locations, depending on the context of a particular role. For example, an individual's home or a residential care home or day centre.

6Cs

Communication

Communication in the setting is important. Without it you cannot build caring relationships or work effectively alongside your colleagues. The role of a care worker requires interaction with a variety of people. Whether they are the people you care for, the people who you work with, or others from outside your setting, such as families and GPs.

As part of your role as a care worker, you will be required to communicate effectively with a variety of people to discover more about them in order to provide high-quality care and support that meets their needs. If you have just been introduced to someone new, how do you know what their likes and dislikes are? And in a **care setting**, how would they like to be cared for by you?

In order to build on your communication skills, first, you will need to find out *why* people

communicate, which is what we focus on in this section; before you go on to learn *how* you can build on skills to meet the communication and language needs, wishes and preferences of the individual you care for. When things get in the way of you communicating effectively, you will need to learn how you can overcome them. You will need to be aware that there are cultural differences when it comes to communication so that you don't cause confusion or offence. You will also need to think about issues around confidentiality because you will be working with the personal and private information of individuals, (such as medical conditions). How can you show you are a good communicator? When do you use communication with others?

This unit will help you to understand how to put these principles into practice and gain a better understanding of why communication is one of the 6Cs in health and social care.

LO1 Understand why communication is important in the work setting

AC 1.1 Identify different reasons why people communicate

What is communication?

When you communicate, you are:

- sending information
- receiving information
- sharing thoughts
- expressing views and ideas
- expressing your feelings.

Communication is a two-way process between you and others. When you communicate, you are sharing thoughts and/or ideas, expressing feelings or sending and receiving information. This is called an interaction.

We communicate every day with our friends, families and our colleagues and we do this for different reasons. Communication is therefore part of our day-to-day lives, and our 'interactions' with other people.

Similarly, in care settings, communication is a key part of your role. It is central to the care and support you provide, it will affect the quality of care you provide and the relationships that you develop with others.

What does communication mean in your role?

In **adult care settings** communication is central to the quality of the care and support you provide and to the relationships that you develop with the individuals you care for, their families and carers, as well as your colleagues and other professionals you may work with.

Ultimately, if you want to be a good care worker, you will need to have good communication skills. This will be key in helping you to build relationships and provide the best possible care and **service** for the individuals you care for.

Key terms

Adult care settings include **residential care homes, nursing homes, domiciliary care, day centres**, an individual's own home or some **clinical healthcare settings**. See page 4 for definitions.

Residential care homes are homes that individuals live in. Care workers will provide meals and assistance with personal care tasks such as washing, dressing, eating.

Key terms

Provision of care means providing care and support to individuals in line with their individual needs, wishes and preferences. This might include providing assistance with household tasks, such as personal care tasks, socialising.

A **day centre** is a setting that provides leisure, educational, health and well-being activities during the day.

Nursing homes are homes that provide the same services as residential care homes but have registered nurses for individuals who have health needs.

An **outpatient mental health clinic** is a service that provides mental health treatments in the community rather than in a hospital setting.

Domiciliary care is where health and social care workers will provide care and support to individuals who still live in their own home but require additional help such as support with household tasks or personal care.

Clinical healthcare settings are places where healthcare professionals such as nurses, doctors, physiotherapists provide direct medical care to individuals such as in a clinic, pharmacy or in a GP surgery.

Reasons for communicating in care settings

People communicate in care settings for different reasons. Below are examples of why people in different roles may need to communicate.

- Adult care workers will communicate with the individuals and families they provide with care and support to form and develop relationships.
- Individuals in care settings may communicate to express their thoughts and ideas about how the activities they participate in could be improved.
- Care team members will communicate with one another to give and receive support.
- Individuals and their families will need to communicate to express their feelings, wishes, needs and preferences.
- Care team members will communicate with one another to obtain and share information in relation to the **provision of care** and support.

In your role you will need to communicate well in order to build meaningful working relationships with your colleagues as well as the individuals you care for and the others involved in their lives. You can do this by being friendly and making sure that they feel comfortable around you. Doing so will mean that they will trust you, feel positive and safe. Good communication skills mean that you can encourage individuals to express how they are feeling, and building that trust means they may share information with you that will allow you to offer better, more informed care. For example, an individual may share with you their concerns about how to manage living at home. This means you can offer care that will be most beneficial or helpful to them.

To get to know the individuals you care for, you will need to be able to communicate with them well in order to find out which methods of communication they prefer to use (see AC 2.2 for more information on communication methods). For example, finding out from an individual how they prefer to communicate in a group situation will result in them feeling able to contribute and more likely to actively interact in discussions. Good communication will therefore produce safe and high-quality care.

If you do not communicate well with the individuals you care for and the others involved in their lives this may lead to misunderstandings and serious failures in the provision of care and support that meets individuals' needs and expectations.

Table 1.1 includes some specific examples of how communication occurs in all settings where care or support is provided across different jobs. Can you think of any others?

Table 1.1 Examples of communication in adult care settings

Care settings	People	Reasons why people communicate
Residential care home	Care worker	In order to find out about an individual's needs; a care worker may need to find out from an individual with a **physical disability** how much support they need to get dressed.
An individual's own home	Personal assistant	In order to ensure the provision of high-quality care and to form working relationships with others; a personal assistant may need to discuss with an individual and their family how they are going to enable the individual to live independently.
Day centre	Activities worker	To enable individuals to share their ideas and thoughts; the activities worker may want some feedback from a group of young people with **learning disabilities** about the music session that they have taken part in.
Nursing home	An individual with **dementia**	To enable an individual to express how they are feeling; an individual who has dementia may need to show a care worker where they are experiencing pain when they move around.
Outpatient mental health clinic	An individual with **schizophrenia**	To learn new skills and information; an individual who suffers from schizophrenia may need to access support and guidance from mental health practitioners over how to manage their medication.
Domiciliary care	Care worker	To exchange information; a care worker may need to learn more about the support a young mother with a physical disability and her son require in order to tailor the support available. The care worker will need to discuss and exchange information with the mother and son.

Key terms

A **physical disability** is a condition that affects and limits the way an individual moves and their ability to perform physical activities. Physical disabilities include being blind or in a wheelchair.

Learning disabilities can be defined as a reduced ability to think and make decisions together with difficulties coping with everyday activities – which affect a person for their whole life. A person with a learning disability may experience problems with budgeting, shopping and planning a train journey.

Dementia is a group of symptoms that affect how you think, remember, problem-solve, use language and communicate. These occur when brain cells stop working properly and the brain is damaged by disease.

Schizophrenia is a long-term mental illness that affects how people think, feel and behave. They may see and hear things that others do not and/or hold strong beliefs that others do not have.

Reflect on it

1.1 Who do you communicate with at work?

Reflect on all the different people you communicate with at work. How many can you think of?

Reflecting on who you communicate with in your work setting can make you more aware about the different people you work alongside and interact with on a regular basis. Good communication is a very important part of working as a team.

Evidence opportunity

1.1 The reasons why people communicate

Identify three people you communicate with in your role and for each one write down two reasons why you communicate with them. You may choose a colleague, an individual, and one of their family members, for example. Think about when, why and how you may communicate with them. Are there any situations that may arise that mean you will communicate with them in different ways? If so, why? It might help if you think of a specific example at work.

Key term

Empathy is the ability to identify with another person's situation and understand their feelings or 'to put yourself in their shoes'.

AC 1.2 Explain how effective communication affects all aspects of your own work

What is effective communication?

In your role, communicating well with the people you care for, their families and your colleagues will be vital. 'Effective communication' will be key, and you will find that it can impact positively on all aspects of your work. As you already know, communication is a two-way process, so before we look at how effective communication will affect your work, let's explore what makes communication effective? Figure 1.1 identifies some key ingredients of effective communication.

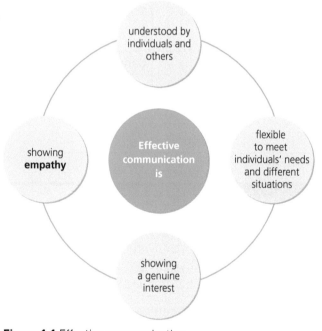

Figure 1.1 Effective communication

How can you communicate effectively?

Below are some tips on how to communicate well and how it can affect your work.

	Dos and don'ts for communicating effectively
Do	Speak clearly so that the person you are speaking to can understand you. If an individual cannot understand you then you will need to adapt the way you speak to ensure the individual can respond and communicate with you.
Do	Be patient and understanding so that the individual does not feel rushed and so that you can build trust.
Do	Show a genuine interest to get to know the individual. This will help you to understand their needs and preferences.
Do	Empathise by seeing things from someone else's point of view. This will allow you to understand how the individual may be feeling and will help to develop an open, honest and, most importantly, compassionate working relationship.
Do	Be aware of the other person's body language and what is being expressed so that you can understand how the individual may be feeling and adapt the way you communicate accordingly.
Do	Maintain good eye contact to show you are listening and understanding. This will also show that you are interested in what the individual is saying. You should be careful, however, as too much eye contact may make the individual feel uncomfortable. Try to assess the situation. Once you have a better idea of how the individual is feeling, you will know how much eye contact is necessary.
Do	Actively listen, not only to what is being said but to the meanings behind what is being said so that you can respond appropriately. For example, an individual may say that they agree with you but at the same time look unhappy; in this situation you could offer the individual another option so that you can check whether they really do agree with you.
Do	Be open and honest in all your communications. This will help with building trust and will ensure that misunderstandings are avoided.
Don't	Forget that you may need to alter the way you communicate with individuals from different cultures because some behaviours can convey different messages in different cultures.
Don't	Look uninterested or allow interruptions as doing so will act as a distraction and it will be more difficult to find out about the individual.
Don't	Rush an individual or speak *at* them as this will make it harder to communicate and for them to trust you.
Don't	Impose your views and preferences on an individual. This will not enable you to build up a good working relationship with individuals.
Don't	Mumble, or speak very quietly, as the person you are speaking to will not hear properly and it could lead to misunderstandings.
Don't	Forget to pay attention to the non-verbal communication used by individuals and what it can mean.
Don't	Ignore the words being spoken. Try not hearing what you want to hear and remember to actively listen (as mentioned above) otherwise, the individual may feel ignored.
Don't	Ignore an individual's feelings, or the different ways an individual may express how they are feeling.

6Cs

C

Compassion

Being kind and considerate towards individuals will show them you **care** and, as a result, individuals will be more likely to work with you and trust you. Showing compassion also involves showing respect for individuals' feelings and views and treating them in a dignified way. This is essential when you communicate with individuals so that they know that you are able to understand how they may be feeling and see things from their point of view. It is important that your intentions are honest and, in this way, they can approach you and learn to trust you with what is important to them. You can show this by taking time out to sit down with an individual and listen to what is worrying them and then reassuring them that they have your support.

Care

Care involves providing individuals in a care setting with a consistent, good-quality level of support. This means you need to take a genuine interest in individuals so that they know you care about them. Doing so will enable you to make a positive difference to their lives. This is essential when you communicate with individuals so that they can actively work with you to achieve what is important to them. You can show individuals you care about them by asking them questions about their likes and dislikes and then ensuring that you remember and take these into account when supporting them with daily activities, their personal hygiene regime, eating, drinking, interests and hobbies.

How does effective communication affect all aspects of your work?

Communicating clearly and making sure that you are understood by the individuals you support, their families, and colleagues is important. As we have discussed, you can do this by being understanding, open and honest. This will build trust and respect and will enable individuals and others to feel comfortable and at ease with you. This is essential for building caring and trusting working relationships. To understand individuals and what they are communicating you need to get to know them. When individuals understand you and what you are communicating they will show you in their unique way; it is important you can spot the signs so that you can continue to communicate with them and provide them with high-quality **care** and support.

To communicate effectively, you will need to think about who you are communicating with and the reasons you are communicating with them. You can then change or adapt the way you communicate based on your observations. This can make a positive difference to individuals' lives and is central for ensuring that the care and support provided meets their personal needs. For example, using photographs alongside discussions when communicating with an individual about where they want to go on holiday can ensure that the individual is making their own choice about where they want to go.

Knowing how to adjust or change your communication to different situations that may arise at work can also mean that you are able to encourage **participation** from individuals and others and show kindness and consideration in your working practices. For example, you may need to do this when an individual's family is anxious or worried about their relative's health or when an individual is finding it difficult to adjust to living in a residential care setting for the first time.

Showing a genuine or honest interest in the individuals you care for will not only reflect your **professionalism** but will also enable individuals and others to trust you and be confident with the care and support you provide.

Empathising with individuals and others (or thinking about how they might feel) can be a very good way of ensuring that they feel they can approach you with any concerns or difficulties that they are experiencing. You should listen carefully to what individuals say or pay attention to the feelings and emotions they express. This can ensure that you respond appropriately and that the experience is a positive one for both of you.

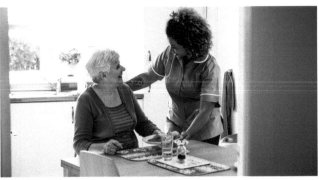

Figure 1.2 What behaviours is this adult care worker demonstrating?

Research it

1.2 Communication skills

Research the skills you need to communicate effectively in care settings.

Take a look at Skills for Care's 'Communication skills in social care':

www.skillsforcare.org.uk/Documents/ Learning-and-development/Core-skills/ Communication-skills-in-social-care.pdf

Key terms

Participation means to take part, or be involved. In this unit, this refers to a way of working that supports individuals' rights to be involved in communications.

Professionalism means demonstrating or showing the knowledge, skills and behaviours expected in your job and showing that you are able to do this successfully and to a high standard.

Effective communication also influences the quality of the teamwork in adult care and healthcare settings because it will encourage clear and consistent ways of working with team members and other professionals such as GPs, nurses, social workers, opticians and dentists as well as avoid misunderstandings.

Communicating effectively means that you and other members of the team can share knowledge, skills and good ideas with each other as well as develop the best working practices to follow. This allows for good teamwork, accurate sharing of information and encourages everyone to learn from one another.

Effective communication in a team involves being honest, respectful, supportive, positive and committed to working with others. This means that your working environment will be a positive one to work in. This will affect how you and others feel when you are at work and therefore mean that you and others will create a nice positive atmosphere to work in, one where you are more likely to offer good-quality care and support.

Evidence opportunity

1.2 Effective communication

Choose one task that you carry out at work on a regular basis. Write an account about how effective communication affects the way you carry out this task.

Remember to provide details about this task and give examples showing how effective communication can impact on how this is done. You may wish to choose a task where you assist an individual to get up in the morning or when you support an individual to take part in an activity. You may also wish to think about this task in relation to non-English speakers, or people communicating using British Sign Language or Makaton. Your daily report (or activity) record could be a useful document to refer to during this activity.

AC 1.3 Explain why it is important to observe an individual's reactions when communicating with them

Reactions, verbal and non-verbal communication

As you will have learned, for communication to be effective in adult care settings, it must be understood by individuals and meet their needs. How individuals respond, both verbally and non-verbally during communications, shows whether they have understood what has been communicated with them. See AC 2.2 for more information.

1.3 High and low pitch and tones

Search the internet for clips to understand what high pitch, low pitch, high tone and low tone voices sound like. That way, you will have a better understanding of what these are and what they may mean when communicating with individuals.

Key terms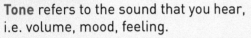

Tone refers to the sound that you hear, i.e. volume, mood, feeling.

Pitch refers to the quality of what you hear, i.e. degree of highness or lowness of tone.

Also see AC 2.2.

The way you and others communicate can be both verbal and non-verbal.

Verbal communication means using words to speak or talk to others. This will also include the **tone** that we use to communicate. For example, speaking in a lower tone may be more appropriate in sensitive situations that require more sympathy such as when an individual is not feeling well; you may need to speak in a higher tone when you are agreeing with an individual's idea for an activity. You may also need to alter your pitch. You may need to speak in a higher **pitch** to make sure you are heard by someone who has a hearing impairment or difficulty. You may need to speak in a lower pitch if you are discussing confidential information in an open environment.

Non-verbal communication refers to all the messages that we convey without words such as our body language and facial expressions, our dress and the way we position ourselves. More specifically, this might include eye contact, how we sit, the movements or gestures that we make with our hands and how close we stand or sit next to someone else.

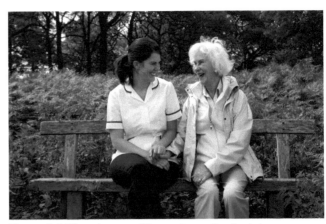

Figure 1.3 What does positive and negative body language look like? How might this individual be feeling? What does their body language reveal? What messages are they sending without saying anything?

For example, if someone makes eye contact, this may mean they are feeling confident in themselves (positive and happy). If they do not make eye contact, this might mean they are feeling unhappy or anxious. If someone sits hunched with their arms crossed, they may be feeling angry, or tense or upset. If someone sits back with their arms open, they may be feeling relaxed, confident and keen to interact with you.

Understanding non-verbal communication is key when observing an individual's reactions. This is because the majority of their reactions will be non-verbal. Remember that everyone is a unique individual and therefore how they use non-verbal communication is personal to them. For example, avoiding eye contact is not always a negative sign, and in some cultures it is actually a sign of respect. It is important to be aware that your own cultural traditions may differ from those of the individuals you care for.

Observing reactions

It is important to observe as well as understand individuals' reactions when you communicate so that you can ensure that you understand how they are feeling. For example, the individual you care for may not tell you that they are feeling worried and upset but you may pick this up by observing their body language – for example, their facial expression may show their anxiety or sadness or they may be turning their body away from you.

The non-verbal messages their body gives out may say more than the words they speak.

If an individual shows they are feeling worried or upset, then you will need to show **compassion** and understanding for how they are feeling. You could for example, say to them 'I can see you are upset, is there anything I can do to help?' or you could take time out to sit with an individual and show them your support in this way.

Treating individuals with dignity and helping their well-being

As individuals have different ways of communicating it is important that you observe their reactions when communicating with them so that you are able to understand what they are expressing and respond appropriately. For example, one individual may say the word 'yes' to express a choice or preference, another individual may point at an object, smile or nod to confirm their preferences.

It is essential that you know how to respond to the unique communication methods that individuals use for not only treating individuals with **dignity** but also for promoting their **well-being** because it involves understanding fully and responding to what they are thinking and feeling. You will explore how to find out about an individual's communication and language needs, wishes and preferences in LO2 (page 12).

Research it

1.3 Well-being and the Care Act 2014

Research the nine well-being principles of the Care Act 2014. What does well-being mean to you?

Care and Support Statutory Guidance – Section 1, Promoting well-being:

www.gov.uk/government/publications/care-act-statutory-guidance/care-and-support-statutory-guidance#chapter-1

SCIE – Care Act 2014, 'How is well-being understood under the Care Act?':

www.scie.org.uk/care-act-2014/assessment-and-eligibility/eligibility/how-is-wellbeing-understood.asp

Identifying changes in the needs of people you care for

Observing an individual's reactions when communicating with them is also essential so you can identify any changes in their needs. For example, a personal assistant who is checking on an individual's comfort may ask the individual how they are feeling as well as observe their facial expression for any signs of pain or anxiety.

It is important for the personal assistant to observe both the individual's verbal and non-verbal reactions to make sure that they have understood the individual's response correctly in answer to their question. Not doing so may mean that the individual's pain or anxiety is not treated and becomes worse and at the same time can lead to the individual feeling frustrated and not listened to.

Think about your reactions and the messages that you communicate

It is important that you are aware of your own reactions and the messages that you may be communicating to individuals and others both verbally and non-verbally. By doing this, you can ensure that only the messages you intend to give out are received. Now read back over AC 1.2 to remind yourself about how *you* can communicate well.

Key terms

Compassion means delivering care and support with kindness, consideration, dignity and respect.

Dignity in a care setting means respecting the views, choices and decisions of individuals and not making assumptions about how individuals want to be treated.

Well-being is a broad or wide-ranging concept that applies to different areas of an individual's life and includes their physical, mental and emotional health. In a care setting, you will be expected to care for people's physical, mental and emotional well-being.

1.3 Observing reactions

Reflect on an occasion when you observed an individual's reactions while communicating with them? What messages did their reactions convey or express to you? How did you adapt or change your communication?

If you have not done this yet, think of a time when you had a conversation with a friend. Did you observe or look at the way they reacted? What messages did you receive from their reactions? Were they interested in what you were saying? Did they look tired? How did you adapt or change the way you communicated?

1.3 Why is it important to observe reactions?

Identify an occasion when you were communicating with an individual and they reacted in an unexpected way. Why did they react in this way? How did you respond? Explain the reasons why it was important that you observed their reactions. Include in your explanation the consequences of not doing so. Could you have responded differently? How?

LO1 Knowledge, skills, behaviours
Knowledge: why is communication important?
Do you know the different reasons you will need to communicate?
Do you know how effective communication affects all your work activities?
Do you know what to look for in an individual's reactions when you communicate?
Did you know that you have shown knowledge of why communication is very important when working in care settings?
Skills: how can you support effective communications in your work setting?
Do you know how to encourage an individual to communicate with you?
Do you know what to do if an individual's family cannot understand what you are communicating and why it is important?
Do you know how you can show people dignity when communicating with them in your work setting?
Did you know that you have just demonstrated skills in encouraging effective communications?
Behaviours: how can you show in your work setting that you are a good communicator?
Do you maintain eye contact when communicating with an individual?
Do you think about who you are speaking to and try to adapt your communication depending on who you are speaking to?
Do you know how you can show that you communicate with compassion in your work setting?
Did you know that you have just shown some of the essential behaviours required to communicate with individuals with different needs and preferences?

LO2 Be able to meet the communication and language needs, wishes and preferences of individuals

Think about a time when you were particularly sad or upset and wanted to talk to a friend. Did you explain your worry or problem to them? How did they respond? Were they helpful? Were they empathetic? How would you feel if they responded in a way that did not take into account how you were feeling?

AC 2.1 Find out an individual's communication and language needs, wishes and preferences

As a care worker it is important that you find out how people like to communicate because different people will communicate in different ways. The easiest way to do this is to ask them, or you could ask colleagues, or their families. It is important that you take the time to find out about how individuals prefer to communicate and what their individual responses mean because you will need to meet these needs and develop the skills to meet them.

Not only do people have different communication and language needs and **preferences** (see page 14 for definition) but their communication needs, wishes and preferences can also be affected by other factors such as illnesses and disabilities.

Different communication needs and preferences

There are different reasons why the people you care for have different communication and language needs, wishes and preferences. Here, we look at just a few of the reasons that you will need to think about and consider.

Think about hearing impairments

If an individual is unable to hear very well, this can make communication difficult for both the individual and for you. It may be that they have lost some of their hearing, or that they cannot hear completely. This may affect their interactions with others. They may feel alone or left out if they are unable to hear what others are saying, or if they cannot hear themselves. It may also mean that they are unable to understand or misunderstand the messages and instructions that you are trying to convey. How would you feel if you were unable to hear or understand what others were saying?

As a care worker, you will need to consider the feelings of someone with a **hearing impairment** (see page 14 for definition), how you can help them and how you can find ways to make communication easier. A young adult who has a hearing impairment may prefer to speak with an activities worker in a quiet and well-lit room where background noise is minimised and natural light enables the individual to see the care worker's face and lip-read what is being communicated.

Research it

2.1 Disabilities and illnesses

Research how disabilities and illnesses can affect the communication, language needs and preferences of the people you care for.

How might a physical disability affect an individual's communication needs? Find out about **aphasia** and **dysphasia**.

How might having an **autistic spectrum disorder** affect an individual's needs and preferences? (See page 14 for definitions.)

How might an illness such as dementia affect an individual's needs and preferences?

Thinking about the ways in which you can meet the communication needs of someone with a hearing difficulty will allow you to support them effectively. For example, you will need to avoid shouting or speaking very loudly because while you may feel like you are simply doing this so that the individual can hear you, they may take this negatively and think that you are shouting at them. Instead, you should speak clearly and slowly.

Think about language

The individuals who you care for may have different language needs. For example, they may not speak English or are unable to understand English. It may be that they have limited or very little understanding of English. This may make it difficult for them to communicate with you, especially if you do not speak their language. A situation like this can also make it difficult for individuals to connect with others in the setting and to form relationships.

Again, it may help you to think about a time when you have been on holiday, or more generally, when you have been in a situation where you did not speak the same language as others and could not understand what others were saying. How did it make you feel?

Individuals may also have different language needs based on who they are speaking to. An older adult who lives independently and speaks both English and Spanish may prefer to speak in English when agreeing their personal goals with their personal assistant but in Spanish when they participate in activities with their family and friends.

Key terms

Preferences are an individual's choices. In this unit, this relates to how they choose or 'prefer' to communicate with others.

Beliefs are ideas that are accepted as true and real by the person who holds them. They could be religious, or political. They may also generally be to do with someone's morals or the way they live, for example 'I believe in treating others how I expect to be treated.'

Values are ideas that form the system by which a person lives their life; often a person's beliefs can develop into their values.

Hearing impairment refers to hearing loss that may occur in one or both ears. This can be partial (some loss of hearing) or complete loss of hearing.

Autistic spectrum disorder is a lifelong condition that affects how a person perceives the world and interacts with others. For example, they may have difficulties interacting and socialising with others.

Aphasia is a condition that affects a person's speech, understanding and use of language. An example of an aspect of this condition may be that they have difficulties putting words together to form sentences.

Dysphasia is a condition that affects how a person understands language and is a less severe form of aphasia. For example, they may have difficulties listening to and understanding what another person is saying.

Culture refers to the particular traditions, customs and values shared by a group people or society.

An **advocate** is a person who speaks on behalf of or represents someone who is unwilling or unable to speak for him or herself, perhaps because of an illness or disability.

As a care worker, you should find out about the language needs of individuals. You can do this by speaking to colleagues, or the individual's family. Finding out about language needs means that you can think about the best ways to support them. Will the individual need a translator or interpreter, for example?

Overcoming any language issues and barriers means that you will be able to support individuals in the best way and that you will be able to understand each other better. It also means that you will help individuals to form relationships with others in the setting and improve their quality of life.

Be aware of differences across cultures

In a care setting, you will come across people from different backgrounds, races and religions. Each culture has their own rules about acceptable behaviours to use when communicating verbally and non-verbally. For example:

- When meeting with an individual for the first time in a care setting, a handshake may be acceptable in one **culture** but not in others.

- Maintaining eye contact as a care worker when you are communicating with an older individual and their family may be appropriate in some cultures but not in others.

- Body language in different cultures can also convey different messages. For example, a nod of the head can indicate agreement in one culture and disagreement in another.

You will need to think about and make sure that you find out about the preferences of the person you care for and their family as this may mean that you avoid causing offence or misunderstandings, and create better relationships. In AC 2.2, we will explore the communication methods that you can use to meet the needs of the people you care for.

Figure 1.4 shows a number of different ways of finding out how individuals want to communicate with you and others.

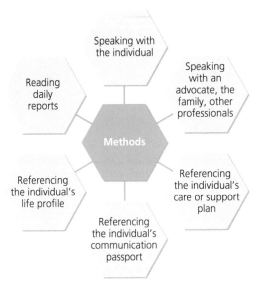

Figure 1.4 Finding out how to communicate with an individual

Research it

2.1 Culture and beliefs

Research how culture and **beliefs** can impact on communication in adult care settings.

Follow the link for Flying Start NHS, for a full explanation of 'Cultural Competence':

www.flyingstart.scot.nhs.uk/learning-programmes/equality-and-diversity/cultural-competence/

Evidence opportunity

2.1 Language needs, wishes and preferences

Identify one individual in your work setting who you communicate with regularly. Show three methods of finding out about their communication and language needs, wishes and preferences. For example, one method may involve asking their **advocate** who knows them well for more information about how they communicate.

Make sure you record and share information

Make sure you record information on an individual's communication, language needs and preferences. It is important that you do this so that it is documented clearly. In this way, your colleagues and others at work who communicate with this individual can do so in a consistent way.

Remember, when you record information about an individual, you must do so respectfully and ensure it remains private and is kept confidential. You will learn more about the practices relating to maintaining confidentiality at work in LO4 at the end of this unit.

AC 2.2 Demonstrate communication methods that meet an individual's communication needs, wishes and preferences

For this AC you will need to show that you are able to use a range of communication methods that meet an individual's communication needs, wishes and preferences. You will be observed when you do this as part of your assessment.

As you have learned, it is important for adult care workers and personal assistants to always find out as much information as possible about how an individual prefers to communicate. It is also important to remember that individuals' needs are different and unique and therefore different ways of communicating are needed for communications to be effective.

There is a wide range of ways or methods of communicating with individuals including non-verbal and verbal communication methods as well as the use of technological aids. You may wish to recap what verbal and non-verbal communication means by reading AC 1.3.

Non-verbal communication methods include the following:

- **Eye contact** – this means the interaction that you make with your eyes and can mean looking towards, away, up, down, opening and closing your eyes. In a care setting, you will need to get to know the individual you are caring for to find out how they prefer you to use eye contact with them.

- **Touch** – this is the physical interaction that you have with others and can include placing your hand over an individual's hand or on their shoulder. In a care setting you may need to do this when the individual you care for is in a distressing situation, for example, in pain or has been told some sad news. Touch can be particularly helpful if the individual has a visual impairment and cannot see very well. In some situations like when you are supporting an individual to walk around the garden, it is more appropriate to let the individual guide you and show you how they want you to support them. Again, it is worth finding out about an individual's preferences when it comes to this.

- **Physical gestures** – this can include things like waving your hand to say hello, spelling out words with your fingers when using sign language.

- **Body language** – this can include facial expressions such as smiling or frowning, nodding your head, leaning your body towards or away from an individual. In a care setting, it is important to maintain positive body language; not doing so may make individuals and others not want to approach you and can also affect how they are feeling.

- **Behaviour** – this can include how you sit such as sitting upright, how you speak (do you speak calmly?), how you move your body (do you ever pace up and down?), gestures (do you ever yawn?). You will need to consider these things when you think about body language.

- **Written** – this can include written words in notes that you may make about an individual's condition, or signs and symbols that represent words and numbers. It can also include letters, reports, emails, the use of **Makaton** and **Braille**.

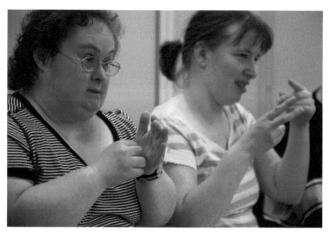

Figure 1.5 Makaton is one form of non-verbal communication

Key terms

Makaton is a method of communication using signs and symbols that is used by individuals who have learning disabilities.

Braille is a method of written communication used by individuals who are blind. Characters (each letter) represented by patterns of raised dots are felt with the fingertips of the individual.

Evidence opportunity

2.2 Communication methods

Select four non-verbal communication methods that you use with two or three different individuals in your work setting. You need to be able to demonstrate how you use these communication methods to meet each individual's specific communication needs, wishes and preferences. You will be observed when doing so. (Permission to do so from each individual may be needed).

Remember to ensure that the methods you use can be understood by the individuals and are in line with how they prefer to communicate and meet their communication needs. You could also record why you chose each method for the individuals.

Verbal communication methods can include the following:

- **Vocabulary** – using words on their own, as part of a phrase or sentence. This can be in different languages. In a care setting, you may need to use simple, straightforward language spoken clearly for those individuals who find it difficult to understand instructions.
- **Tone** – spoken words may be loud, assertive, quiet, calm, friendly or positive. When working with individuals, you will need to think what tone is most suitable based on the situation.
- **Linguistic tone** – how you use language to express what you mean, such as the strength of a vocal sound made by a person in a communication, for example, quiet or loud.
- **Pitch** – you may speak in a high-pitched voice when excited, or a low-pitched voice when coming to the end of a sentence and when discussing matters that are confidential. See AC 1.3 for more a more detailed explanation of the use of pitch.

Technological aids are developing all the time as a means of helping individuals with speaking or hearing difficulties to communicate. There is a wide range of aids available to suit different needs. Technological aids can include the following equipment:

- **Voice Output Communication Aids (VOCA)** – these help individuals to communicate by speaking recorded messages, and display words and symbols on a screen.
- **Hearing aids and cochlear implants** – these help to improve an individual's hearing.
- **Mobile phones** – these can also be helpful as some mobile phones include features like 'increased magnification' for an individual with sight loss (the words and pictures on the phones can be bigger) and hearing aid compatibility so that it is easier to hear for those with hearing difficulties.
- **PCs, tablets, laptops** – include software applications designed to enable individuals with a range of needs to communicate more effectively such as an app that lets you choose a pre-recorded voice or records your own voice saying the words.

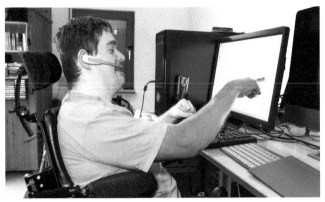

Figure 1.6 Using technology to communicate

Reflect on it

2.2 Tone and pitch

Reflect on a talk that you have had with an individual or observed with an individual. How were linguistic tone and pitch used and why?

Research it

2.2 Technological aids

Identify three technological aids that can be used with individuals with a range of different communication needs and preferences. For each one, research their purpose, how they are used and the benefits to communications. You might want to visit the following websites.

Communication Matters:

www.communicationmatters.org.uk

Sense:

www.sense.org.uk/content/about-us

Key terms

Vocabulary means the words that are known and used by a person.

Pitch means the quality of a vocal sound made by a person in a communication, e.g. low or high.

Technological aids refer to electronic aids that enable a person to communicate and interact.

Other communication aids available to support effective communication can include the following:

- **Picture Exchange Communication System (PECS)** – these are used by individuals with autism spectrum disorder to communicate with others using pictures. For example, pictures can be exchanged by individuals for items they would like such as a book or something to eat as well as to answer questions such as 'What do you want to wear today?'. These pictures can also be presented in the form of a communication book or board that is personal to the individual and can be used solely with them. PECS encourages individuals who have difficulties communicating with others to approach others to initiate communications.

- **Talking Mats** – these are an application used by individuals with dementia who have difficulties with their verbal communication to enable them to communicate using a combination of pictures and symbols with text. For example, the individual could be given options of different activities available and the individual could then choose the ones they would like to participate in as well as those that they wouldn't. Cue cards or picture cards could be used instead where technology equipment, i.e. tablets or PCs, are not available.

- **Objects of reference** – these are used by individuals who may find it difficult to understand spoken words or photographs. Objects of reference are items that represent to the individual an item, a person, an activity and/or a place. So, you may use different objects of reference for the same item for two different individuals, e.g. a plate can mean lunchtime to one individual whilst a sandwich may mean lunchtime to another.

- **Communication passports** – these are used by individuals who have difficulties communicating with others to provide information about themselves such as their likes, dislikes or medical condition. These may

be used, for example, by the individual when accessing a college course for the first time or during a stay in hospital.

AC 2.3 Show how and when to seek advice about communication

Individuals' communication and language needs, wishes and preferences are very diverse and can also change. Knowing how and when to seek advice about communication is therefore very important for ensuring communications with individuals are effective.

How to seek advice about communication

Every adult care setting will have developed its own procedures for how to seek advice about communication, including the people and relevant organisations to approach depending on your specific job role and responsibilities. For example, internal sources of advice (those in the setting) may include your manager or the senior support worker, and external sources of advice (that can be found outside the setting) may include the individual's advocate or organisations such as the Royal National Institute of Blind People (**RNIB**) or the **Alzheimer's Society**.

Evidence opportunity

2.3 How and when to seek advice about communication

Show how you use your work setting's procedure for seeking advice about communication for one individual. You could also reference the individual's care plan and, more specifically, the section in it about communication.

You must, however, ensure that the individual's privacy and personal details are kept confidential (for example, their name must not be visible).

Give an example of a situation when you might need to seek advice.

When to seek advice about communication

Knowing when to seek advice about communication is also very important. There are specialist organisations that will have the expertise so it is important to approach them if you don't know what is best to do. Not doing so in a timely manner could lead to individuals feeling devalued and frustrated. Misunderstandings and confusion could also arise.

Examples of when you need to seek advice about communication could include when:

- an individual cannot make themselves understood
- an individual cannot understand what is being communicated
- there has been a change in an individual's communication needs
- specialist advice is required, for example how to use an individual's communication aid.

Case study

2.3 Seeking advice about communication

Riya is new to care and has recently begun working as a domiciliary care worker providing care and support to older adults living in their own homes. Her main tasks and responsibilities involve promoting individuals' independence, dignity and choices, providing assistance to individuals with personal care as well as assisting with preparation for meals and drinks throughout the day and carrying out household tasks such as laundry, washing up and vacuuming.

On a Tuesday morning, Riya visits Stan who has recently had a stroke. Stan enjoys speaking with Riya and tells her all about his week every time he sees her. Riya finds it very difficult to

understand everything that Stan is saying to her because since his stroke he has difficulties in finding the right words and expressing himself when speaking to others.

Riya feels very embarrassed about not being able to understand him and does not want to tell him how she is feeling because it may upset him or make him think that she is unable to understand him because she is new to care work.

Questions

1 What should Riya do? Why?
2 What are the consequences of Riya not taking any action?
3 Who can she go to in her work setting?
4 What services outside of her work setting may be able to provide her with information, advice and support?

Reflect on it

2.3 Advice about communication

Reflect on an occasion when you or someone in your work setting has sought advice about communication. When did they seek advice and why? What were the benefits of doing so?

Key terms

RNIB stands for the Royal National Institute of Blind People. This is a UK charity that provides information, advice, practical and emotional support to people affected by sight loss.

Alzheimer's Society is the UK's leading dementia support and research charity for people affected by any form of dementia in England, Wales and Northern Ireland.

L02 Knowledge, skills, behaviours
Knowledge: do you know how to find out and meet an individual's communication and language needs, wishes and preferences?
Why is it important that you communicate in positive ways with individuals? Do you know about the different communication methods you can use?
Do you know what records can be used to find out more about an individual's communication and language needs?
Do you know the sources of advice in your care setting for finding out about an individual's wishes and preferences? Why is it important to know what sources of advice about communication are available?
Did you know that you have shown knowledge of how to get to know an individual and be able to communicate with them effectively?
Skills: how can you demonstrate effective ways of communicating with individuals?
How can you find out about an individual's communication and language needs, wishes and preferences?
How can you promote individuals' rights when communicating with them in your work setting?
Do you know how to use your body language to show you are listening to an individual?
Do you know how to use the tone of your voice to show an individual you understand how they are feeling?
How can you act responsibly when seeking advice about communication for an individual?
How do you know how and when to seek advice about communicating with an individual?
Did you know that you have just demonstrated how to seek advice about communication, and also demonstrated the use of verbal and non-verbal communication skills?
Behaviours: how can you show that you can demonstrate courage when seeking advice about communication on behalf of an individual?
How can you show that you are committed to supporting an individuals' communication needs, wishes and preferences?
Do you know how to adapt your verbal communication to meet an individual's communication needs?
Do you know how to speak up for an individual in a sensitive way?
Do you know how to seek advice in a confident manner?
How can you show courage when seeking advice about the communication needs for an individual?
Did you know that you have just shown some of the essential behaviours required when seeking advice about communication for an individual?

6Cs

Courage

Courage is required when speaking up for an individual. Not doing so may put the individual at risk and may mean that their communication and language needs, wishes and preferences remain unmet. For example, if you notice that a colleague is not using an individual's communication aid with them it is important that you do not ignore this but report it immediately to ensure that all communications with individuals are effective.

LO3 Be able to reduce barriers to communication

Getting started

Think about a time when you have been outside your care setting, perhaps at a party or in a noisy environment when you were with a friend? How did the environment affect your communication?

Could you hear each other speak and understand one another? Did you go somewhere else where you could hear each other?

AC 3.1 Identify barriers to communication

There are times when communications are not effective. Barriers are things that will get in the way of you being able to communicate effectively with individuals, or them being able to communicate with you.

It is important, therefore, that you think about what barriers could exist and learn what you can

do to overcome them. Put yourself in 'the shoes' of the individual and the difficulties they may have communicating. What barriers are there for the individual? What barriers are there for you?

Think about barriers like those mentioned in Table 1.2 but also think about things that you are doing that may present barriers. Thinking about the barriers that exist will mean you can then think about how you can overcome them.

Table 1.2 Barriers to communication

Reasons for ineffective communication	Examples of barriers to communication
The environment	• **Noise** – a room that is too noisy means that it is difficult to listen or hear properly and you can become distracted by others in the room. • **Distractions** such as other people being in the environment or telephones ringing can also hinder communication and may also mean individuals may not feel comfortable sharing their thoughts and feelings with interruptions and others around. • **No privacy** may prevent the safe sharing of information. • **Bad light** – poorly lit rooms prevent lip-reading or being able to make eye contact, see each other's body language and facial expressions. It may also mean that individuals are unable to read documents that they may need to look at. • **Cluttered** – a room with too much (or tall) furniture may prevent reading of facial expressions and making eye contact. It may also mean that people in wheelchairs, for example, may struggle to communicate if they cannot see over tall tables. You will need to think about all the different things in the environment that could be a barrier to effective communication between you, the people you care for, their families and friends as well as the people you work with.

→

Table 1.2 Barriers to communication *continued*

Reasons for ineffective communication	Examples of barriers to communication
The adult care worker or personal assistant	• **A lack of time** to spend communicating with the individual means you cannot find out as much or get to know the individual as you would like. • **Tiredness** can lead to communications being poor because your concentration and listening skills may suffer. This in turn may mean that you misinterpret what is being communicated. • **A lack of training** on how to communicate effectively may mean that you may not have the skills to communicate in the ways that you should. • **A poor understanding of an individual's communication and language needs** and preferences may mean that you cannot tailor the methods you use to communicate to the individual's needs. • **Differences in culture** or beliefs may mean that you cannot understand each other or have certain **prejudices** and **stereotypes**. It can also mean that you have to alter the way you interact with individuals from different cultures and faiths. For example, a handshake in one culture may be seen as respectful but not appropriate in another because of the contact made. • **Aggression** can make it very difficult to communicate with individuals because you will both not feel relaxed or comfortable. This makes it difficult to think, say and express how you feel. • **Language** can also be a barrier if you use 'specialist' language that individuals cannot understand. For example, you may be used to using terms and acronyms such as 'BP' for blood pressure or 'LDs' for learning disabilities but the individuals you work with may not understand these, and find them confusing. You could revisit AC 2.1 (page 13) to recap on cultural differences or look at Unit 209 on equality, diversity and inclusion. You should think about all the ways in which you and your communication skills could be a barrier to effective communication.
The individual	• **Difficulties when communicating with others** who they do not know can mean that it is difficult for them to convey thoughts, feelings and more private or confidential information. • **A lack of trust in their own abilities** when communicating, or some people may generally not be very good at communicating. • **Poor experiences of ineffective communications**, for example they may have experienced a care worker or other professionals talking over them, about them, rather than to them during a meeting about their care. • **Complex spoken and written communication and language needs and preferences** such as sensory impairments, speech impairments, learning disabilities and dyslexia can mean that more time is required to communicate and adaptations need to be made to how you communicate. You will need to think about all the barriers that the individuals you care for are facing when it comes to communication.

Prejudice is a negative opinion that you may have of someone which is not based on experience or interaction.

A **stereotype** is an oversimplified idea of what you think someone or something will be like, based on perhaps their culture or beliefs. For example: all young people are lazy; all older people develop dementia.

Reflect on it

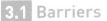

3.1 Barriers

Reflect on the different people you communicate with in your work setting. What barriers are there to communicating effectively with each person? For the individuals you work with, you may find it useful to refer to their communication profiles and care plans.

Evidence opportunity

3.1 Barriers to communication in your setting

List the different barriers to effective communications that exist in your work setting. Consider the individuals, your colleagues and other health and social care professionals you work with.

AC 3.2 Demonstrate how to reduce barriers to communication in different ways

For this AC your work practices will be observed; you will need to be able to demonstrate that you know how to minimise and reduce barriers to communication in a range of different ways.

Once you have identified what the barriers to communication are, it will then be necessary to find ways to minimise or overcome them so that effective communications can once again take place. There are many different methods of reducing communication barriers depending on the type of barrier, your knowledge and skills of effective communication and the different approaches that can be used. Overcoming barriers to communication will enable and empower both you and the individual to communicate to the best of your abilities. Below are examples of the methods that can be used to reduce a range of different types of barriers to communication.

The environment

Noise: communication in a very noisy meeting room can be improved by removing the causes of the noise. For example, you can:

- switch off the air-conditioning unit
- close the windows
- close the door.

If you cannot avoid the noisy environment, you will need to make sure that you still communicate clearly, by perhaps speaking in a slightly louder tone, and use gestures and signing if needed, so that the individual can understand you. You may even need to use written communication.

Poor lighting: communication in a room that has poor lighting can be improved by improving the lighting. For example, you can:

- use brighter lights
- reposition furniture
- ensure communications take place by the windows where it is brighter.

If you cannot avoid being in a room where the light is poor, you will need to make sure that the individual is able to understand you. You will need to speak clearly so that they can hear you and also listen to what they communicate. If they cannot see your facial expressions, then it may be that you could change the tone of your voice to express what you are feeling. Likewise, if you cannot see the individual very well, then you should pay attention to the tone of their voice to understand how they may be feeling. You may need to record the conversation.

Other distractions, such as other people nearby, can mean that sharing private information is difficult. In this scenario, you could try to book a quiet room in advance where you can ensure that

Research it

3.2 **Reducing barriers**

Research ways of reducing communication barriers in the environment. You might like to look at the following website for useful tips

Royal College of Nursing, First Steps, Barriers to communication:

http://rcnhca.org.uk/top-page-001/barriers-to-communication

any sensitive or confidential information is shared safely. If it is not possible to book a private room, you could perhaps delay the meeting slightly or reschedule it for another time so that the individual may feel comfortable.

If the environment is not suited to people who use wheelchairs, it may be that you need to adapt the environment accordingly. Installing a ramp will allow individuals to access a building easily; adjusting the height of counters and tables will help wheelchair users so they can use them comfortably.

The adult care worker or personal assistant

Communication between an adult care worker and an individual that is rushed can be improved by:

- the adult care worker allowing sufficient or enough time to meet with the individual to find out the individual's specific communication and language needs, including how these will impact on all communications
- the adult care worker looking at their diary and rescheduling a meeting for a time when they will be able to devote enough time to the individual.

Communication between a personal assistant and an individual that involves misunderstandings can be improved by:

- the personal assistant finding out from the individual the communication methods they prefer to use
- the personal assistant seeking advice from a colleague or someone who knows the

individual well and can provide guidance on how to avoid misunderstandings and promote positive communications.

The individual

Communication with an individual who has difficulties when communicating with others can be improved by:

- the individual making others aware of their specific communication and language needs, wishes and preferences directly
- making available their communication profile, care or support plan that provides further information
- finding out about the individual's culture and speaking to those who know the individual well about how to communicate
- finding out about how other illnesses and conditions may affect an individual's communication, such as:
  - dementia (so that you know to speak using short sentences to avoid confusion)
  - **Asperger's syndrome** (so that you know to use clear language)
  - learning disabilities (so that you communicate using a combination of signs and gestures and give individuals time to respond to questions and interactions)
- learning a little about the language an individual speaks or consider using an interpreter or a translator
- speaking clearly with an individual who has a hearing impairment, checking that hearing their aids (if used) are working, organise a hearing check-up, using written communication or signing
- using verbal communication with an individual who has sight loss and using the tone of your voice and touch as and when appropriate
- using specialist services such translators, interpreters and signers who can support individuals. Translators can help with translating written communication from one language to another and interpreters with spoken language. Signers can interpret communications through lip-reading and

signing using British Sign Language. Individuals with learning disabilities can make use of Makaton, which is a way of communicating using signs and symbols, and individuals with sight loss can use Braille.

Communication with an individual who has had a poor experience of communication with others can be improved by reassuring the individual that you are a skilled and effective communicator and then encouraging them to experience positive communications with you.

Slowly building a trusting and respectful relationship with an individual is the basis of all good communication.

Case study

3.2 Reducing communication barriers

Sangan has been providing one-to-one support to Michael, a young man who has Asperger's syndrome. Asperger's affects Michael's ability to communicate and interact with other people. Michael has difficulties understanding what others are saying, following conversations with other people and finds it difficult to interpret other people's non-verbal communication such as their body language, including their sense of humour, feelings and emotions.

Michael has many interests and tends to tell people he meets what they are but avoids interacting with them fully. In addition, Michael prefers to avoid eye contact with others and appears to get anxious when eye contact is maintained with him and when he is being asked questions about himself.

Michael has been invited to a family gathering as it is one of his nephew's birthdays and he is anxious about attending this social occasion as he knows there will be lots of people there who know him.

Discussion points

1 How can Michael's communication needs make communications with others difficult?
2 What strategies can Sangan use to reduce these barriers to communication?
3 What are the benefits of effective communication when working with individuals?

Key term

Asperger's syndrome is a disability that affects how individuals interact with others, i.e. individuals may have difficulty understanding and relating to other people and taking part in day-to-day activities.

Reflect on it

3.2 Impact and consequences

Reflect on or think about the impact of not reducing barriers to communication. What are the consequences for each of the following:

- the individuals requiring care or support
- the adult care worker
- personal assistant
- the team?

Evidence opportunity

3.2 Reducing barriers to communication

Select three barriers to effective communication that exist in your work setting and that you included in your list for AC 3.1. For each one show two different methods that you can use to reduce these barriers. For example, you may seek support from a professional or specialist service or you may make changes to the environment. You will be observed demonstrating these methods in your work setting.

Dos and don'ts for overcoming communication barriers	
Do	Speak clearly, repeat if necessary, paraphrase and reword. Give the individual time to respond – you need to show you can be patient and considerate.
Do	Actively listen – recap your learning for AC 3.3 for more information about this.
Do	Use appropriate language, address individuals by their first name only if they prefer to be addressed in this way.
Do	Show that you are genuinely interested by using appropriate body language and gestures such as leaning towards the individual and nodding.
Don't	Mumble, cover your mouth, use slang and acronyms because this may make understanding what you are communicating difficult.
Don't	Use complex or inappropriate language.
Don't	Invade the individual's 'personal space' as this may make them feel uncomfortable.
Don't	Impose your own experiences, values and beliefs on individuals. Be respectful of the experiences, values and beliefs of others.

AC 3.3 Demonstrate ways to check that communication has been understood

For this AC your work practices will be observed; you will need to be able to demonstrate that you know how to use different ways of checking with an individual that communication has been understood. You will need to identify and reduce barriers to communication, as this is an important part of your job's role when working with individuals. Being aware of an individual's ability to understand what is being communicated is also very important. You will need to make sure that the individuals in your care truly understand the things that you are communicating to them. You can do this by using a variety of different methods.

1. Ask the individual

Asking the individual if they have understood what has been communicated is one way of checking whether the communication methods you have used are effective and have been understood. If the individual does not respond or looks away this could be a sign that the communication has not been understood.

If it is not possible to ask the individual then those who know them well such as an advocate, a colleague or another health or social care professional could be useful sources of information. You will find out more about the range of information sources available to enable more effective communication in AC 3.4.

Use the right language and words

Open and closed questions: open questions encourage individuals to communicate and are used when you want to find out information such as 'Tell me about your day' or 'How did you feel about the support you received this morning when getting dressed?' Closed questions enable 'Yes' or 'No' answers, or encourage short, factual answers, for example 'Do you like your course?', 'What time is it?', 'Where are you going?'

Appropriate language: as you have learned, this will also improve understanding and avoid communications being misunderstood.

Ask the individual to recap: if the individual can repeat and explain what you have just communicated to them, then this is a good way to know that your communication has been understood.

Key term

Open questions usually begin with 'What?', 'Why?' or 'How?' in order to encourage the expression of opinions and feelings. This is different to 'closed questions' which normally start with 'Who?' or 'Where?' and encourage short, factual answers.

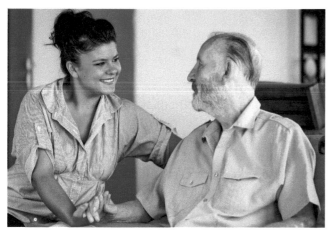

Figure 1.7 How do you ensure that you actively listen to individuals?

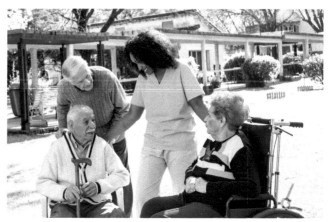

Figure 1.8 Why is it important to the well-being of individuals that they feel listened to and heard?

2. Observe the individual

Observing individuals when communicating with them is a useful way of checking whether they have understood what has been communicated to them. For example, if a personal assistant is communicating with a young person who has hearing loss and the young person does not respond to their questions being signed or begins to lose interest then this could be an indicator that the individual has not understood what is being communicated to them.

3. Practise active listening

Actively listening to individuals when communicating with them enables communication to be fully understood by identifying the true meaning behind the words and gestures used. As you will have learned, this involves observing and checking the messages that are being communicated both verbally and non-verbally. For example, you (or the 'active

Key terms

Paraphrasing is a way of repeating what has been said or heard using different words.

Active listening is a communication technique that involves understanding and interpreting what is being expressed through verbal and non-verbal communication.

listener' in this case) could **paraphrase** what an individual has told them, to ensure that they have fully understood what is being communicated. You could ask them open questions to clarify their understanding, for example using questions that begin with 'How' or 'Tell me'. This will also help you to obtain more information and gain a better insight into the individual's opinions and feelings. You could sit forward to show them you are interested in what they are saying and let them finish what they are saying to you. You can make sure that your facial expressions show that you are interested by smiling when appropriate and maintaining eye contact.

If the individuals feel that you are truly listening to them, they are more likely to trust you and tell you confidential and sensitive information that will, in turn, benefit them and better inform the care that you offer them. Think about how you would feel if you were explaining something important and your carer was not listening.

SOLER, a theory developed by Gerard Egan, can be used to describe key techniques that are essential for **active listening**:

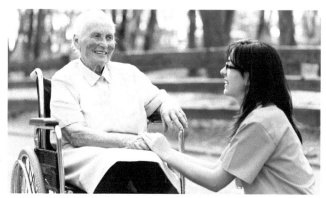

Figure 1.9 What messages are being communicated?

- **S**it squarely: think about how to position yourself in relation to the individual you are communicating with to show you have a genuine interest.
- **O**pen posture: think about how to maintain an open posture, for example do not cross your arms.
- **L**ean: think about the way you can lean towards the individual you are communicating with to show your interest, but take care not to invade their personal space.
- **E**ye contact: think about how and when to maintain eye contact to show you are listening i.e. not too little this may show you are not interested, or too much as this may make the individual feel uncomfortable.
- **R**elax: think about what effect *you* being relaxed can have on the individual, for example it can show that you have time for them.

All these methods for checking that communication is understood require sufficient time being made available. You will also require a good knowledge and understanding of the individual's specific communication and language needs and preferences. You will need to know which methods are most effective with different individuals, and this is a skill that you will develop over time. It is important that you remember to use the right approach when putting these methods into practice, then to follow up with any individuals where communication was not fully understood the first time. Be aware that there are cultural differences when it comes to body language. Always keep this in mind when communicating with individuals, to avoid causing offence or misunderstanding.

Evidence opportunity

3.3 Checking communication has been understood

Show two different methods that you use to check that communication has been understood. Remember that you will be observed. You could also support this by listing the different methods you use to check that communication with a diverse range of individuals in your work setting has been understood. Which methods work well? Which methods could be improved?

Reflect on the consequences of you not checking that communication has been understood by an individual. How could this impact on your working relationship with the individual? Could this affect other people in your work setting?

AC 3.4 Identify sources of information, support and services to enable more effective communication

Adult care settings contain a range of sources of information and support to enable more effective communications to take place, for example:

- people who know the individual well such as the individual's **key worker**
- records such as the individual's care/support plan and communication profile.

Sometimes when there is a change in an individual's needs, perhaps due to the onset of a health condition such as a stroke, then additional information and expert support may be required from external organisations. Specialist communication professionals and services can be useful sources of information, support and advice and can help with reducing barriers to communication and enabling effective communication to take place. These include:

- Professionals such as **translators** and **interpreters** where there are barriers around language, for example when an individual's first language is not English, and you are unable to speak their first language. You may also need to consult with a sign language, or Braille or Makaton, expert. You should discuss what services are available with your manager.

- **Speech and language services**/therapists or psychologists who work in speech and language services. They may be needed when there is a change in an individual's health (e.g. physical or mental health) that affects their communication.
- Advocate workers who work in **advocacy services** that can help individuals to speak

up for themselves when they are unable to because of a learning disability or a lack of confidence, for example.

- Specialist organisations who can provide additional support and access to services for individuals' specific communication needs include for example the Stroke Association and the National Autistic Society. There are organisations for most illnesses or conditions and they will be able to give you expert advice about specific conditions.

Key terms

A **key worker** is a person who works closely with the individual to understand their needs, wishes and preferences and who is specifically tasked with working closely with the individual.

Translators are professionals who convert written communication from one language to another.

Interpreters are professionals who convert spoken/oral or sign language communication from one language to another.

Speech and language services are providers of specialist communication information and support such as translation, interpreting, advocacy, speech and language services.

Advocacy services support individuals to speak up when they are unable to; they represent the individual's best interests.

Evidence opportunity

3.4 Sources of information, support and services

Find out from your work setting three internal and three external sources of information, support and services that are available to enable effective communication. Discuss

with your manager the procedure you must follow to access these. For example, you may look at the organisation or setting's contact records with local services available. Ensure you record all of this as evidence in your portfolio.

Reflect on it

3.4 Information, support and services

Read the statistics below.

'Nearly 20% of the population experience communication difficulties at some point in their lives.'

Source: Law, J. et al (2007) *Communication Support Needs: a Review of the Literature*, Scottish Executive Social Research

'88% of long-term unemployed young men have speech, language and communication needs.'

Source: Elliott, N. (2009) *An Investigation into the Communication Skills of Long-Term Unemployed Young Men*, University of Glamorgan

Reflect on this and record your reactions. Why is it important that you are aware of the range of information, support and services that can enable more effective communication and how you can access these? What would be the consequences of not doing so?

Reflective exemplar	
Introduction	I work as a personal assistant with Jo, a young man who has learning disabilities and lives on his own in a flat. My duties involve supporting Jo to use public transport to travel to and from his workplace and go shopping every week for food and household goods.
What happened?	Last week when I was supporting Jo with food shopping in the supermarket, one of the cashiers recognised Jo, approached him and standing very close to him said 'Hello' loudly. Jo jumped back and shouted, 'No, no' and then placed his hands over his ears.
	I supported Jo to move to a quieter area away from the till and asked him if he was all right. Jo kept his head down and shouted out again, 'No, no'. I reassured Jo and explained that we could remain in this quiet area until he was ready to continue to shop. Jo kicked the shopping basket over and ran out of the supermarket.
	When I returned to the office I discussed the situation with my manager and sought her advice about how this communication could have been improved; including the different communication methods I could have used.
What worked well?	I read Jo's body language and supported him to move to a quieter area; this removed him from the situation and gave him time and space to calm down.
	I reassured Jo; this ensured Jo felt supported.
What did not go as well?	I used a lot of verbal communication and mentioned the words 'continue to shop' – perhaps Jo may have misunderstood what I was saying, perhaps he was distressed, he may have thought that I wanted him to continue to shop.
	I did not explain to the cashier how she could have communicated with Jo more effectively; this could prevent this situation from occurring again.
What could I do to improve?	As I could see Jo was distressed, I should have communicated with him by using non-verbal communication methods only. I need to read through Jo's communication profile and support plan again and ensure I understand the full range of communication methods he uses and prefers in different situations. I will ask my manager if I am unsure about anything.
	I should have demonstrated to the cashier how to communicate with Jo quietly, by observing her space and positioning and by using non-verbal communication methods.
Links to unit assessment criteria	ACs 2.3, 3.1, 3.2

L03 Knowledge, skills, behaviours

Knowledge: do you know how to identify barriers to communication?

Do you know the reasons why you may be having difficulties communicating with an individual? Do you know how to reduce any barriers?

Why is it important to check that communication has been understood by an individual?

Do you know what sources of information are available if you are finding it difficult to communicate with an individual in the care setting where you work?

Did you know that you have just answered questions about how to identify barriers and where to find support available in relation to communication?

Skills: how can you ensure that your communications are effective?

How do you ensure that you treat each person you communicate with in your work setting as an individual?

Do you know how to reduce barriers that arise in relation to communications?

Do you know how to check that your communications have been understood?

Did you know that you have just shown some of the skills that are required by effective communicators?

LO3 Knowledge, skills, behaviours
Behaviours: how do you ensure you take into account individuals' unique needs and preferences when communicating with them?
Do you know how to show your respect for an individual's culture and reduce any barriers here?
Do you know how to show you are patient when communicating with an individual who is having difficulties understanding you?
Do you know how to show the provision of high-quality support when communicating with an individual?
Did you know that you have just shown some of the essential behaviours that are required when communicating with individuals who have different communication and language needs?

LO4 Be able to apply principles and practices relating to confidentiality at work

Getting started

Think about a time when you have written an email to a friend with private information, or told a friend a secret that you did not want others to know. How would you feel if that information was passed on without your permission? Would it be okay if the information had been passed on because your friend thought they were thinking only the best for you?

AC 4.1 Explain the term 'confidentiality'

Confidentiality is an important principle for those working in care settings with children, young people and adults as you will come across personal, private and sensitive information in your role. It underpins every aspect of their job roles, duties and responsibilities. As a health and social care professional, this will mean that you will need to:

- respect the personal information about the individuals and their families
- respect the individuals and their families' rights to privacy
- share information only with those who need to know
- get permission from the individual before you share information

Key term

Confidentiality means to keep something private or secret. Confidentiality is important in an adult care setting because it respects an individual's rights to privacy and dignity, it will instil trust between you and others, it promotes an individual's safety and security and it shows compliance with legislation such as the Data Protection Act 1998 (replaced by the GDPR 2018, see Unit 206, Handle information in care settings).

- instil trust between you and the individuals and/or their families
- share personal information only with others when there is a reason to do so.

Evidence opportunity

4.1 What does 'confidentiality' mean?

Share with a colleague your understanding of the term 'confidentiality'. Find out from your colleague their understanding of what this term means. Provide an explanation of this term in the context of your job role and work setting.

Reflect on an occasion when you shared personal information about yourself with another person. How did it make you feel? Do you feel that your information was respected and treated confidential? If so, how? You can either record this as written evidence or as a professional discussion with your assessor.

AC 4.2 Demonstrate confidentiality in day-to-day communication, in line with agreed ways of working

For this AC, you will be observed demonstrating confidentiality in your day-to-day work practices; you will also be expected to demonstrate that your working practices are in line with your care setting's agreed ways of working. Demonstrating confidentiality requires adult care workers and personal assistants to follow the **agreed ways of working** as set out in their confidentiality policy and procedures in their work settings. Legislation such as the Data Protection Act and the Freedom of Information Act is also relevant because they set out how to work with personal information about individuals and their families. Further information about relevant legislation is provided at the end of this unit.

Confidentiality in day-to-day communication refers to all personal information that is held about or obtained from individuals and their families such as name, address, date of birth, employment history, current and past health conditions, care and support needs. It includes all personal information that has been shared verbally, in writing, electronically or in other formats such as photographs, signs and symbols.

There are occasions when you may need to pass on information and this is discussed in AC 4.3.

Key terms

Agreed ways of working are the policies and procedures set out by your employer for your work setting. In this unit, the agreed ways of working that we discuss are to do with communication.

Consent means when someone agrees to something. Here you will need to obtain 'consent' (or agreement) or permission from an individual or their representative if the individual is unable to.

6Cs

Commitment

Commitment means to be dedicated. In a health and social care setting, this means commitment to improving the experience of people who need care and support, ensuring it is person-centred. In this section in particular, you will need to show commitment to maintaining the confidentiality of individuals' personal information at all times. This is important for building good, honest and open relationships with individuals. The 'dos and don'ts' table below has useful tips on how you can show your commitment to maintaining confidentiality, as well as what not to do.

Dos and don'ts for maintaining confidentiality in care settings	
Do	Only share individuals' personal information with those who have authorisation or those who are allowed to know it, for example your manager. If there is a health emergency then a GP or hospital consultant may request personal information about an individual's health. You will need to seek guidance from your manager about this or they may need to speak directly with your manager who will only disclose the information that is required.
Do	Make sure individuals' records are stored securely in the care setting. This means, store individuals' communication profiles in a locked cupboard when the profiles are no longer being used.
Do	Make sure individuals' written records are completed in a private area, i.e. complete individuals' daily reports in the office and out of view from others.

→

\	Dos and don'ts for maintaining confidentiality in care settings
Do	Make sure that individuals' electronic records are only accessed by those who have permission to do so, i.e. by ensuring all personal information held about individuals in electronic files is password protected.
Don't	Share individuals' personal information with other individuals in the care setting unless you have permission or **consent** (see page 32 for definition) to do so from the individual. If the individual is unable to consent, then you must have permission from their representative, in other words do not disclose personal information about individuals to others accidentally such as mentioning that an individual is diabetic and therefore cannot have a piece of chocolate cake like everyone else.
Don't	Discuss individuals when out in public places. In other words, do not discuss individuals when outside of the care setting as others may overhear. However, it may be that a situation has been upsetting and you feel you need to share this. If you do talk about them then you must do so in a way that any personal, private information is kept confidential. Never mention names, personal details, appearance, where the individual is from or anything that may reveal the identity of the individual. The best approach is to not reveal personal information about individuals or discuss them in a negative way. This will not only mean that you are following confidentiality rules and guidelines, but it will also mean that individuals, as well as colleagues and those outside the workplace, know that you can be trusted and relied upon.
Don't	Discuss individuals with other individuals you care for. Think about how you would feel if people you knew discussed you with others. Again, creating and maintaining trust between yourself and the individual you care for is key to your relationship and the care that you offer them.
Don't	Leave individuals' records out when not in use as these may be accessed by those who do not have authorisation to do so.
Don't	Give confidential details over the phone if possible. If you do need to give details over the phone, then check the identity of the person who has called you. You may need to take their number and call them back so that you are able to take some time to check the identity of the person requesting information.
Don't	Speak about individuals where other members of staff can overhear you.

Research it

4.2 Confidentiality

Research the confidentiality rules for care settings explained in 'A guide to confidentiality in health and social care' produced by the Health and Social Care Information Centre (HSCIC) in 2013:

http://content.digital.nhs.uk/media/12822/Guide-to-confidentiality-in-health-and-social-care/pdf/HSCIC-guide-to-confidentiality.pdf

Evidence opportunity

4.2 Confidentiality and policies and procedures (agreed ways of working)

Discuss your work setting's confidentiality policy and procedures with your assessor. Record the key points of your discussion and show through your work practices three different examples of how you maintain confidentiality in your day-to-day communications, the individual's consent form could be one of them. You will need to demonstrate how you maintain confidentiality to your assessor, for example by seeking permission from your manager and the individuals involved.

You will need to demonstrate confidentiality in your work practices. This might be through an observation or from a witness statement from your manager.

Reflect on the three examples you used to show how you maintained confidentiality in your day-to-day communications. What skills did you use? What skills did you apply well? What skills could you improve? Ensure you keep a record of your reflections.

6Cs

C

Competence

Competence refers to effectively putting your knowledge and skills into practice. Doing so will show that you are able to provide high-quality care and support to individuals. In this section, you can show that you are competent by demonstrating confidentiality in your day-to-day communications with individuals and others who you work with. The 'dos and don'ts' tables on pages 33 and 35 provides helpful tips on some of the ways in which you can protect the confidentiality of those you work with.

AC 4.3 Describe situations where information normally considered to be confidential might need to be passed on

'Need to know'

Individuals have the right to have all personal information held about them kept private, however sometimes there may be occasions when it is necessary to share their personal information with others **in confidence**. This process of sharing confidential information with others is referred to as doing so on a **'need-to-know'** basis. This means that only relevant information is shared with those who require it.

Key terms

🔑

'**In confidence**' in a care setting, means to trust that the information will only be passed on to others who need to know.

'**Need to know**' means that you should only give away information that is absolutely necessary in order to protect an individual's privacy and ensure their safety.

Research it

4.3 'Need to know'

Research the procedures in place in your work setting for when confidential information can be shared on a 'need-to-know' basis.

Examples of situations where confidential information may need to be passed on

Below are some examples of situations where confidential information will need to be passed on. Can you think of any others?

- An older adult is found unconscious in their home by a domiciliary care worker and is taken to hospital. In order to treat the individual effectively, the hospital consultant will require personal information about the individual such as whether the individual has any current health conditions and whether they are taking any medication.

- A young person who visits a mental health drop-in centre and wishes to have lunch will need to inform the staff there about their allergy to nuts so that their dietary needs can be met and they can be kept safe from becoming unwell.

- An adult who lives in a residential care setting shares information with their key worker that they observed a visitor shout at another individual who lives in the same care setting. The adult will need to be informed that the care worker is required to pass this information on 'in confidence' to their manager who will in turn inform adult care services in order to protect the individual and any others from any further harm or abuse.

- A young person who tells their personal assistant that a friend of theirs stole some goods from the local shop will need to be informed that it is the personal assistant's duty to pass this information on to their manager in the first instance. The manager may then need to inform the police. If so, the young person will be informed of all actions taken and why they are required.

Obtain consent

If you need to pass on information about individuals to others, you must make sure that you tell the individual. In some cases you will need to inform the individual in advance and obtain their consent. This may be the case when, for example, a court or tribunal (where a dispute is settled) has requested information. When an individual lacks capacity and is unable to give consent then permission must be sought from their representative.

A personal assistant is employed directly by the individual with care or support needs or by a family member when the individual does not have the capacity to be the employer. If you are a personal assistant, you will have a contract of employment that will set out your rights and responsibilities

as an employee including who you can share information with, such as doctors, and when this may be required, such as during hospital appointments. Sometimes, however, it may be necessary for you to share confidential information without your employer's consent. For example, if you identify that your employer is being abused you have a duty to report this to the council's safeguarding board.

Check the identity of anyone you give confidential information to

As you are dealing with confidential information, it is important to check the identity of anyone who has requested the information, especially people who you do not know outside the setting. This is to ensure that any confidential information is not then passed on to others to misuse.

Dealing with family members or relatives

Remember that just because someone is related to the individual, it does not mean that they are automatically entitled to see the individual's records. You must ensure you have consent from the individual.

	Dos and don'ts when dealing with others
Do	Explain the reasons why you are unable to give out information to family members.
Do	Explain that you understand their situation.
Do	Reinforce the rights of their relative.
Don't	Feel pressured to give family members information just because they are related to the individual and even if they have the individual's interests at heart.
Don't	Avoid speaking with family members.
Don't	Be afraid of repeating yourself in relation to why you are unable to give out information.

Evidence opportunity

4.3 When confidential information may need to be passed on

Discuss with your assessor three different occasions where confidential information about individuals was passed on in confidence to others. For each situation include details of the reasons why the information was required, how the information was passed on, and to whom. The discussion could either be recorded, you could discuss this with your assessor or your manager could provide a witness testimony.

Reflect on it

4.3 Confidential information

Reflect on the importance of sharing confidential information about individuals when providing care and support. What are the consequences of not doing so?

AC 4.4 Explain how and when to seek advice about confidentiality

How to seek advice

Each work setting will have its own confidentiality policy and procedures that set out the process to follow for how and when adult care workers and personal assistants can seek advice about confidentiality. For example, this may involve speaking with the manager or team leader (if an adult care worker) or the employer (if a personal assistant). The thing to remember is that you should ask your manager if you are unsure about any confidentiality issues.

Although each work setting will have developed its own confidentiality policy and procedures, there are some key information points that will be included:

- purpose of or the reasons behind the policy/procedures about confidentiality
- principles that underpin the confidentiality policy and procedures
- the information that will be held by the organisation and the reasons why
- how information held is accessed
- how information will be recorded
- how information will be stored
- how information will be disclosed
- how breaches of confidentiality are reported
- the underpinning legislative framework.

Evidence opportunity

4.4 How and when to seek advice about confidentiality

Obtain a copy of the confidentiality policy and procedures for your work setting. How does this compare to the key areas identified in the template above?

Discuss with a colleague the procedure for seeking advice about confidentiality in your work setting and the reasons why you might do this.

When to seek advice

As you will have learned, there are occasions where information normally considered confidential might need to be passed on. It may also be necessary to seek advice about confidentiality if:

- the adult care worker or personal assistant is unsure if they are able to disclose personal information about an individual
- you do not know the identity of the person requesting the information, for example a social worker who telephones the work setting and requests information about an individual
- you are at a care or support meeting where the individual's family and other professionals are present.

Seeking advice can also help to reinforce and reassure the adult care worker or personal assistant that the work setting's confidentiality policy and procedures have been fully understood and complied with.

Evidence opportunity

4.4 When to seek advice and why

Discuss with your manager when it may be necessary to seek advice about confidentiality in your work setting and the reasons why.

Case study

4.4 Maintaining confidentiality

Sylvia is 70 and has lived at Holm residential care home for three years. Her niece, Alison, lives close by and is a regular visitor to the home. Alison has established a monthly support group in the home for the relatives of the individuals who live there, and volunteers once a week supporting the activities co-ordinator.

This morning Sylvia slipped over on the stairs coming down for breakfast and injured her leg. An ambulance was called and it was decided to take her to hospital. As Sylvia was leaving in the ambulance, she told her key worker that she does not want Alison, her niece, to know that she has been taken to hospital as she does not want

to worry her. The key worker was unable to discuss this with Sylvia as there was no time.

In the afternoon, Alison visits the residential care home and asks where Sylvia is.

Questions

1 What would you say to Alison?
2 Would you have a duty to maintain Sylvia's confidentiality?
3 Would you have a duty to keep Alison informed about her relative?
4 Imagine if you were Sylvia's key worker. What would you have said to her in response to her saying that she does not want her niece to know that she's been taken to hospital because she does not want to worry her?

LO4 Knowledge, skills, behaviours
Knowledge: why is confidentiality important when providing care and support?
Do you know what confidentiality means?
Do you know how it can affect individuals if you do not maintain their personal information confidentially?
Do you know when you may need to pass on confidential information and the reasons why?
If you do need to seek advice about confidentiality, do you know how and when to ask?
Did you know you have shown understanding of what confidentiality means and why it is important to individuals who have care or support needs?
Skills: how do you promote the importance of confidentiality in your work setting?
Do you make sure that when you complete documents your handwriting is clear and legible?
Do you make sure that what you have written can be read and understood easily, in case your colleagues need to access and read the documents?
Do you know how to keep personal information shared verbally about individuals confidential?
Did you know that you have just shown that you have some of the skills needed to promote confidentiality in your work setting?
Behaviours: how do you show your commitment to confidentiality?
Do you date all your documents?
Do you make sure that they are anonymised? In other words, do you make sure that the individual's name is not included?
Did you know that you have adhered to or followed some of the requirements of the Data Protection Act 1998?

Suggestions for using the activities

This table summarises all the activities in the unit that are relevant to each assessment criterion.

Here, we also suggest other, different methods that you may want to use to present your knowledge and skills by using the activities.

These are just suggestions, and you should refer to the Introduction section at the start of the book, and more importantly the City & Guilds specification, and your assessor who will be able to provide more guidance on how you can evidence your knowledge and skills.

When you need to be observed during your assessment, this can be done by your assessor, or your manager can provide a witness testimony.

Assessment criteria and accompanying activities	Suggested methods to show your knowledge/skills
LO1 Understand why communication is important in the work setting	
1.1 Reflect on it (page 6)	Complete a spider diagram of the different people you communicate with or write a reflective account.
1.1 Evidence opportunity (page 6)	Provide a written account and address the points. Remember to include when you communicate with them as well as why and how.
1.2 Research it (page 9)	Carry out some research in your work setting to find out the different skills you and your colleagues use to communicate effectively. Make notes detailing your findings.
1.2 Evidence opportunity (page 9)	Write an account about how effective communication affects the way you carry out one task that you carry out on a regular basis. Remember to address the points outlined in the activity. You could also write a reflective account.
1.3 Research it (page 10)	Write a statement about high and low pitch and tones based on the clips you have watched, and when you may need to use them in your setting.
1.3 Research it (page 11)	Having researched the well-being principles think about the importance of understanding the meanings behind an individual's reactions. Provide a short written account to detailing your thoughts.
1.3 Reflect on it (page 12)	Write a short reflective account detailing the reasons why it is important to observe an individual's reactions when communicating with them. You will find it helpful to address the questions in the activity.
1.3 Evidence opportunity (page 12)	Write an account answering the questions. You could write a personal statement or reflective account more generally about your experience of an occasion when it was important to observe an individual's reactions when communicating with them, and explain why it was important.
LO2 Be able to meet the communication and language needs, wishes and preferences of individuals	
2.1 Research it (page 13)	Write a short account of what you have found out about disabilities and illnesses that may affect communication, language needs and preferences.
2.1 Research it (page 15)	Write notes on what you have discovered from your research about how culture and beliefs can impact on communication. How do these affect how you communicate? Or you could write a reflective account about your own culture and beliefs.
2.1 Evidence opportunity (page 15)	Show three methods of finding out about their communication and language needs, wishes and preferences. For example, one method might involve asking their advocate, who knows them well, for more information about how they communicate. You will need to show your assessor.

Suggestions for using the activities	
2.2 Evidence opportunity (page 16)	Show your assessor through your work practices how you use non-verbal and verbal communication methods to meet an individual's communication and language needs, wishes and preferences. You may also like to record why you chose each method for the individual.
2.2 Reflect on it (page 17)	Write a short reflective account. Or you could explain to a colleague the talk that you had with an individual and how linguistic tone and pitch were used and why. Make notes to detail your discussion.
2.2 Research it (page 17)	Write notes about how the use of technology aids can support an individual to communicate.
2.3 Evidence opportunity (page 18) 2.3 Case study (page 19)	Show your assessor through your work practices how and when you seek advice about communication. You could also explain to your assessor how and in which situations you have sought advice about communication. A case study has been included to help you.
2.3 Reflect on it (page 19)	Discuss with a colleague a time when they sought advice about communication, when, why and what they thought were the benefits of doing so. Make notes to evidence your discussion. Or you could write a reflective account about the consequences of not seeking advice about communication. You might find it useful to refer to your setting's policies and procedures to see what they say about this.
LO3 Be able to reduce barriers to communication	
3.1 Reflect on it (page 23)	Discuss with a colleague the different people you communicate with and what barriers you have come across. Provide a short reflective account to evidence your discussion or a reflective account addressing the questions in the activity.
3.1 Evidence opportunity (page 23)	List the different barriers to effective communication. You could also tell your assessor about the barriers to communication that exist. Or complete a spider diagram of the different barriers to communication.
3.2 Research it (page 24)	Make notes detailing what you found out from your research.
3.2 Case study (page 25)	Read through the case study and provide a written account detailing the answers. Discuss the points with your assessor.
3.2 Reflect on it (page 25)	You might like to write a short reflective account about the impact of not reducing barriers to communication and what this might mean for individuals, you as an adult care worker, someone in a personal assistant role or your team.
3.2 Evidence opportunity (page 25)	Select three barriers to effective communication that exist in your work setting and that you included in your list for AC 3.1. For each one, show two different methods that you could use to reduce these barriers. Show your assessor through your work practices how you reduce barriers to communication that arise. Remember, the observation could be a generic observation by your assessor of your practice to reduce barriers, or be an account in a witness statement from your manager.
3.3 Research it (page 27)	You might like to write notes to document the findings from your research about tips for communicating with individuals with hearing loss. You could share these with a colleague.

➜

Suggestions for using the activities	
3.3 Evidence opportunity (page 28)	Show two different methods that you use to check that communication has been understood.
	You'll need to show your assessor through your work practices how you use different methods to check that communication has been understood.
	You could also support this with a written account listing the different ways you use to check communication has been understood. You could then reflect on the consequences of not checking that communication has been understood.
3.4 Evidence opportunity (page 29)	Find out from your work setting three internal and three external sources of information, support and services that are available to enable effective communication. Discuss with your manager the procedure you must follow to access these.
	Ensure you record all of this as evidence in your portfolio.
	You could also complete a spider diagram of the different sources that exist both within and outside of your work setting.
3.4 Reflect on it (page 29)	Write down your thoughts on the statistics that you have read, and record your reactions. Explain why it is important that you are aware of the range of information, support and services that can enable more effective communication and how you can access these. What would be the consequences of not doing so? You could also explain this to your assessor.
LO4 Be able to apply principles and practices relating to confidentiality at work	
4.1 Evidence opportunity (page 31)	Discuss with a colleague an occasion when you shared personal information about yourself with another person. Address the points outlined. You could either record all of this as written evidence or as a professional discussion with your assessor.
	You could also write a personal statement or reflective account about your experience of the meaning of the term 'confidentiality' in relation to your work role and setting.
4.2 Research it (page 33)	Write notes detailing what you have learnt from 'A guide to confidentiality in health and social care settings'.
4.2 Evidence opportunity (page 33)	Discuss your work setting's confidentiality policy and procedures with your assessor. Record the key points of your discussion.
	Show your assessor through your work practices three different examples of how you maintain confidentiality in day-to-day communication in your work setting. This might be through an observation or a witness statement from your manager.
	You could also support this by writing a reflective account about three different examples when you maintained confidentiality in your day-to-day communications. Address the questions in the activity and ensure you keep a record of your reflections.
4.3 Research it (page 34)	Make some notes about the procedures in place in your work setting for when confidential information can be shared on a 'need-to-know' basis. You might like to recap these to a colleague and ask your manager any questions you may have.

→

Suggestions for using the activities	
4.3 Evidence opportunity (page 35)	Tell your assessor about three different situations where information normally considered to be confidential might need to be passed on in your work setting. You could record this discussion or your manager could provide a witness testimony.
	You could support this by writing a personal statement or reflective account about your experience of different situations that might arise in your work setting where confidential information might need to be passed on.
4.3 Reflect on it (page 36)	Write a short reflective account about the importance of sharing confidential information about individuals when providing care and support. What are the consequences of not doing so?
4.4 Evidence opportunity (page 36)	Obtain a copy of the confidentiality policy and procedures for your work setting. How does this compare to the key areas identified in the template?
	Address the points in the activity, discuss with a colleague and provide a written account to evidence this. You can produce this procedure in a flow chart to show what you must do. You could also write a personal statement or reflective account about your experience of when and why to seek advice about confidentiality in your work setting.
	Or you could discuss the points with your manager who could provide a witness testimony. You could also discuss with a colleague the procedure and different steps to take for seeking advice about confidentiality in your work setting and the reasons why. Provide a written account to evidence your discussion.
4.4 Evidence opportunity (page 36)	Discuss with your manager when it may be necessary to seek advice about confidentiality in your work setting and the reasons why. They will be able to provide a witness testimony.
4.4 Case study (page 37)	Read through the case study and discuss the points with a colleague. Make sure you provide a written account detailing your responses and discussion.

Legislation	
Relevant Act	**It states that:**
Data Protection Act 1998	information and data must be: processed fairly and lawfully; used only for the purpose it was intended to be used for; be adequate, relevant, accurate and up to date; held for no longer than is necessary; used in line with the rights of individuals; kept secure; and not transferred to other countries without the individual's permission.
General Data Protection Regulation (GDPR) 2018	In May 2018 the General Data Protection Regulation came into force. It provides detailed guidance to organisations on how to govern and manage people's personal information.
Freedom of Information Act 2000	individuals have the right to apply for access to information held by a wide range of public bodies, such as local authorities and hospitals.
Care Act 2014	local authorities must provide comprehensive information and advice about care and support services in their local area. This information and advice must be provided using methods and formats that meet individuals' needs and can be understood.
Equality Act 2010	employers and providers of services for individuals with disabilities have to make reasonable adjustments when these are required. For example, by making information available in large print for individuals with sight loss and installing a hearing loop system in a meeting room.
Human Rights Act 1998	individuals' human rights, such as the right to security and freedom of expression, are protected.

Resources for further reading and research

Books

Butler, S.J. (2004) *Hearing and Sight Loss – A Handbook for Professional Carers*, Age Concern

Caldwell, P. and Stevens, P. (2005) *Creative Conversations: Communicating with People with Learning Disabilities*, Pavilion Publishers

Ferreiro Peteiro, M. (2014) *Level 2 Health and Social Care Diploma Evidence Guide*, Hodder Education

Moss, B. (2015) *Communication Skills in Health and Social Care* (3rd edition), Sage Publications Ltd

Weblinks

www.actiononhearingloss.org.uk Action on Hearing Loss – information and factsheets on communicating and supporting people who are deaf, deafblind or have a hearing loss

www.alzheimers.org.uk Alzheimer's Society – information on communication methods and strategies to use with individuals who have Alzheimer's disease

www.autism.org.uk The National Autistic Society (NAS) – information on communicating with individuals on the autistic spectrum

www.rnib.org.uk Royal National Institute of Blind People (RNIB) – information on communicating with individuals who have sight loss, are blind or partially sighted

www.scie.org.uk Social Care Institute for Excellence (SCIE) – e-learning resources on effective communication skills and how to apply them

www.stroke.org.uk The Stroke Association – information, support and services for individuals who have had strokes

Personal development in care settings (207)

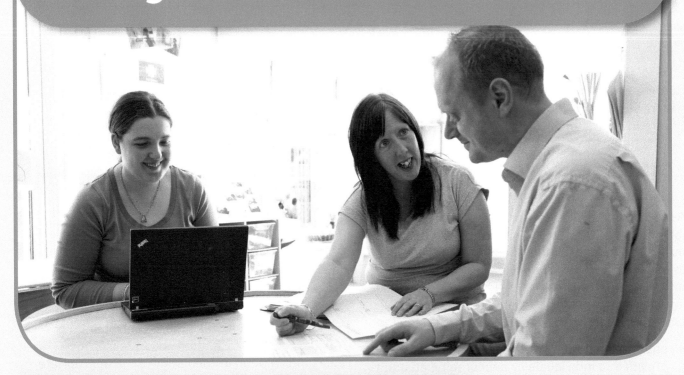

About this unit

Credit value: 3
Guided learning hours: 23

Personal development is not just about developing your knowledge, skills and practice at work. It is also about you getting to know yourself, developing a better understanding of who you are, and how what you think, feel and do impacts on others.

In this unit, you will have an opportunity to explore your own role, **duties** and **responsibilities**. You will learn about the standards, regulations and agreed ways of working that influence how you carry out your role. You will also increase your awareness of personal **values**, **attitudes** and **beliefs**, and learn how to ensure that these do not affect the quality of your work.

Personal development involves being able to reflect on your work activities and situations that arise at work and understanding the reasons why this is an important skill to have (as this will help you to develop your knowledge, skills and practice). During the course of the unit you will also understand how to assess your own knowledge, skills and understanding in order to meet the required standards. You will also have the opportunity to understand how you agree, contribute and record your own personal development plan (PDP) by working alongside others, and what sources of support you can access. Finally, you will understand the importance of taking feedback on board and how you can record your progress in relation to personal development.

Learning outcomes

LO1: Understand what is required for competence in your work role

LO2: Be able to reflect on your work activities

LO3: Be able to agree a personal development plan

LO4: Be able to develop your knowledge, skills and understanding

LO1 Understand what is required for competence in your work role

AC 1.1 Describe the duties and responsibilities of your role

As you enter the adult care profession and setting (or a new role within it) you will be informed of the **duties** and **responsibilities** that you will be required to carry out in your role. All roles in a care setting, including the one you are in, will have a set of knowledge, skills and behaviours that are required and expected from workers. These are essential for:

- ensuring that high-quality care and support is provided to individuals by encouraging all adult care workers to work in consistent ways

- making clear what is expected from adult care workers by ensuring all adult care workers understand what their day-to-day work tasks involve

- ensuring that all adult care workers show the correct **attitudes**, **values** and **behaviours** (such as dignity and respect) towards the individuals they care for.

As part of your role you are required to carry out specific tasks. These are described in your **job description** as duties. Your job description will also set out the different responsibilities you have as part of your role. Examples of duties may include providing support to individuals to learn new skills, recording and reporting information. Examples of responsibilities may be to provide support to individuals that helps to empower them (to take more control of their lives), to record information accurately or to report information immediately to the appropriate person.

 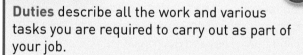

Job description: support worker

Duties

- To provide assistance to individuals when required with care tasks, which can include: showering, maintaining their personal hygiene, preparing meals, managing money, shopping and attending health appointments.
- To maintain daily records, including care plans.
- To attend team and support meetings as required.
- To undertake training required.

Responsibilities

- To respect the individual's right to make their own choices and refuse assistance with tasks.
- To promote the individual's independence, privacy and dignity at all times.
- To promote effective communication with individuals.
- To carry out all tasks using safe practices and in a safe environment.
- To ensure confidentiality is maintained at all times.
- To ensure all records are completed accurately, in a timely manner and kept up to date.

Figure 2.1 Duties and responsibilities for a support worker

The duties and responsibilities you have will vary and depend on the following:

- **The type of organisation you work for** – for example, residential care or **domiciliary care**.
- **The size of the organisation you work for** – this also means that the type of **induction** and initial training you have will vary. For example, in a large organisation you may have a formal induction process and training sessions where you will gain an understanding of the setting, the agreed ways of working and its policies and procedures. However, in a small organisation, or if you are working as a personal assistant, you may learn much of what you will do 'on the job', in other words, as you are doing your job.

- **What your job involves** – for example, providing care to different individuals, planning and carrying out group activities.
- **Your experience of working in the health and social care sector** and the role you have been employed to carry out. For example, you may be new to working in care or you may have years of experience.

Key terms

Domiciliary care refers to care provided to an individual who lives in their own home. This can include assistance with getting dressed, taking medication and preparing meals.

Induction means an introduction to a new organisation or setting, or a new system of working.

How you carry out your responsibilities will depend largely on you, your personality, your approach to your work and your passion and interest in carrying out your job to the best of your ability.

Your ability to carry out your role well is referred to as '**competence**'. If you are competent then you can show that you have the correct and expected knowledge, skills, attitudes, values and behaviours and can apply these when you are carrying out your job. If you are not competent then you will not be able to carry out your job role well or effectively and you will not therefore be able to provide high-quality care and support.

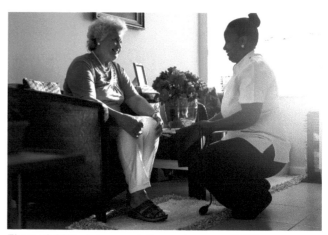

Figure 2.2 What do your duties and responsibilities say about you?

6Cs

Competence

Applying the knowledge and skills you have gained in your role is central to providing high-quality care and support.

As mentioned, you can show that you are competent in your role by effectively carrying out the duties and responsibilities that you are assigned. This includes being aware of and complying with the policies and procedures in your setting and ensuring you follow best practice to provide the best support you can.

Constantly thinking how competent you are in your role, and thinking of ways to improve it, will also enable you to become a better care worker as you are continually trying to progress and achieve high standards of practice and care for individuals.

There are also other legal requirements that inform your duties and responsibilities and these are explored in AC 1.2.

Reflect on it

1.1 Are you competent?

Reflect on the knowledge, skills and behaviours expected from you in the care setting where you work. Are you competent? How may this influence the care and support you provide to individuals?

AC 1.2 Identify standards, regulatory requirements and agreed ways of working that may influence your knowledge, understanding and skills to carry out your work role

What standards are in place for adult care workers?

The way you carry out your duties and responsibilities in the care setting where you work is guided by a set of **standards** that establish the knowledge, skills and values that will help you carry out your duties and responsibilities well and to a high standard.

Below are some examples of the different sets of standards that are in place for those who work in the health and social care sector. There is overlap in what these standards ask of care workers but it is important that you know them so that you have an understanding of the types of things that you need to do in order to follow best practice and provide high-quality care.

Codes of conduct and practice

Codes of conduct and practice are agreed ways of working for professions such as healthcare and social care workers and other organisations that provide services such as care and support. The Code of Conduct for Healthcare Support Workers and Adult Social Care Workers in England reflects best practice and although it is not a legal requirement, it is recommended that it be followed. It established the standards of conduct, behaviours and attitudes that can be expected from care workers and support workers.

It states that healthcare support workers and adult social care workers must:

- be accountable by making sure they can answer for their actions or omissions (oversights), for example by being honest about when things have not gone well and mistakes have been made
- promote and uphold the privacy, dignity, rights, health and well-being of the individuals who use health and care services and their carers at all times, for example by supporting individuals' and carers' rights when meeting with them
- work together with their colleagues to ensure the provision and delivery of high-quality, safe and **compassionate** healthcare, **care and support**, for example by showing your kindness and respect when supporting individuals' preferences
- communicate in an open and effective way to promote the health, safety and well-being of the individuals who use health and care services and their carers, for example by involving individuals and their carers when planning their care and support
- respect an individual's right to **confidentiality**, for example by only disclosing their personal information with those who need and require it
- be committed to improve the quality of healthcare, care and support through **continuing professional development**, for example, by regularly attending training
- uphold and promote **equality**, **diversity** and **inclusion**, by treating people as individuals and respecting their unique needs and preferences.

Skills for Care and Skills for Health (2013) 'Code of Conduct for Healthcare Support Workers and Adult Social Care Workers in England'

Key terms

Standards may include codes of conduct and practice, regulations and minimum standards.

Compassionate care and support refers to providing care and support with consideration, kindness and while supporting individuals' rights such as privacy, dignity, respect.

Confidentiality refers to keeping individuals' personal information private and only disclosing it to those who need to know it.

Continuing professional development refers to the process of identifying, documenting and monitoring the knowledge, skills and experience that you learn and apply at work.

Equality refers to ensuring equal opportunities are provided to everyone irrespective of their differences such as age, ability, background or religion.

Diversity refers to recognising, respecting and valuing people's individual differences.

Inclusion refers to involving people in their care or the services they use so that they are treated fairly and not excluded.

6Cs

Communication

When working in an adult care setting, you will need to ensure that you develop good communication skills to enable you to be an effective communicator as this is essential for developing working relationships. In your role, you will need to ensure that you can communicate well with the individuals that you care for, their families or carers, and colleagues. Your role and responsibilities will require you to communicate in various ways, both verbal and non-verbal, for example one of your duties may be to assist an individual with eating and drinking. Even a task such as this will require you to communicate well with the individual, to find out what their preferences are for food and drink, whether they feel comfortable, whether they would like assistance with cutting the food or if they can do this on their own (see Unit 203, Communication in care settings).

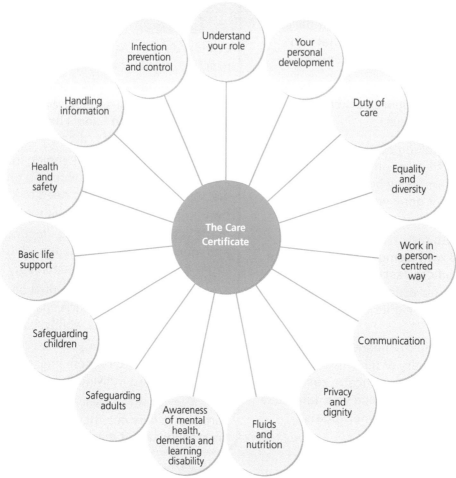

Source: *The Care Certificate Framework (Standards)*, Health Education England, Skills for Care and Skills for Health

Figure 2.3 The Care Certificate's standards

Reflect on it

1.2 Codes of conduct

Reflect on the code of conduct or practice that you follow in the care setting where you work. What does it say about the standards that are expected from you? How does it compare to the code of conduct for healthcare support workers and adult social care workers?

The Care Certificate

This is a set of 15 standards commonly used alongside the Code of Conduct for Healthcare Support Workers and Adult Social Care Workers.

It established the standards that health and social care workers are expected to follow in their day-to-day work to be able to provide high-quality care and support.

Workers are introduced to these standards as soon as they begin work; as part of the introduction to their role and the care setting where they work.

The Care Certificate's 15 standards are identified in Figure 2.3.

Minimum standards

The minimum standards refer to the knowledge and skills that are required by all health and social care workers to carry out their tasks to a standard beyond which the provision of care must never fall.

The Care Quality Commission's (CQC) fundamental standards describe the minimum standards that all those who access adult care services can expect. Some examples of the fundamental standards are listed below.

- **Person-centred care** – adult care workers must provide care that meets individuals' unique needs and preferences.

- **Dignity and respect** – adult care workers must treat individuals with dignity and respect at all times and this includes respecting their privacy and promoting their independence.
- **Consent** – adult care workers must ensure individuals or their representatives have given their consent before providing them with care and support.
- **Safety** – adult care workers must promote individuals' safety at all times and not put them at risk of any danger or harm.
- **Safeguarding** from abuse – adult care workers must ensure that the care and support provided is free from abuse.
- **Food and drink** – adult care workers must ensure that individuals are provided with sufficient food and drink to maintain their health and **well-being**.
- **Premises and equipment** – adult care workers must ensure that the equipment used in the provision of care and support to individuals is safe to use, kept clean and stored away safely when not in use.
- **Complaints** – adult care workers must ensure that they follow their care setting's agreed ways of working when individuals complain about their care.

National Occupational Standards

The Health and Social Care **National Occupational Standards** describe:

- the required knowledge, skills and values for health and social care workers in the UK
- best practice in different areas of work
- the basis of training and qualifications, for example the Level 2 Diploma in Care which you are studying is a qualification that is based on the National Occupational Standards that describe the knowledge and skills required of adult care workers
- the standards that each worker in every role in the health and adult social care sector must meet, for example the job of a care assistant will include promoting, monitoring and maintaining health, safety and security in the workplace; promoting effective communication and relationships;

contributing to the protection of individuals from abuse; enabling individuals to maintain their personal hygiene and appearance and enabling individuals to participate in recreation and leisure activities.

If you find that you are not meeting the required standards then it is important that you reflect on why this is. It is your responsibility to make sure that you take action to change things and improve your working practices. You can do this by speaking to your manager, getting advice from them and letting them know of any changes that you plan to make. You can also speak to colleagues to find out if they have any useful feedback. There is more on feedback in AC 4.4.

What regulatory requirements are in place for adult care workers?

Rules or regulations that are set in law also influence the way that adult care workers can carry out different tasks in the care setting where they work. The Care Quality Commission (CQC) is the independent **regulator** of health and adult social care provision in England.

- The CQC checks that the care and support services provided are safe, effective, caring, responsive to people's needs and well-led, and then documents its findings in a report that is then made available for the public to see and read.

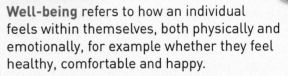

Key terms

Well-being refers to how an individual feels within themselves, both physically and emotionally, for example whether they feel healthy, comfortable and happy.

National Occupational Standards ensure that adult care workers provide good care and support and that best practice is followed.

Regulator is a term used to describe an independent body such as the CQC that inspects, monitors and rates adult social care services in terms of their safety, effectiveness, care and management.

- The CQC was established under the Health and Social Care Act 2008 (Regulated Activities) Regulations 2014 and includes a set of regulations that influence the day-to-day practice of adult care workers. For example:
    - **Regulation 10: Dignity and respect** – under this regulation, adult care workers are required to treat individuals with dignity and respect at all times when providing care and support including treating them fairly, respecting their privacy and promoting their independence.
    - **Regulation 12: Safe care and treatment** – under this regulation, adult care workers are required to have the necessary competence to ensure individuals' safety is maintained, and danger, harm and abuse prevented.
- Not all services are regulated by the CQC – for instance, friends of the individual's family or one of their neighbours might provide informal care to an individual. However, the CQC requirements are still good practice in such cases and should be followed.

Other relevant regulations that influence how adult care workers carry out their day-to-day work have been established by the Health and Safety at Work Act 1974 and include:

- **The Control of Substances Hazardous to Health Regulations 2002** – influence the safety of adult care workers' work practices in relation to handling substances such as cleaning substances that may be dangerous to their health. For example, these require adult care workers to wear protective equipment such as aprons and gloves when using cleaning substances, by ensuring cleaning substances are locked away securely after use to prevent them being used by individuals who may not understand how to use them safely.
- **The Management of Health and Safety at Work Regulations 1999** – influence adult care workers' work practices by requiring, for example, that they take reasonable care of their own health and safety and those of others such as individuals and visitors, and

report any health and safety concerns they have.
- **The Manual Handling Operations Regulations 1992** – influence adult care workers' work practices by requiring that they follow the care setting's agreed ways of working for safety at all times and make use of equipment such as hoists provided to carry out their work safely.

You will learn more about these regulations and how they influence adult care workers' work practices in Unit 210, Health, safety and well-being in care settings.

What 'agreed ways of working' are in place for adult care workers?

In addition to the standards and regulatory requirements that are in place for adult care workers, all care settings have 'agreed ways of working'. You will be expected to know what these are and show that you are able to follow them while you carry out your day-to-day work.

Agreed ways of working can include:

- **policies** such as safeguarding adults, health and safety, risk assessment
- **procedures** such as moving and handling, assistance with personal hygiene
- **guidance** such as how to support an individual with their mobility or how to communicate with an individual who has specific communication needs
- **best practice** such as how to involve individuals and their families in care and support planning or how to promote healthy eating with individuals.

All of these things are in place to ensure that you are able to carry out your role to a high standard and offer the best care possible to individuals. These standards, codes of practice and regulations are very important because they make it lawful to work in a way that protects individuals from danger, harm or abuse. However, simply knowing about the relevant standards, regulations and agreed ways of working required is not enough because you will also have to demonstrate the skills you have and put your knowledge into practice as part of your job.

You will notice that there is some overlap in the areas across the different standards, regulations and agreed ways of working, and it may even be a little tricky to work out exactly which parts of your role they relate to. However, it is important to remember that they all inform your work, from treating individuals with dignity and respect in personal care routines, to the way you handle meal times, to ensuring a safe environment is maintained, to how you record and store their data. These standards, regulations and agreed ways of working really do matter.

Research it

1.2 Keeping up to date with standards, regulations and legislation

You must stay up to date with all changes to standards and regulations, as well as legislation, so that you can ensure you are following best practice and continually improving your way of working. Below are some useful websites you may like to visit:

The Government's website:

www.gov.uk

The Health and Safety Executive's website:

www.hse.gov.uk

The Care Quality Commission's website:

www.cqc.org.uk

Evidence opportunity

1.2 Standards, regulatory requirements and agreed ways of working

Find out about the agreed ways of working that are in place in the care setting where you work. You will find it useful to speak with your manager and colleagues about how these agreed ways of working influence your day-to-day work. Now identify two standards and two regulations and describe how they influence your work role.

Produce a leaflet that shows your findings.

AC 1.3 Describe how to ensure that your personal values, attitudes or beliefs do not obstruct the quality of work and working practice

What do we mean by values, attitudes and beliefs and why is it important to be aware of them in a care role?

Your values, attitudes and beliefs are unique to you and part of who you are and so they will influence your role as an adult care worker including what you do and how you do it. In a care setting, you will be working with a wide array of people who will come from different backgrounds, many of whom may have similar values, attitudes and beliefs to you and many of whom may have different ones to you. They may, for example, come from a different cultural or educational background, you may share different political beliefs or have different attitudes towards various things.

Much of our role involves working very closely with the people for whom we provide care and support, our roles are based on close interactions and relationships. Because your beliefs, values and attitudes make up so much of the person you are, they will inevitably play a role in the relationships that you have not only outside but inside the setting and will also influence your work. You may find that you tend to speak more with individuals, and the families of these individuals, with whom you have things in common, and so take a greater interest in their choices and preferences. You may find you spend less time with the people you have different values to, which may also mean you are also less sympathetic or empathetic in your care because you are not seeing things from their point of view. You might not even realise you are doing this but it may show in your work. (We will look at some examples of how to address this later in this unit.)

It is for this reason that you will need to be aware of your own values, beliefs and attitudes because they will impact on your role and the people you care for. Being aware of them will ensure that you consider whether your own thoughts and beliefs influence individuals positively or negatively. You will then be able to address those issues if you feel that there are any differences between you and individuals that you care for that are getting in the way of you providing the best support possible. It may mean that you need to perhaps think about your own values if they affect an individual in a negative way.

It is important to remember that you may not necessarily agree with the individuals you care for, or believe in their lifestyle choices. But you should respect them and empathise so that you can fulfil your responsibility of providing high-quality care. This is also part of providing **person-centred practice**. See page 53 for more on how can you ensure that your personal values, attitudes and beliefs do not obstruct the quality of your work and working practice. You could also refer to Unit 209 on equality, diversity and inclusion, AC 2.2.

Values

Your values are what you believe to be important to you. Values guide how you live your life and the decisions you make. Values are usually formed through your childhood and adult life and may change as you mature and you have different experiences. For example, as a child you may have believed that spending time with your family was very important. As an adult spending time with your friends and a partner may have become more important than spending time with your family. Your values as an adult may in turn impact positively on

the individuals you provide care and support to by ensuring that in your role you promote individuals' independence and opportunities for them to meet and socialise with their friends.

Attitudes

Your attitudes are your personal ways of expressing through the way you act what you think and feel; they can reflect your values and beliefs. Your attitude to different situations, people and ideas develops through experiences you have and begin to develop in childhood. For example, you may have a positive attitude to work because you lived in a household where you and your brothers and sisters were brought up by a single parent who had three part-time jobs. As you were the eldest, you were expected to find a job to help your parent support the family. Your attitude towards employment may in turn have a positive influence on the young adults you provide care and support to by ensuring that you encourage them to believe in their own potential and abilities and to strive for the area of work they want to be in.

Your attitudes can also reflect negatively on your work practices. For example, you may believe in a healthy lifestyle and lead one yourself and so find it difficult to care for an individual who is obese and not interested in changing their lifestyle to a healthier one regardless of the health risks this brings.

Beliefs

Your beliefs are personal to you and what you regard to be true. They can sometimes be shared with others who belong to a similar group or culture. Beliefs can be political, religious, cultural or moral and are formed throughout your life. For example,

---

Key term

Person-centred practice refers to a way of working that takes into account the individual's whole person and focuses on an individual's specific needs, abilities, preferences and wishes. You may also wish to refer to Unit 211 on person-centred approaches.

Reflect on it

1.3 Values

Reflect on what your values are. Talk to your family and friends and find out what their values are. How do they compare to yours? Are there any similarities or differences between the values you hold and those that your family and friends hold?

Research it

1.3 Attitudes and beliefs

Research the different attitudes and beliefs that two different cultures may have. You will find it useful to use the internet for your research but remember you can also speak with the people you know such as your family, friends and your work colleagues.

Think about how attitudes and beliefs may impact positively on adult care workers' practices in care settings.

you may believe in God and pray every day or you may believe that it is very important you exercise or use your right to vote. Your personal beliefs may impact positively on the individuals you provide care and support to by ensuring that you respect the personal beliefs of others and understand that their beliefs may be different to your own.

How are your personal values, attitudes and beliefs formed?

Everyone is different and therefore holds their own unique personal values, attitudes and beliefs. These are formed and developed during our lives from childhood to late adulthood and can be influenced by:

- **The people in our lives** – such as family, friends and teachers. How family and friends behave towards you will in turn influence how you behave towards others. If your family and friends show you care and kindness then you are likely to act in this way towards others. If your teachers provided you with a positive educational experience then this is likely to influence your values and beliefs about the importance and benefits of a good education.

- **Religion** – such as Christianity, Hinduism, Islam, Sikhism, Buddhism or Judaism. These are some of the religions that are practised in the UK and have specific beliefs and practices associated with them. If you follow one of these religions and their associated practices then this will influence what you believe to be 'right' and 'wrong' (your moral values) as well as what you eat and drink and how you dress.

- **Life events** – such as starting school, starting employment, moving out of the family home, marriage, divorce, death of a family member or friend. These examples of 'events' can occur in our lives and impact significantly on the values, beliefs and attitudes we develop. How we survive these events will in turn influence whether we see them as positive or negative experiences and will be reflected in how we come across to others when we are supporting them through the same life events.

- **The media** – such as television, the internet, newspapers and music. What you see, read and hear about in your life can influence the values, beliefs and attitudes you form. For example, a television programme about what

individuals value as they get older, which stresses the importance of contact with others and companionship, can in turn influence your relationships with older people by making you more aware of what is important to them.

Information and stories that you may read about on the internet and in newspapers about best practice in the adult care sector can influence the practices you follow in the care setting where you work.

Listening to music can enable you to experience its many benefits, namely relaxation and expression of how you think and feel. This may in turn lead you to supporting individuals to follow their music interests or providing music as a therapeutic activity.

How can you ensure that your personal values, attitudes and beliefs do not obstruct the quality of work and working practice?

As you have learned we are all different and have unique backgrounds, experiences and influences in our lives that will in turn influence what we think and feel and how we behave towards others. You may know individuals and colleagues in the care setting where you work that share your values, attitudes and beliefs but there may also be individuals and colleagues who you work with that do not. It is very important that differences (that may arise between individuals or colleagues) do not impact negatively on the quality of your work and working practice.

You can do this by:

- Being aware of how your personal values, attitudes and beliefs can affect the way you think, feel, interact and behave towards others.

  - For example, you believe maintaining contact with family is important. An individual you provide support to has chosen to live on his own and not return phone calls and letters received from his family. It is important you do not insist that he makes contact with his family if he does not want to as it is his right to make his own choices. Instead, you must respect his right not to. You may discuss with him the reasons why, but only if he wishes to do so with you.

- Being aware of the personal values, attitudes and beliefs that individuals and others you work with hold.

- For example, you get to know an individual who you have recently started providing support to and have found out a little more about their background, needs, views, preferences, values, attitudes and beliefs. You find out that this individual enjoys being around their friends and particularly young people who are of a similar age and that going out in the evenings in the local area where she grew up is very important to her. When providing this individual with support when going out into their local area it is important that you listen to their views and opinions and take into account their values and beliefs; not doing so may mean that the individual chooses to not go out or socialise with other young people of their age.

- Being respectful of the differences between your own, individuals and others' values, attitudes and beliefs, and having a person-centred approach.

  - For example, you work within a team of five carers, one senior carer and a manager and you are all from different backgrounds and cultures. It is important that all of you work to the values of the organisation, respect one another's differences and all of you recognise the valuable contributions each of you makes to the care and support services that are provided to individuals and their families. Not doing so may mean that you do not work well together and therefore are unable to provide high-quality care and support. When working with individuals, make sure that you do not let your own beliefs influence their choices and preferences, either directly through your words, or indirectly, perhaps through your body language. For example, you may inadvertently suggest by a nod that you agree with a person's actions. Instead, you should ensure that you are giving them their right to make their own decisions, and positively supporting them in doing this.

Evidence opportunity

1.3 Values, attitudes and beliefs

Identify two personal values, two attitudes and two beliefs that you hold.

Write a description, using examples of the different ways that you ensure that each of these does not obstruct the quality of your work and your working practice.

In pairs, share your descriptions and write down their similarities and differences.

LO1 Knowledge, skills, behaviours
Knowledge: what does being competent in your job role involve?
Do you know what the standards and regulations are that influence your competence to carry out your job?
Do you know what duties and responsibilities you are required to carry out as part of your job?
Do you know why you must not let your personal values, attitudes and beliefs affect the quality of your work?
Did you know that you have just answered three questions about being competent in your job?
Skills: how can you show that you are carrying out the duties and responsibilities of your job?
Do you know how to follow the agreed ways of working for carrying out your tasks?
Do you know how not to allow your own personal values, attitudes and beliefs to influence your work?
Did you know that you have just answered two questions about how you demonstrate your competence at work?
Behaviours: how can you show the personal qualities you have when carrying out your job?
Do you know how to carry out your duties and responsibilities consistently and in accordance with your job description?
Do you know how to follow standards, regulations and agreed ways of working to the best of your ability?
Do you know how to show respect and support for values, attitudes and beliefs that are different to your own?
Did you know that you have just answered three questions about some of the essential behaviours that are expected of all competent adult care workers?

LO2 Be able to reflect on your work activities

Getting started

Think about a time when you have had to deal with a tricky or difficult situation. For example, you may have had to console a friend who was going through a difficult time. After the conversation, did you look back and think about how you handled the situation? Did you think about what went well and what you could improve on next time if faced with a similar situation?

AC 2.1 Explain why reflecting on work activities is an important way to develop knowledge, skills and practice

What is reflection?

To reflect means to think. Being able to reflect is an important skill to have as part of your work role. It involves thinking honestly about your practice, both the positives and negatives, and not being afraid to question your practice. When you reflect, you:

- take a 'step back' from your day-to-day activities and spend time thinking about a work activity you have carried out or a situation you have experienced
- examine in detail the reasons why and how you carry out your work practices
- assess the knowledge and skills you have and the behaviours you show including their impact on you, the individuals you provide care and support to and others
- identify your strengths and weaknesses
- identify areas of your work practice that can be improved
- develop different ways of working that can improve your working practice
- develop new areas of learning such as different or new approaches to situations that may arise.

Reflection can be thought of as a continuous cycle. Gibbs' reflective cycle (1988) (Figure 2.4) is often used by adult care workers for reflecting on their work activities. It shows the different stages in the reflection process and the questions you should be asking yourself.

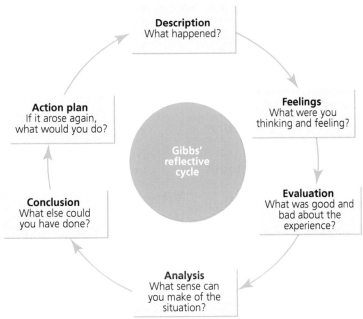

Source: Gibbs, G. (1988) *Learning by Doing*, Further Education Unit, Oxford Polytechnic: Oxford

Figure 2.4 Gibbs' reflective cycle

Another reflective tool is Driscoll's (2000) reflective cycle, which includes three stages when reflecting on your own work practice:

1 **What?** This is a description of the situation and its purpose is for you to reflect on specific aspects of that experience. You can reflect on:

- What is the purpose of reflecting on the situation that happened?
- What happened?
- What did I see?
- What did I do?
- What didn't I do?
- What did others do?
- What was my reaction?

2 **So what?** This is the analysis of the situation you experienced and its purpose is for you to consider the learning that arises out of the reflection process you've undertaken. You can reflect on:

- So what feelings did I experience during the situation?
- So what feelings did I experience after the situation?
- So what if any were the differences between my feelings during and after the situation?
- So what was the impact of what I did and/or didn't do?
- So what have I identified are my strengths in my practice?
- So what have I identified are my development areas in my practice?
- So what feelings did others experience during and after the situations?
- So what if any were the differences between others and my feelings during and after the situation?

3 **Now what?** This is the proposed actions to implement following your learning and its

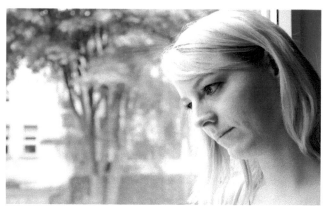

Figure 2.5 Do you have the skills to be a good reflector?

purpose is for you to implement the learning you've gained into your practice. You can reflect on:

- Now what are the implications for my practice if I implement the new learning?
- Now what are the implications for my practice if I do not implement the new learning?
- Now what are the implications for others?
- Now what have I learned about my practices?
- Now what information and support do I need to carry out these proposed actions?
- Now what would I do differently if a similar situation arises again?
- Now what can I do to ensure I continue to improve my practice?

Why is reflection important?

Reflecting on your work activities does not just happen once a week or at the end of the month, it is a continuous process that you will use throughout your career and in the different roles you undertake. Reflecting on your work activities is an important way to:

- **Get to know yourself** – the personal qualities you have, the areas of knowledge, understanding, skills and behaviours you have and those you need to develop. Gaining a greater understanding of who you are will help you to recognise how your practices influence others. This will also lead you to know more about the individuals you provide care and support to so that you can ensure that you adapt your working practice to meet their unique needs and preferences.

- **Develop yourself** – by identifying opportunities to address the gaps that there may be in your knowledge, skills and behaviours. For example, you may do this by accessing additional training from the care setting where you work or working closely with a more experienced colleague. Doing so will improve your competence and your work practice.

- **Develop best practice** – by finding out about the working practices and approaches that are not working you and your colleagues will then be able to develop new ways of working and approaches that will have a positive influence on the **care** and support that you provide to individuals. Keeping a close check on these new ways of working will help you to then identify best practices that you and your colleagues can apply in your day-to-day work activities.

Essentially, it is only by reflecting that you can look at a situation and decide if you need to change your approach or actions, either during the situation or the next time you are faced with a similar one.

Reflect on it

2.1 Reflect on a situation

Think about a situation in the setting. How did you handle the situation? How did this affect the individual for whom you provide care? How did they feel as a result? How about their families or carers? What about your colleagues? What went well? What did not go so well? What would you do differently next time? What can you improve? How will you improve? Will you need any training to develop any skills, for example?

6Cs

Care

Caring consistently and enough to make a positive difference to individuals' lives is essential to your role. Reflection is a key part of caring for individuals. For example, an individual may have taken offence at something you said even though you did not mean any harm. However, you will make sure that next time you are careful not to mention the same topic so you do not cause any hurt. It is because you genuinely care and are concerned for their well-being that you reflect and think about how you can improve your practice next time.

\	Dos and don'ts for reflecting each day
Do	Think about your successes and the things that you have done well so that others can learn from them. Thinking positively can also improve your performance and positively affect your behaviour when you are around individuals.
Do	Take some time to step back and decide how you will approach the situation you are faced with to ensure you have thought this through and it is a sensible approach.
Do	Take some time at the end of the day to reflect on what has happened during that day (what has gone well and what you could improve). Making this a part of your daily routine for improving your role can therefore improve the experiences of the people you care for.
Don't	Focus on the weaknesses and things that have not gone well as this will leave you feeling demotivated. Instead, you should actively look to learn from any errors and mistakes so that you do not make them again and individuals do not suffer as a result.
Don't	'Dive in' thinking that you have other individuals to tend to and so don't have time to think properly about a situation as this may lead to mistakes and may make the individual feel that their needs are not important to you.
Don't	Think that you are too busy or too tired to reflect at the end of the day, Reflection will enhance and improve your life in the care setting by improving your work practices.

Reflection is good practice. Just by doing this, you are showing that you are a mature and competent care worker who is striving to increase in knowledge, develop their skills and provide best practice by continually finding ways to improve. Reflecting will allow you to learn from what went well as well as what did not go so well.

As human beings, we often tend to focus on our mistakes, weaknesses and the things that we did not do well, or the things that we could improve. For example, you may have run a 10K race, and did not finish in the time that you wanted to, and so you may dwell on the finish time rather than all the effort you put into training or the fact that you did better than your previous race.

However, it is important that you also think about the things that you did well. Focusing on your strengths will mean you can tell colleagues about what went well, which will encourage good practice across the team. It is also a good way to remain positive and remain confident with the knowledge that while things might not go perfectly all the time, other situations have gone well. It is also a reminder that you are a competent worker able to provide high-quality care and support.

Evidence opportunity

2.1, 4.2 Reflection and development

Identify two areas of your knowledge and two skills you would like to develop further.

In pairs, discuss how you can use reflection to develop these knowledge areas and skills and why this is important. You can think about the benefits to how you carry out your duties and responsibilities in the care setting where you work and to the quality of the care and support you provide. After your discussion, write about the benefits of reflecting on your practice and how it can help develop your knowledge and skills further.

AC 2.2 Assess how well your knowledge, skills and understanding meet standards

As you learned earlier on in this unit (AC 1.2) the way you carry out your duties and responsibilities in the care setting where you work is guided by standards that are required and expected from you. These standards include codes of conduct, regulations and National Occupational Standards that set out the knowledge, understanding, skills, behaviours and competence required from you and all adult care workers.

It is very important that you keep a close check on how well your knowledge, skills and behaviour match these standards and regularly monitor that you are meeting them fully to ensure that you are:

- continuing to develop in your work role
- ensuring the well-being of the individuals you provide care and support to
- maintaining safe practices.

You can assess how well your knowledge, skills and understanding meet these standards by:

- **Reflecting** – spend time thinking about the knowledge, skills and understanding expected from you, to what extent you meet the standards expected from you, what needs to happen to ensure you meet these standards fully, how you can make improvements to your knowledge, skills and understanding.
- **Evaluating** – spend time assessing how your attitudes and behaviours impact on your work practices and working relationships in the care setting where you work. Assess whether you have been successful in ensuring that your values and beliefs do not impact on the quality of your work, the successful work activities you have carried out and how they have impacted on the quality of the care and support provided.

Other ways to increase your knowledge, skills and understanding to meet standards

As a care worker, you should not only refer to the various standards that we have discussed to ensure that your practice is informed by these, but you should also ensure that you are constantly reassessing your knowledge, skills and understanding to ensure that they are up to date and meet any changes in standards and practice.

Your setting and colleagues are not the only sources that you can use to ensure that you are up to date. You will also need to make sure that you are paying attention to what is happening around you and how health and social care issues are being reported in the media. For example, you could ask if you could observe or 'shadow' a senior colleague who is experienced, or is able to demonstrate good practice to see how they perform in their role and learn from their expertise. This will allow you to increase your knowledge in areas in which you may not be particularly confident. Obviously, you will need to consider whether you have time to do this and it may be that there are areas that your colleague could also improve on. But it is a good way to learn, especially from people who may have more experience than you and are doing different work activities to you so that you can learn about how you can also carry out these activities. Do not be afraid to ask for these opportunities, or for advice and feedback on how you are doing. Colleagues and those senior to you want the best for their care workers, individuals and the setting, and a motivated and enthusiastic workforce that seeks such opportunities only helps the setting to maintain high standards by having people who are able and competent in their roles.

Training outside of the setting is also a good way to ensure that you are up to date with your skills, and to gain new ones. You can then also share this knowledge with colleagues which will again encourage good practice.

Issues around social care are often a topic of debate in government, and there are often changes to legislation which will be documented in the news. Or there may be TV shows that focus on issues in the health and social care sector. The news often tends to cover some of the more negative issues in care homes but it is important that you use this as motivation to ensure that you are doing your best to ensure good practice. You may also read about various stories in newspapers and magazines and all of this should help you to be a more informed worker who has a good knowledge and understanding of what is happening currently.

It is also your duty as a care worker to keep up to date with best practice by researching textbooks, journals and the internet to learn about new theories, data and statistics and new thinking when it comes to the care sector. Again, not only can this positively impact the care you are able to offer, but it can also mean that you are a source of great information for colleagues. As part of your research you can also approach external agencies and charities that may have a better understanding than you do, of dementia for example. You may want to gain a greater understanding of any new developments in this area and may ask if they can offer you information, leaflets, or direct you to any other useful sources of information.

You can ask for feedback from colleagues, individuals and families in order to assess how you are doing. This can be formally, through appraisals and meetings with colleagues, or questionnaires for individuals and families, or informally in a conversation. You may find that you receive both compliments and criticism but it is important you take both constructively and learn from both. See AC 4.4 for more information on feedback.

Whichever way you choose to research, make sure that you always question the source and where the information has come from to ensure it is reliable. In an age of social media and 24-hour news channels, we are often bombarded with information that can at times be overwhelming. Some sources of information are more fact-based, others are more opinion-based. It is therefore always important to ask yourself if the source is reliable, i.e. who is offering this information and why?

Reflect on it

2.1, 2.2, 4.2 What went well?

Identify one work task that you have carried out well in the care setting where you work. Reflect on the reasons why this work task was successful. Reflect on the impact it had on the care setting where you work and on all the different people involved; remember don't forget to include yourself!

1.2, 2.2 Knowledge, skills, understanding and standards

Identify two standards that you have learned about and that influence your knowledge, skills and understanding in your job role. Provide three examples of the knowledge, skills and understanding you have developed and describe how they match these two standards.

You can produce a PowerPoint presentation of your findings.

AC 2.3 Demonstrate the ability to reflect on work activities

In AC 2.1, we discussed what is involved in reflection, the various stages and why it is important. You may wish to return to AC 2.1 to recap on this in order to understand how you can demonstrate this when reflecting on work activities. Remember that you will be observed reflecting on these work activities.

Showing that you can reflect on your work activities involves developing the following skills and qualities:

- self-awareness – how your behaviours impact on individuals, others and your work practices
- honesty – being honest with yourself about what has worked well (and what has not) and how to develop a more positive attitude
- **commitment** – striving to improve the quality of your work practices.

There are two different methods that you can use for reflecting on your work activities:

1 Reflecting on a work activity after it has happened – this is known as 'reflection on action'. If you use this method to reflect, then you will need to be committed to learning from the experience and then taking the necessary actions for making improvements.

2 Reflecting on a work activity while it is happening – this is known as 'reflection in action'. If you use this method to reflect, then

6Cs **C**

Commitment

In a care setting, this refers to your dedication to providing the best care for the individuals for whom you are responsible. It means continuously reflecting on how you can improve your work practices in order to improve the experience of the people who need care and support. You can do this by thinking about the various things we have discussed in this section. Remember: during or following a work activity, you can think about the things that went well (and the things that you can improve on). How will you improve your work practices? How can you ensure a safer environment? How will you communicate better? It is in this way that you can show that you are committed to being a reflective care worker, one who is constantly striving to be the best they can be.

Courage

Courage refers to your dedication to doing the right thing at the right time so that the individuals in your care and whom you support are kept safe. It can often be courageous to acknowledge that you did not do something so well, to take some criticism and know that you need to improve and learn. There is nothing wrong with admitting that you could be better at something. After all, you have your interests and the best interests of the people you care for at heart. Improvements mean that you are progressing, that you are getting better.

Remember, do not just focus on all the things that did not go well. Also think positively – about all the things that you are doing well. This will help you continue to do the things you are doing well and become better at the things that you are not!

you will need to be able to 'think on your feet' and take the necessary actions for making improvements while it is happening. Taking actions quickly requires **courage**.

The reflective exemplar below provides you with an opportunity to explore in more detail how adult care workers in care settings reflect on work activities and the benefits of doing so. In the exemplar, the activities worker reflects on their work activity after it has happened.

Research it

2.3, 4.2 'Reflection on action' and 'reflection in action'

Research the 'reflection on action' and 'reflection in action' concepts that were developed by Donald Schön.

Produce a spider diagram of the skills you need to reflect on your work activities – both after and while they are happening.

Reflective exemplar	
Introduction	I work as an activities worker in a day care centre with older adults. The activities I carry out with individuals encourage them to develop new skills, interests and provide them with opportunities to meet other people. The activities I carry out will depend on individuals' needs, likes and preferences. They include one-to-one activities such as playing Scrabble and individuals talking about their backgrounds; group activities such as cooking and gardening as well as going out, for example, to the local garden centre and to a coffee shop for a coffee and a slice of cake.
What happened?	Yesterday, I carried out a cooking activity with a small group of three individuals. The four of us met last week to plan what the activity would involve. We discussed what to cook and everyone agreed that they wanted to bake some biscuits. We agreed on a recipe to follow and what ingredients we would need. We made a shopping list of all the ingredients needed based on the recipe we had found, what equipment we would need – we made a list of all the equipment needed. We also checked we had the right equipment in the cupboards. We then discussed everyone's roles – everyone agreed that they wanted to bake their own biscuits and that we would all go shopping together the day before the activity. Cleaning up after the activity was agreed to be everyone's responsibility. In addition, I agreed to have overall responsibility for the activity and provide any help with carrying out the activity if individuals required this.
	The cooking activity went very well, everyone seemed to enjoy themselves and the group worked well together. Once the biscuits had cooled down, these were placed on separate plates ready to taste with a nice cup of tea. When the tea was ready and everyone sat round the table I noticed that one of the individuals in the group did not eat any biscuits. I offered her one of the biscuits she had made. She pulled a face and ran out of the room. I was left feeling very confused because the session had gone so well.
What worked well?	I was so happy that everyone was so enthusiastic about taking part in both planning and taking part in the cooking activity. The small group worked very well together and the biscuits produced were delicious!
What did not go as well?	One of the individuals in the group did not want to taste any of the biscuits, not even her own. It was disappointing that she didn't join in this part of the activity with the rest of the group, particularly as she had taken so much care in producing the biscuits.
What could I do to improve?	After the cooking activity, I met with the individual who did not want to taste any of the biscuits and she explained that she did not want to do so because she had spotted one of the members in the group dipping her finger into the cake mixtures before they were placed in the baking tins.
	After what happened, I think next time I will need to provide a lot more information to the group about food hygiene, its importance and how we can show good practices while carrying out cooking activities. I will need to make some time to include this as part of the planning process every time I carry out a cooking activity. I think I will also speak with the manager of the day care centre to see if we could jointly arrange some formal food hygiene training for all the individuals who take part in the cooking activities.
Links to unit assessment criteria	ACs 2.1, 2.3, 4.2, 4.4

Evidence opportunity

2.3, 4.2 Reflect on a work activity and how it has improved your knowledge, skills and understanding

Identify a work activity you have recently carried out in the care setting where you work. Using the learning you have gained in this unit about the reflection process, reflect on the work activity and write down the reflection process you followed. Then answer the following questions.

1 What have you learned about yourself?
2 What knowledge have you gained?
3 What skills have you gained?
4 What changes do you plan to make to the way you work? Remember that changes may not always be needed.

LO2 Knowledge, skills, behaviours
Knowledge: why is reflection important?
Do you know what reflection is and why it is important?
Do you know how reflecting on work activities can improve your work practice?
Did you know that you have just showed your knowledge of the meaning of reflection and why adult care workers use it to improve their work practices?
Skills: how can you show that you are able to reflect on your work activities?
Do you know how to assess whether your knowledge and skills meet the standards expected of you?
Do you know how to make improvements to your work practices?
Do you know how to evaluate how effective your reflection skills are?
Did you know that you have just demonstrated some of the skills required to be a good reflector?
Behaviours: how can you show the personal qualities you have when you are reflecting on and assessing your work activities?
Do you know how to reflect honestly on your work activities and assess your performance?
Do you know how to show that you are committed to improving your work practices through reflection?
Did you know that you have just demonstrated a few of the essential behaviours required to be an effective reflector?

LO3 Be able to agree a personal development plan

Getting started

Think about a time when you set yourself a personal goal. Perhaps this was to get fit and run a half marathon. How did you go about planning your training for this? Did you set yourself a time frame and short-term goals before the marathon? Did you go to anyone for advice and support? Who was this?

AC 3.1 Identify sources of support and how they can be used for your learning and development

To develop yourself personally and professionally also involves being supported to do so. In the care setting where you work support may come from a wide range of sources which you will be able to use for your own learning and development. These include:

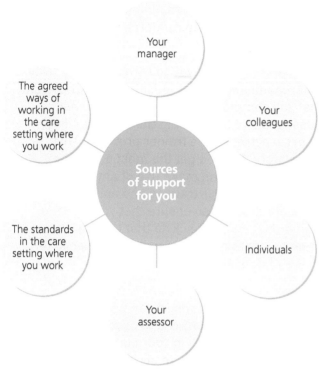

Figure 2.6 Sources of support for your personal development

- formal and informal support
- supervision and appraisals
- support from both inside and outside the setting.

Formal and informal support within the organisation

Supervision and appraisals

Your manager will meet with you to assess your performance at work. This process is referred to as formal **supervision** and is there to support you with planning and monitoring your personal development. For example, in the care setting where you work you may have regular performance reviews where you discuss and evaluate your performance at work with your manager.

Supervision means you have regular meetings with your manager where you will have an opportunity to discuss any issues and receive feedback on what has been going well, and what improvements you need to make. Because these meetings may happen only every few weeks it is a good idea that you note down things that you want to discuss beforehand. This is a

Key terms

A **supervisor** refers to the person in your work setting that oversees your work and assesses your performance at work; this is usually your manager.

A **mentor** refers to a person in your work setting who has more experience than you and can provide you with guidance and advice in relation to your job role and responsibilities. This person, however, is there to offer advice more informally than your manager. If there is an issue, for example, that you are not sure how to address with your manager, you could talk to your mentor first.

good opportunity to discuss specific cases and individuals you are working with. You can also use these opportunities to demonstrate how well you are doing by noting down all the ways in which you have shown good practice and reflected on your work. You could share reflective accounts that you have written to demonstrate this. You can also discuss career progression and whether you have identified any sources of support and training courses you would like to undertake.

Your manager may also arrange some regular formal support meetings for you and your colleagues to discuss any issues you are experiencing in your professional environment. They may even organise **mentoring** sessions where you will be able to speak with a more experienced colleague and get advice on the issues you are facing at work as well as advice on career development. (Also see AC 4.1 for more information on mentoring.)

Appraisals are another source of formal support and involve your employer (not necessarily your manager) assessing your performance in your job role with you over a much longer period, e.g. one year. It provides you with the opportunity to discuss and reflect on your work performance: to identify your strengths; areas for development; what improvements you need to make and how you can progress in your role with training and development opportunities.

Colleagues

Your colleagues can be the source of both formal and informal support. They can share best practice with you and provide you with their honest views about your strengths and work practices. They can also be the people you turn to when you need advice or guidance about your day-to-day work activities. This might be through the formal meetings discussed above, a more informal catch-up at lunch or coffee break, or even some advice or words of encouragement when you are doing your job.

Individuals

Individuals can be a useful source of support as they will very often show you how your work practices have impacted on them. They can also provide you with their views about the care and support they have received.

Training

Training (both formal and informal) is an important way to build new skills, understanding and improve your current practice.

- You may receive training from your manager in how to complete an activity, or this may come from colleagues.
- It may be that your manager has organised some formal training inside the care setting, where a professional trainer visits you at the setting.
- Training can be 'on-the-job' where you learn new skills as you do your job (as an ongoing process) although you may have 'training days' dedicated to this. See the section on 'Sources of support outside the setting (formal and informal)' on the next page for more information on training.
- There may be online courses that you can do. Although these may be more theoretical, they can still give you an idea of how to apply that theory to your work practices.

To get the most out of training, ensure that you understand what skills you will learn and ask your manager any questions you may have before you attend. It is also worth making notes during the training and keeping any material that you are given for future reference. Telling colleagues about the training once you have completed it can help reinforce what you have learned.

The trainer may ask you to complete an activity beforehand and ask for feedback. It is important that you complete all the activities set, ask questions and take part in the presentations or extra activities the trainer provides. This will ensure that you get the most out of the course and you can make use of any feedback offered during your training and apply it to your work practices. Also ensure that you give the trainer honest feedback so that they can make improvements and improve the experience for those who receive the training next.

Assessor

Your assessor can support you with further development and verification of your knowledge, skills and behaviours in your current job role. They can provide you with access to useful information about best practice and can work closely with you so that you are able to provide evidence of your competence at work.

Standards

The standards in the care setting where you work can be useful sources of information about the level and quality of work practice you will need to provide as evidence in order to be considered as a competent adult care worker. As you have read, these can also be used as the basis for when you are reflecting on your work activities.

Agreed ways of working

The agreed ways of working in the care setting where you work can be useful sources of information and guidance for ensuring that you carry out your duties and responsibilities in accordance with your job description, legislation and the standards that the care setting where you work expects from you.

> **Reflect on it**
>
> **3.1** Sources of support
>
> Reflect on the sources of support that you have in the care setting where you work. Which ones have you made use of? Why?

Sources of support outside the setting (formal and informal)

Support for your personal development can also come from people and organisations outside of the care setting where you work and can even be online:

- **Trainers** – as discussed, training plays a key role in your learning and development. Training can be both in the setting and outside the setting. It may mean that you go to a training provider outside of the setting. They can share their knowledge and skills in specific areas of work such as in dementia care, planning activities and completing manual handling risk assessments.
- **Your family and friends** – you must not forget the support you receive from your family and friends. For example, financial support when you are studying or help with other personal responsibilities when working long shifts.
- **Online forums** – these provide support and suggestions for how to overcome difficulties you may be experiencing. They are also places where people can share best practice and useful resources such as books and websites they have come across to help further develop their work practices (remember, you must check that these are reliable sources and think about where the advice is coming from).
- **E-learning** – short courses and study delivered online can be a good way of further developing your knowledge around key aspects of your work practices.

You may need support from this wide range of sources in relation to a specific area of your practice, for example when you are learning a new work activity or completing a task in a different way because there has been a change in an individual's needs. You might also need their support when you want to acquire or gain new knowledge in a specialist area such as dementia care or you may want to update your knowledge of changes to legislation that have arisen and that will impact on your working practices.

It is important that you make the most of all the support available to you to make progress on your learning and development journey.

Research it

3.1 External sources of support

Research the external sources of support that are available to you outside of your care setting. You will find it useful to speak with you manager and colleagues about this. Do you know how to access them? Discuss these with your manager when you next review your personal development plan.

Evidence opportunity

3.1 Sources of support for learning and development

Identify three sources of support that you have used. For each one identify one way that you have used it for your learning and development. Produce a poster with your findings.

Self-directed learning is particularly important if you are not working in a setting with other colleagues or are self-employed. For example, if you are a private carer or a carer employed directly by the individual with care or support needs, you can obtain feedback directly from the individual and/or their family about how your care or support is being experienced and how you are perceived as a carer. In addition, you could keep your knowledge up to date by reading, watching real-life documentaries in care settings and researching lessons learned from research undertaken.

AC 3.2 Describe the process for agreeing a personal development plan and who should be involved

What is a personal development plan (PDP)?

Now that you know about the different sources that are available to support you with your learning and development we will consider how you can use these sources of support to agree your own **personal development plan** (PDP) (definition on page 67).

In some care settings, PDPs are also known as 'personal learning plans' (PLPs) or 'personal development reviews' (PDRs). What are they known as in the care setting where you work?

A personal development plan is a formal record of your learning and development, and identifies:

- the knowledge, skills and behaviours you have
- your strengths as well as the areas you need to improve
- your plans for the future including how you would like to develop in your job
- the learning and support you need to improve your practice and develop in your job and career.

It is for this reason that it is vital that you have a PDP in place.

Who should be involved when agreeing a PDP?

You will agree your personal development plan by discussing this with your manager or supervisor during the appraisal process. This is because personal development plans not only take into account your learning and development needs, but also the needs of the care setting where you work. This is to ensure that you carry out your work tasks competently, in line with your job description and your care setting's standards and agreed ways of working.

Your manager (who may also be your employer) or supervisor will ask you to plan for this discussion by reflecting on your own development, achievements and areas for development.

As part of your planning you should involve other people.

- **The individuals** – their comments about the care you provide can help you to reflect on your strengths and areas for improvement.
- **The carers** – their views on the support you provide to them and their relatives can help you to reflect on your abilities and behaviours.
- **Advocates** – advocates speak up for individuals and they are independent of the care setting where you work and so can be a useful and

objective (unbiased) source of information about the quality of support you provide.

- **Team members** – your colleagues who work with you on a day-to-day basis can provide you with a good insight into your strengths and the areas of your work that require further development.
- **Other professionals** – as part of your role you may be required to contact other professionals who are external to the care setting where you work, such as GPs, dentists and pharmacists. You can reflect on the working relationships you have developed with them; perhaps you have received comments from them about the quality of your work, such as, your communication skills or the care and support you provide?

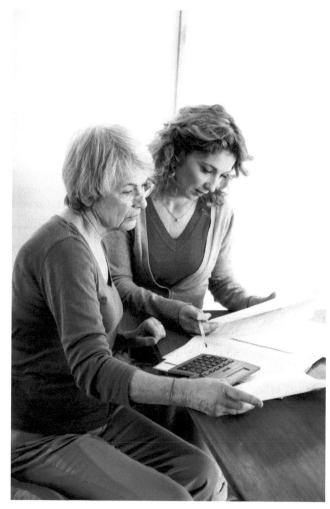

Figure 2.7 What does your personal development plan look like and who is involved in the process?

Reflect on it

3.2 Who do you involve when agreeing your PDP?

Reflect on who you would involve and why when agreeing your personal development plan. What value will they add to your learning and development?

Key term

A **personal development plan (PDP)** may have a different name but will record information such as agreed objectives for development, proposed activities to meet objectives, timescales for review.

Process for agreeing your PDP

The process involved for agreeing a personal development plan involves the following seven key steps.

1 Identify the skills and knowledge that are required to carry out your job role well – your job description that details your duties and responsibilities will be used as the basis of your discussion with your manager or supervisor.

2 Identify the skills and knowledge you have at present – you will need to gather the information you have collected from the people you have involved in your planning.

3 Identify any gaps you might have in your skills and knowledge (and what will be required to bridge the gaps) – you will need to discuss and agree these with your manager and supervisor.

4 Set goals for how to fill these gaps – you will need to discuss with your manager what you would like to achieve as well as what your manager expects from you. See the following section on SMART goals. These will reflect your own goals and those of the setting in which you work.

5 Agree the ways you can bridge the gaps in your skills and knowledge – depending on your agreed goals. You will need to agree how you are going to do this, such as through attending a training course or working alongside a more experienced member of the team.

6 Agree when these gaps will be met – you and your manager will discuss and agree on what needs to be addressed urgently and what doesn't and then set realistic timescales for achieving these in the short term (six months), the medium term (one year) and the long term (two years).

7 Review your goals on a regular basis and plan your new goals for the future – you will need to discuss and agree these with your manager or supervisor in order to recognise what you have already achieved and what you would like to aim for next. This should document both your own and your manager's assessment of your learning and development. This is also an opportunity to update your PDP and record any training that you may have undertaken, for example. You may also need to change milestones and goals if you find they are not working. An appraisal is a good time to discuss your personal and professional development although you should be discussing this on an ongoing basis when meeting with your manager.

SMART goals

It is important that the goals you include in your personal development plan are SMART. This means that they must be:

Specific: they must be clear and state exactly what you want to achieve. For example, an individual may be feeling low in themselves and have very little confidence as a result. Your aim may be to promote the individual's well-being so that they can regain their confidence, feel better in themselves and start socialising with others again.

Measurable: they must have milestones or clear end-points so that you can measure how you are progressing and know when you have reached a certain goal. For example, an individual may have undergone an operation and is unable to eat by themselves or go to the toilet and dress themselves. Your goal may be to ensure that they can independently do these things in the next six months. A marker or a measurable goal may be when they are able to have their first meal on their own with very limited assistance from you in the next two months, the next marker may be when they are able to go to the toilet unassisted in the next three months.

Achievable: you must be able to achieve them, in other words they must be part of your role. For example, you may decide to focus on work activities that are agreed as part of the scope of your job role and so can be achieved as part of the day-to-day support that you provide to individuals. If you see that you are on your way to achieving goals, this will serve as great motivation for achieving and progressing further. This will not only impact positively on the individuals you care for, because they experience better care as a result of your improved practice, but it will also impact positively on you and your colleagues, Also, organising them into short-, medium- and long-term goals ensures that they are more achievable. For example, a short-term goal may be to help an individual with their personal care as they go through dementia. A medium-term goal may be to go on a course and train to find out more about dementia care. A long-term goal may be to support one other inexperienced colleague in this process. It may also include thinking about your long-term career plans, which might be to progress to a supervisor role.

Realistic: the goals you agree should be achievable in the timeframe that you are set and in the scope of your job or you will agree on training that will enable you to achieve the goal. For example, you would not be expected to provide medical advice, such as that a GP would normally do.

Timely or time-based: there should be a clear timeframe for when you are expected to achieve the goal, and clear milestones to aim for. That way, you and your manager can work towards these and plan any training and development needs within that schedule. Timeframes should be realistic and

give you the best chance to meet them successfully (allowing you to feel encouraged to progress and meet the other goals that you are set).

AC 3.3 Contribute and agree to your personal development plan

The most important person involved in your personal development plan is you. Demonstrating that you are willing to contribute to your personal development plan is the key to its success. You can contribute to your personal development plan by:

- **planning** – shows that you have prepared for a discussion with your manager or supervisor and indicates that you are keen to learn, improve your knowledge, skills and practice
- **reviewing** – being keen to review and update your personal development plan on a regular basis shows that you have a good insight into your progress regarding your learning and development
- **listening** – shows that you take seriously all comments, views and opinions received about the support you provide from all those involved in the personal development planning process. It shows that you are committed to making improvements to your practice.

As you draw up your plan make sure that it is highlighting all the things we have discussed above. In other words, ask yourself, is it outlining all my short-, medium- and long-term career goals? Will I be able to achieve these goals in these timeframes? Is the training relevant to what I want to achieve?

Figure 2.8 on page 69 is an example of a personal development plan. Part one outlines strengths, weaknesses, opportunities and what may stop you progressing further. It should also be dated, have your name and that of the setting.

Evidence opportunity

3.1, 3.2 Sources of support and the process for drawing up a PDP

Produce a one-page information handout about the different people who can support you with agreeing a personal development plan at work. Include one example of how they can support you, and produce a step-by-step diagram or flow chart to describe the process for agreeing your personal development plan.

Reflect on it

3.3 Your PDP and you

How do you show your manager or supervisor that you are keen to contribute to your personal development plan? What are the consequences of not doing so?

Part two outlines what you want to achieve in your role and how you will be supported. Perhaps this will include support from your manager or some training. It will also cover how you will show you have achieved your goal and a target for when you will review this. It could have a section for manager's responsibilities. Part three outlines short, medium and long term, which is a good way to break down your goals. Part four covers whether and how you have achieved your goals and whether you need to update or revise them.

Personal development plan

Name: Organisation:

Date PDP completed:

Part 1 – Personal analysis

What are my strengths?

What are my weaknesses and the areas that I need to further develop?

What opportunities are there available to me that can help me learn and develop?

What threats are there that may affect my plans to learn and develop?

Part 2 – Setting goals

What do I want to learn?

What do I have to do?

What skills do I want to gain?

What support will I need?

What other resources will I need?

How will I assess and evidence my achievement?

How will I show I have achieved this?

What is my target date for achieving this and reviewing my progress?

Part 3 – Personal objectives

What are my short-term goals for the next 12 months?

What are my medium-term goals for the next two to three years?

What are my longer-term goals beyond three years?

Part 4 – Review

Goal	Outcome – did I achieve this, and by agreed timescales?
1.	1.
2.	2.
3.	3.
4.	4.
5.	5.

Figure 2.8 Personal development plans vary in style and structure. This is just one example of a PDP. What does your PDP look like?

As well as making contributions it is also important that you agree to your personal development plan. As you have learned, planning your personal development involves meeting your learning and development needs but also those of the care setting where your work. This means that sometimes the goals that are set may not always be your preferred goals as they may reflect the care setting's needs first and foremost. It is important to not be disappointed should this happen but instead you must focus on working closely and positively with your manager or supervisor so that you can draw up a personal development plan that meets your needs and those of the organisation you work for.

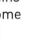

Case study

3.1, 3.2, 3.3 Agreeing a personal development plan

Marilyn works as a reablement worker providing support to individuals to live independently, often following an illness or accident. Marilyn enjoys her job and particularly enjoys working alongside other professionals such as **social workers** and **physiotherapists** as well as supporting individuals to cook and take part in activities such as swimming and going to the gym.

Marilyn has requested a meeting with her manager to discuss her personal development plan as she feels that some of her learning needs have changed since these were documented in her plan. During the meeting with her manager Marilyn explains how she has achieved her goal to improve her record keeping in relation to when she visits individuals in their homes. Marilyn's manager disagrees because she feels that this goal was only set a week ago and that it is difficult therefore to assess how Marilyn has improved. Marilyn's manager suggests that they review her plan again at the end of the month as originally agreed.

Marilyn is left feeling disappointed and explains to her manager that her main goal is to become a senior reablement worker and how record keeping is an essential skill and how she is worried now that she does not have the ability to progress in her career.

Questions

Imagine you are Marilyn's manager.

1 How would you respond to Marilyn's concerns?
2 What sources of support could Marilyn access?
3 Do you think Marilyn understands the process for agreeing her personal development plan?
4 Identify three key aspects of the process for agreeing a personal development plan.

Key terms

Social workers assess, commission and co-ordinate care services and seek to improve outcomes for individuals, especially those who are more vulnerable. They may work in multi-disciplinary teams and can specialise in areas such as mental ill health, learning disabilities, care for older people or safeguarding.

Physiotherapists are professionals who help people affected by injury, illness or disability through exercise, manual therapy.

Evidence opportunity

3.3 Contributing to your PDP

Discuss with your assessor the contributions you have made to your own personal development plan. For each contribution you have made, discuss why it is important to you. Write down notes to document your discussion.

LO3 Knowledge, skills, behaviours
Knowledge: what is a personal development plan?
Do you know who you can use for support for your learning and development?
Do you know why you have a personal development plan, the process for agreeing one and who should be involved?
Did you know that you have just answered two questions about the meaning and importance of personal development plans?
Skills: how can you show that you can agree your personal development plan?
Do you know how to prepare yourself for agreeing your personal development plan?
Do you know the process to follow for agreeing your personal development plan and how to contribute to it?
Did you know that you have just answered two questions about some of the skills you have when contributing and agreeing to your personal development plan?
Behaviours: how can you show the personal qualities you have when agreeing your personal development plan?
Do you know how to listen effectively to others' views about your work practice?
Do you know how to show that you are keen to improve your practice?
Did you know that you have just answered two questions about a few of the essential behaviours that are expected of all adult care workers when agreeing their personal development plan?

LO4 Be able to develop your knowledge, skills and understanding

Getting started

Think about a time when you learned something new. It may be when you learned to play a new sport or mastered a new recipe, or even read a book where you learned about a topic of which you previously had no understanding. Imagine if you had not read that book. How would you be aware of the issues around that topic? How did it improve your knowledge? How did learning a new sport help you? Did it help you become fitter and more active?

AC 4.1 Describe how a learning activity has improved your knowledge, skills and understanding

Types of learning activities

As you know there are many different sources of support for your learning available to you both within and outside of the care setting where you work. Being an effective learner means being in control of your own learning. There are many different types of learning activities to choose from:

- **Training** usually takes place in the care setting where you work and is usually carried out by more senior team members which can include your manager or supervisor. It is usually focused on specific work areas, for example it can help you to update your knowledge on safeguarding or further develop your practical manual and handling skills. Whatever the training, you will need to ensure that this is relevant and will enable you to improve your knowledge, skills and understanding.

- **Learning programmes** can take place in the care setting where you work or outside of the care setting, such as in a college or in a virtual online learning environment. A qualified person such as a teacher, tutor or assessor usually delivers the programme. Learning programmes can be useful for improving your knowledge, understanding and further developing your skills, for example on diabetes care or even about the Level 2 Diploma in Care you are currently undertaking.

4.1 Training

Research other examples of training that adult care workers undertake on a regular basis in the care settings where they work. The internet and the manager in the care setting where you work will be useful sources of information.

Create a poster with your findings.

- **Mentoring programmes** take place in the care setting where you work. They are led by a more experienced member of the team and involve providing support to someone who has less experience, for example by guiding you in how to overcome a difficult situation you have experienced at work or supporting you to plan for a new work activity.

- **Coaching programmes** also take place in the care setting where you work. They are led by a member of the team who is experienced and competent in a specific skill or work area. They can provide training, for example on carrying out a risk assessment or supporting an individual who has specific communication skills.

- **Reading and information sharing** can take place both within and outside of the care setting where you work. For example, your manager may provide you and your colleagues with a legislation update or you may read an article in the newspaper about what high-quality care and support looks like and you may discuss this with your colleagues.

- **Reflection** can take place both within and outside of your care setting, both during and after situations and experiences. For example, you may reflect on how you can adapt your communication with an individual who is not responding to you positively or you may reflect on your work achievements after your appraisal.

- **Visiting other settings** and speaking to care workers based there can increase your knowledge and understanding of how other settings function and learn about their ways of working. You will of course need to ask your manager and gain permission from them in order to do this. Your manager will then need to get permission from the setting, and arrange a suitable time and for someone to show you around.

- **Individuals and their families**. It is also important to remember that you will be constantly learning from the individuals that you care for on a daily basis. This may include simply learning something new about their lives or preferences. It might be something as simple as finding out that they do not like to have broccoli in their lunch, which will enable you to make sure that this is not in the meals they are given. By learning directly from individuals, you can ensure you tailor your practice to their needs.

Showing how a learning activity has improved your knowledge, skills and understanding

It is important that you are able to show how a learning activity has improved your knowledge, skills and understanding. Below is an example of how you may be able to do this.

If you attend a training day on moving and handling individuals, the trainer may have covered the following.

- What does it mean to 'move and handle' in a care setting?
- How do we support individuals while doing this?
- How do we show compassion and ensure the individual is not in any discomfort?
- Demonstrations and practical activities.

In order to show how this learning activity has improved your knowledge, skills and understanding, you might want to think about what you learned. Did you learn any new skills? Did you improve any current ones you had? Do you have a better understanding of the topic as a result of the training? What do you still need to learn? Do you need further training? Do you feel you can undertake these skills in the setting? You could include this in your reflective account and share this with your manager.

4.1 Learning activities and knowledge, skills and understanding

Think about a learning activity you have recently completed. Produce a leaflet that describes: the learning activity; why you did it; what learning you gained and how it improved your knowledge, skills and understanding. If you have completed a training evaluation form as part of any internal training, then you may wish to use this as evidence to help you evaluate your learning.

The importance of developing your knowledge, skills and understanding

As we discussed in AC 2.2 and 3.1, it is important that you continually strive to develop your knowledge, skills and understanding by ensuring that you are up to date with any recent developments in health and social care. This means going to the library to access journals, researching on the internet, ensuring you are keeping up to date with any developments in the news and speaking to colleagues inside the setting. Being an informed care worker who is constantly doing this as well as using learning activities such as training to develop their knowledge, skills and understanding will only benefit your setting, improve your practice and thus the lives of the individuals you care for.

AC 4.2 Describe how reflecting on a situation has improved your knowledge, skills and understanding

You learned about reflective practice and what being a good reflector involves earlier on in this unit (see AC 2.1 and 2.2) and it would be worth recapping that section. There are many different situations that may arise in the care setting where you work.

2.1, 2.3, 4.2 Reflecting on situations

Reflect with your colleagues on two different situations that have arisen in the care setting where you work. Take it in turns to identify one example of the learning gained by reflecting on each situation.

For example:

- an individual may learn a new skill
- an individual's family may provide their support during a group activity
- an individual may want to try a new activity
- an individual may refuse to take part in an activity
- an individual's family may disagree with the choices their relative has made in relation to their care or support
- an individual may have a fall.

Reflecting on a situation that has taken place in the care setting where you work can improve your knowledge, skills and understanding by:

- making you more aware of your own abilities and limitations
- making you more aware of the knowledge, skills and understanding you have and those you need to gain or improve on
- helping you to identify suitable learning activities to meet your learning needs
- improving your work practice.

Not setting time aside to reflect means that you risk your performance at work becoming poor in quality; this in turn will impact on the quality of the care and support you provide to individuals. You may also place these individuals at risk of danger, harm or abuse through poor working practices. This can have serious consequences for their lives and your career.

2.1, 2.3, 4.2 Reflection and how it can improve knowledge, skills and understanding

Describe to your assessor a situation that has arisen in the care setting where you work, then write a reflective account about it. Describe how reflecting on it has improved your knowledge (one example), skills (one example) and understanding (one example).

You may reflect on a situation that involved an individual's family disagreeing with you and the team about their relative's care. As a result of reflecting on and thinking about this situation you may know more about the individual's needs and preferences. Your skills in relation to working with individuals' families may have improved as well as your communication skills in sensitive or difficult situations. In addition, your understanding of other people's perspectives (and how to support them) may have developed.

You might like to think of it in these terms:

- As a result of reflecting and thinking about this situation, I now know more about …
- My skills have improved as a result of …
- I can now do …
- I understand that I must …

AC 4.3 Explain the importance of continuing professional development

Continuing professional development (CPD) refers to the process of tracking and documenting the skills, knowledge and experience that you gain both formally and informally as you work, beyond any initial (induction) training. It is a record of what you experience, learn and then apply. In other words it means looking at the skills and what you are learning in your role, making sure that you are keeping a record of what training and learning you have undertaken, for example by keeping records of any certificates you have received for courses you have undertaken and putting together a CPD folder that includes these. You can also include other evidence such as reflections and witness statements from those who have observed your practice.

CPD also involves continually looking at opportunities and ways to further your development by outlining any new training that you need or other ways to develop, perhaps through mentoring sessions. As a result, you have a clear idea of how you are progressing, your goals and where you are headed in the long term in terms of your career. You might like to refer to the section on training in AC 3.1. If you do not do this, then you may not realise that you are using work practices that are out of date, your skills and knowledge will not develop further as a result and this will mean that you will not be able to provide individuals with up-to-date, good-quality care.

Maintaining, reviewing and updating your professional development throughout your career is important because doing so will:

- **improve your knowledge and understanding** – your knowledge of specific areas of work will increase because you have clearly outlined the areas you want to increase your knowledge and understanding in
- **improve your skills** – your skills will develop because you have clearly outlined these and identified ways to improve and gain new skills, for example through training. This is not just professional skills and qualities such

as being an effective communicator, but also includes developing the personal qualities of compassion and empathy that are required in your role

- **improve your work practice** – thinking about your practice, how you are progressing and constantly thinking about ways to improve will mean your practice is more likely to meet the required standards such as those that we discussed in AC 1.2

- **help you apply new working approaches** – as you think about your practice, you may identify new ways of working, you will gain an understanding of new and effective working approaches and how to ensure that these will also impact on individuals in a positive way

- **help you adapt your practice** – as you develop, you will learn about best practice and how to apply it, including using different skills to change the way you practise to ensure it remains up to date

- **help you develop in your job role** – you will increase in confidence when applying the knowledge and skills you have learned; this may lead you to explore different job roles and positions, for example the role of supervisor

- **provide you with an opportunity to reflect** – your self-awareness of your knowledge, skills, behaviours will increase, meaning that you will know what you are doing well and what you need to improve in order to develop further.

AC 4.4 Describe how feedback from others has developed your knowledge, skills and understanding

You have already learned about the importance of maintaining your continuing professional development so that you can continue to maintain and develop existing and new areas of knowledge, skills and understanding.

Feedback may come from people inside and outside the setting. It may be that it is a simple 'good work' or 'well done' that you receive from your manager or your colleague at the end of the day. It could also be given in a team meeting or supervision session that you have with your manager.

Feedback involves **others** providing you with:

- **Viewpoints** – these can be very useful as they may well be different to your own and encourage you to see things from others' perspectives. This may be criticism that points out the things that you are not doing well, but it is important that you take this constructively. See 'How to handle feedback and criticism' on page 76.

- **Their experiences** – these are invaluable as every person is unique and has gone through different things, both in and outside the setting and so their experiences will inform the advice they are able to offer and this experience will also inform their practice.

- **Information and advice** – these are very important for ensuring that you continue to develop in your work role as it may be information about a topic that you are unfamiliar with or advice about good practice.

In the care setting where you work you may receive feedback from a range of different people. For example:

- The **individuals** who use (or 'commission' their own) health or social care services may also be a useful source of information in the sense that they will be able to provide you with a direct account of how your care and support has influenced their lives. Their feedback may be formal or informal, they may make comments about the care or support you provide while you are assisting them with a daily activity. They may also thank you for your support or give you ideas for what other support they would like from you.

- The **families, carers and advocates** of the individuals you work with may share with you their opinions about your knowledge, skills and behaviours. They may provide you with verbal feedback about, for example, what the individual has said about the way you interact with them or in relation to the difference your support has made to the lives of individuals' families and carers. Advocates may comment on the working relationship that you have with them, for example.

- Your **supervisor, line manager or employer** may provide you with feedback in relation to how you are carrying out your work activities, the skills you have demonstrated competently and those you still need to develop. The feedback can be both formal and informal, verbal and in writing. It will most certainly form part of you agreeing your personal development plan.

- **Team members** such as the chef, domestic, laundry and maintenance staff, may provide

you with feedback based on their observations of you providing support with individuals. This may be quite informal and perhaps during a coffee or lunch break.

- Other **colleagues** may provide you with useful feedback about your personal qualities and areas for further development, for example. Some may be more objective because they may not know you as well as others.

- Other **professionals** you work with such as the nurse, GP, trainers, may feed back to you about how well they think you work with them to support individuals. They may also notice the working relationship you have developed with individuals, and comment on your personal qualities, knowledge and skills.

How to handle feedback and criticism

As shown in the above list, you will receive feedback from a wide range of sources and of different types. It is important that you use the feedback that you receive in constructive ways. For example, if it is information and advice on best practice about how to complete a certain task from a senior colleague, for example about a moving and handling procedure, it is important that you take this on board, and use their expertise to guide you. You may even ask to observe a practical demonstration. The point is to use their feedback to develop your knowledge, skills and understanding in this area.

If, for example, the advice that you receive points out some of the weaknesses in your performance and is therefore more critical, it is important again to use the criticism to improve your practice rather than lower your self-esteem. You should not feel upset when someone in the workplace points out a way that you could improve, or highlights an error. You may not even agree with it, but it is important to think about the criticism and learn from it. However, remember that you should continue to also think about your strengths and remember that everyone makes mistakes, has weaknesses and will receive criticism. It is not just you. If you feel that a comment someone makes about your performance has no basis, then you can always ask them to give you more detail and explain their reasons so that you are able to understand fully what you may be doing wrong and can change your practice as a result.

In summary, feedback is only useful if you take it on board!

To make the most of the feedback you receive from others, remember to be:

● open to all feedback received – to both the positives and negatives

● positive and willing to learn from it
● a good listener, patient and showing respect for the opinions of others
● prepared to act on it.

Read the 4.3, 4.4 Case study and think about how Lucinda has used the feedback she has received from others.

Case study

4.3, 4.4 Receiving and using feedback

Lucinda is a support worker and as part of her job role supports and enables individuals to express their views, wishes and choices when they are unable to do so because of an illness or injury. Lucinda's role also involves ensuring that individuals remain as involved as possible in all decisions which affect them.

Lucinda supported Frank, who has recently been diagnosed with Alzheimer's, to meet with his social worker to discuss his current and future care needs. Lucinda arranged for the meeting to take place in Frank's flat so that he would feel relaxed.

Once the social worker had arrived, Lucinda supported Frank to make everyone a cup of tea and then started the discussions by saying that Frank had written an account a few days earlier about what he enjoys most about his life, what he would like to change, his fears, hopes and dreams. Frank handed his written account to the social worker and smiled. The social worker asked him a few questions about what he had written; Lucinda checked with Frank that he had understood the question and then suggested to him he take his time to respond. The social worker wrote down his replies and explained that she would now need to go and find out about

the services that are available in the local area to meet Frank's needs and then would arrange another meeting.

The next day Lucinda received a phone call from the social worker who explained that she liked the way she had used Frank's love of writing as a way of him expressing his views, thoughts and wishes and thought that this was very effective. Lucinda thanked her for the feedback. Lucinda also received a letter from Frank thanking her for her support the day before.

Later that afternoon, Lucinda attended a team meeting. Lucinda shared the feedback she had received with her colleagues and manager; she also answered their questions about how a written account can be a useful way for some individuals to express themselves. The team praised Lucinda on her achievements.

Questions

1 Who did Lucinda receive feedback from?
2 Describe Lucinda's attitude towards the feedback she received.
3 Would you describe Lucinda as providing support to Frank with compassion? Why?
4 How did Lucinda use the feedback she had received?

6Cs

Compassion

Being able to deliver support with compassion involves doing so with kindness, consideration, dignity and respect. This is a key part of your role, as you will be working with various individuals. However, it is important not to just be compassionate when working with individuals, but to be compassionate also in your relationships with families and your colleagues, even as you offer advice or point out a weakness. For example, you could mention to a colleague that they had carried out a task well but had also made a mistake, and make suggestions on how to improve it. This means that you are thinking about how they may receive the feedback and offer positive as well as negative feedback. Of course, you may not always be able to offer positive feedback, but it is important to be clear about your reasons so that they understand why they are being criticised. This is also showing compassion in your interactions.

Evidence opportunity

4.4 Receiving feedback

Discuss with your assessor two occasions when you received feedback. Consider what the positives were. Were there any negatives? What did you do with the feedback you received? Why? (Remember that feedback can be formal or informal.)

AC 4.5 Demonstrate how to record progress in relation to personal development

You will need to demonstrate how you record your progress in relation to your personal development; your practices will be observed.

Reflect on it

4.5 How is your PDP stored?

Reflect on your personal development plan and the arrangements that are in place in the care setting where you work for its security. How do you access it? When you update it, where do you do this? Where is it stored?

Evidence opportunity

4.5 How to record progress

If you have completed a personal development plan, read through the last entry made. Does it accurately reflect your progress to date? If not, how do you plan to update it? Discuss all of this with your assessor or manager. If discussing with your manager, this can be evidenced using a witness testimony.

Your personal development plan is a continuous record of your development at work. It is an important record because it:

- helps you to reflect on your practice
- identifies your achievements, strengths and abilities
- provides an up-to-date picture of what you have learned and how you have applied it
- provides useful information on what you aim to achieve and how you are going to do it
- reminds you to continue to develop your knowledge, skills and understanding.

Personal development plans can take many forms; in some care settings, they are recorded electronically, in other care settings they are recorded on paper and held in a file. Personal development plans contain personal information about you and therefore must be updated in private and stored securely when not in use.

LO4 Knowledge, skills, behaviours
Knowledge: why is it important to develop knowledge, skills and understanding?
Do you know how a learning activity has improved your knowledge, skills and understanding?
Do you know why it is important to reflect on situations that occur in your work setting?
Do you know why it is important to update your CPD and the consequences of not doing so?
Do you know how feedback has developed your knowledge, skills and understanding?
Did you know that you have just answered four questions about what continuing professional development involves?
Skills: how can you show that you are developing your knowledge, skills and understanding?
Do you know how to reflect on learning activities and situations you have experienced?
Do you know how to obtain feedback from others?
Do you know how to record the progress you have made in relation to your personal development?
Did you know that you have just answered three questions about some of the skills you have in relation to reviewing and updating your continuing professional development?
Behaviours: how can you show the personal qualities you have when maintaining your professional development?
Do you know how you can use learning activities and reflections in situations to develop as a professional?
Do you know how to use your experiences and learning and apply these consistently to your work practices?
Do you know how to respond positively to others' feedback?
Do you know how to maintain confidentiality when recording your progress in relation to the development of your knowledge, skills and understanding?
Did you know that you have just answered four questions about some of the essential behaviours that are expected of all adult care workers when developing their own knowledge, skills and understanding?

Suggestions for using the activities

This table summarises all the activities in the unit that are relevant to each assessment criterion.

Here, we also suggest other, different methods that you may want to use to present your knowledge and skills by using the activities.

These are just suggestions, and you should refer to the Introduction section at the start of the book, and more importantly the City & Guilds specification, and your assessor who will be able to provide more guidance on how you can evidence your knowledge and skills.

When you need to be observed during your assessment, this can be done by your assessor, or your manager can provide a witness testimony.

Assessment criteria and accompanying activities	Suggested methods to show your knowledge/skills
LO1 Understand what is required for competence in your work role	
1.1 Evidence opportunity (page 44)	You could write about your duties and responsibilities at work. You could cover how your responsibilities are different to those of a colleague.
	You could also discuss your job role, duties and responsibilities with your assessor. Use your job description as the basis of your discussion.
1.1 Reflect on it (page 46)	You could make notes to answer some of the questions in the activity.

→

Suggestions for using the activities	
1.2 Reflect on it (page 48)	Complete a spider diagram of the different standards, regulatory requirements and agreed ways of working that may influence your work role. Include examples of all three. Then make some notes to answer the questions in the activity.
1.2 Research it (page 51)	Visit the websites and make some notes about anything new that you have learned from your research. Share this with a colleague.
1.2 Evidence opportunity (page 51)	Complete the activity and produce a leaflet that covers your findings.
	You could also produce a presentation of the standards, regulatory requirements and agreed ways of working that influence your work role.
1.3 Reflect on it (page 52)	Complete the activity. You could also think about the questions in relation to the people you work with. Write a reflective account about this.
1.3 Research it (page 52)	You may like to note down your findings and thoughts.
1.3 Evidence opportunity (page 54)	Write a description of two personal values and two attitudes that you hold, and the different ways you ensure that each of these do not obstruct the quality of your work and practice as instructed in the activity.
	You could also discuss with your assessor the different ways you ensure that personal values, attitudes and beliefs do not influence the quality of your work. Include examples of the methods you use.
	You could also write a reflection about an occasion when you ensured that your personal values, attitudes and beliefs did not influence the quality of your work.
LO2 Be able to reflect on work activities **LO1 Understand what is required for competence in your work role** **LO4 Be able to develop your knowledge, skills and understanding**	
2.1, 4.2 Research it (page 56)	You could produce a poster or make notes about your findings.
2.1 Reflect on it (page 56) 2.1 Reflect on it (page 57)	Write a short reflective piece answering the questions in the activities.
2.1, 4.2 Evidence opportunity (page 58)	Complete the activity. Write about the benefits of reflecting on your practice and how it can help develop your knowledge and skills further. You could include the reasons why and examples of why it is an important way to develop your knowledge, skills and practice.
	You could also produce a presentation that explains the reasons why reflecting on work activities is an important way to develop your knowledge, skills and practice.
2.1, 2.2, 4.2 Reflect on it (page 59)	Write a short reflective account addressing the questions in the activity.
1.2, 2.2 Evidence opportunity (page 60)	Produce a PowerPoint presentation of your findings as instructed.
	You can show your assessor how you assess how well your knowledge, skills and understanding meet different standards.
	You could also show product evidence of your personal development plan to support your observation work.
	You could also include a witness testimony to support your observed work practices.
2.3, 4.2 Research it (page 61)	Produce a spider diagram and explain the concepts of 'reflection on action' and 'reflection in action' to a colleague. You could also write notes about your findings.

Suggestions for using the activities	
2.1, 2.3, 4.2, 4.4 Reflective exemplar (page 61)	The reflective exemplar will help you to understand how to reflect on work activities.
2.3, 4.2 Evidence opportunity (page 62)	You could write answers to address the questions. You could show and speak to your assessor to show how you reflect on your work activities.
	To support the skills you have demonstrated, you could also show your personal development plan.
	You could also include a witness testimony to support your observed work practices.
LO3 Be able to agree a personal development plan	
3.1 Reflect on it (page 64) 3.1 Research it (page 65)	Complete a spider diagram of the different sources of support that you can use for your learning and development. Remember to include examples of the support available both within (as the Reflect on it activity asks you to explore) and outside the care setting where you work (as the Research it activity asks of you).
	You could also discuss with your assessor the different sources of support available to you that can be used to support your learning and development, both in and out of the care setting where you work.
3.1 Evidence opportunity (page 65)	Produce a poster detailing the three sources of support you have used for learning and development.
	Alternatively, you could write a short piece about this.
3.2 Reflect on it (page 67)	Write a short piece detailing who you would involve when agreeing your PDP and what value they will add to your learning and development.
3.1, 3.2 Evidence opportunity (page 68)	You could produce the handout and step-by-step diagram or flow chart as instructed.
	You could, alternatively, write a personal statement about the process to follow for agreeing your personal development plan.
	Or you could produce a presentation that describes the process for agreeing a personal development plan. Remember to also include all those people who should be involved in the process.
3.3 Reflect on it (page 68)	You could write a short reflective piece.
3.3 Evidence opportunity (page 70) 3.1, 3.2, 3.3 Case study (page 70)	Discuss with your assessor how you contribute and agree to your personal development plan. The case study will help you.
	You could also show product evidence of your personal development plan to support your observed work.
	You could also include a witness testimony to support your observed work practices.
	You could also provide a written account to evidence your discussion.
LO4 Be able to develop your knowledge, skills and understanding	
LO2 Be able to reflect on work activities	
4.1 Research it (page 72)	You could develop a poster to detail your findings, or you could discuss these with a colleague and write some notes to evidence your discussion.
4.1 Evidence opportunity (page 73)	You could produce a leaflet as instructed in the activity. Or you could put together a PowerPoint presentation.
2.1, 2.3, 4.2 Reflect on it (page 73)	Write a reflective account of a learning situation you have experienced. Reflect on how it has improved your knowledge, skills and understanding. Remember to address all three areas.

→

Suggestions for using the activities	
2.1, 2.3, 4.2 Evidence opportunity (page 74) 2.1, 2.3, 4.2, 4.4 Reflective exemplar (page 61)	You could describe this to an assessor and then write a reflective account. You could also collect a witness testimony to support your reflective account. You could also use your personal development plan as (a work product) evidence. The reflective exemplar will help you to understand how to reflect on work activities.
4.3 Research it (page 74)	Discuss your findings. Write down some notes to evidence your discussion.
4.3 Reflect on it (page 75)	Write a short piece about the consequences of not maintaining your CPD and how this will affect the others mentioned in the activity.
4.1, 4.3 Evidence opportunity (page 75) 4.3, 4.4. Case study (page 77)	Write a case study about the activity. Remember to consider how you applied your learning in the setting. The case study on page 76 might help you. Or you could write a personal statement addressing the points in the activity. Include the reasons why continuing professional development is important. You could also produce a presentation that explains the importance of continuing professional development for carrying out your job role.
4.4 Evidence opportunity (page 78) 4.3, 4.4 Case study (page 77)	You could discuss this with your assessor. You could also write a reflective account to evidence your thoughts. You should also try and address the questions in the activities for AC 4.4. You could also collect a witness testimony to support your reflective account, and work product evidence such as evidence from your CPD folder of the feedback you have received from others, e.g. thank you cards from individuals, emails and letters from individuals' relatives and emails. The case study on page 76 will help you to think about how feedback can be obtained and used for your learning and development.
4.5 Reflect on it (page 78)	Write a short reflective account.
4.5 Evidence activity (page 78)	You could discuss this with your assessor and demonstrate how to record progress. If you discuss this with your manager, they will be able to provide a witness testimony. You could also support your observed work with product evidence such as your personal development plan, including any updates you've made.

See AC 1.2, page 50 for information on legislation relevant to this unit.

Resources for further reading and research

Books

Ferreiro Peteiro, M. (2014) *Level 2 Health and Social Care Diploma Evidence Guide*, Hodder Education

Knapman, J. and Morrison, T. (1998) *Making the Most of Supervision in Health and Social Care*, Pavilion

Schön, D. (1983) *The Reflective Practitioner: How Professionals Think in Action*, Temple Smith

Weblinks

www.cqc.org.uk Care Quality Commission (CQC) – information about CQC's regulations and the fundamental standards

www.gov.uk The UK Government's website for information about current legislation including health and safety

www.skillsforcare.org.uk Skills for Care – resources and information on the Care Certificate and the Code of Conduct for Healthcare Support Workers and Adult Social Care Workers in England

Equality and inclusion in care settings (209)

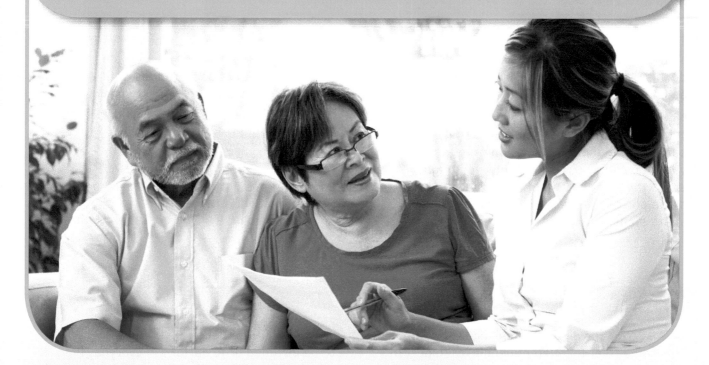

About this unit

Credit value: 2
Guided learning hours: 17

Supporting **equality**, **diversity** and **inclusion** in care settings is essential for delivering good, safe, quality care and creating a positive, caring and fair environment. Making sure that people are treated equally and fairly, in a way that takes into account their individual needs, is an essential part of your role.

In this unit, you will learn about the importance of equality and inclusion. You will find out how you can work in an inclusive way, and how to access information, advice and support about diversity, equality and inclusion.

You will learn about the meaning of equality, diversity and inclusion, the reasons why these concepts are important to your role as an adult care worker and how they can enable

you to reduce the likelihood of **discrimination** occurring.

Being able to practise in an inclusive way involves you complying with relevant legislation and codes of practice, both of which you will find out about in this unit including how you can apply them on a day-to-day basis. You will be able to practise your skills for showing respect for individuals' beliefs, culture, values and preferences and positively challenging discrimination when it occurs.

Of course, you won't be able to do all this without the correct information, advice and support about diversity, equality and inclusion. Knowing how to do so and when is another important area of knowledge you will develop in this unit.

Learning outcomes

LO1: Understand the importance of equality and inclusion

LO2: Be able to work in an inclusive way

LO3: Know how to access information, advice and support about diversity, equality and inclusion

LO1 Understand the importance of equality and inclusion

Getting started

Think about how you would describe yourself to someone who didn't know you. You might like to do this in terms of your age, background, physical appearance, personality, likes and dislikes.

Now think about three people who you know very well such as your friends or family. For each person, describe what they have in common with you. For example, you might share the same interests or enjoy going to the same places. Why is it important to you that you share similar interests?

For each person you have described, think about how they are different to you. For example, they might be from different backgrounds or live in a different area to you. They might speak a different language to you. Why do you think these differences are important? Do you value how they are different to you? Do you appreciate their differences? In what ways?

Thinking about this will help you to think about some of the things that we will discuss in this learning outcome and unit.

Key terms

Diversity means different types and variation. This could refer to different people, or things. In a health and social care setting for example, you will come across various different people, from different or 'diverse' backgrounds and needs. They may be different, for example, because of where they come from, how they dress and their age.

Equality means treating people fairly and valuing them for who they are. It means not to think of anyone as being less important than someone else. In a health and social care setting, this also means making sure that everyone is entitled to the same rights and opportunities.

Inclusion means being included or involved, for example being part of a wider group, or a group of friends. In a health and social care setting,

this means ensuring that all individuals are able to be included or to partake in everyday life regardless of any differences. This can create a sense of belonging.

Social inclusion means providing opportunities for individuals to participate and be involved in their wider communities so that they feel included, have a role and are part of society. This might be through accessing public transport, socialising with friends, accessing a course at a local college or participating in a local cultural event.

Discrimination means treating people unfairly or unlawfully, because they have a disability, or are of a different race, gender or age, for example.

AC 1.1 Explain what is meant by diversity, equality, inclusion and discrimination

What does diversity mean?

As we have discussed above, diversity essentially means different types, or variation. The UK is a 'diverse' country with people from different

countries, family backgrounds, views and ways of living. The different people that live in the UK all contribute to society in their own ways. People vary in terms of their gender, abilities, height, weight, age, sexual orientation, race and beliefs. Everyone is entitled to their own values, beliefs and cultures; these may be similar or different to those of others but it is important that they are all recognised as important.

Thinking positively about diversity

Living alongside people who are from different backgrounds and contribute different experiences can be a positive experience because each person brings with them their own cultures, beliefs and experiences that provide us with the opportunity to learn about new and different aspects of their cultures. This is true whatever your nationality, religion, race, gender or sexuality. This information can in turn lead to new ideas and beliefs about living together.

The world is vast, with people who have different ways of living. Just imagine for a minute what the world would be like if we all lived separately, if we never knew about other cultures and other ways of living. What would it be like if we never interacted with people who looked a bit different to us, or believed in something a bit different to us? What if we could never travel to other places? Why do you travel to other places? Is it to see new places, or is it also to experience different cultures and experience how other people live? What if we never came across people who live a different way of life to us, or who think in a different way to us? How would we ever understand how they think and feel?

We are living through a pivotal time in history, a social revolution, especially with regard to the rights of lesbian, gay, bisexual, transgender and queer (**LGBTQ**) people. This renewed awareness of the importance of diversity and equality has led to same-sex marriage being legalised in the UK in 2014 and the first same-sex marriages taking place in 2014, as well as increasingly open discussion of women's rights and issues around historical abuse. These discussions are now occupying an important place on the political stage and are crucial to social change.

It is important in your role that you try to have a positive and open attitude towards diversity as you will come across different people from various backgrounds. As we all come across people who are different to us in our daily lives, it is important that we respect their rights to have different values, beliefs and cultures that may be different to our own.

Diversity in the setting

The people that you will work with, as well as the individuals you will care for, in the setting will reflect the societies that we live in, and you will come across people from different countries and walks of life. The setting will therefore reflect the diverse and vibrant country that we live in.

Adult **care settings** are also different and varied in terms of the services they provide, the staff they employ, their location and size. The individuals who live in these care settings or who access their services are different in terms of their backgrounds, needs, abilities, interests and preferences. They will have their unique personal experiences, and attitudes. The adult care workers who work in these care settings are also different in terms of their experiences, values, behaviours, skills and knowledge. It is this diversity that makes adult care settings such interesting places to work in.

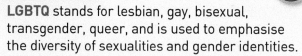

Key terms

LGBTQ stands for lesbian, gay, bisexual, transgender, queer, and is used to emphasise the diversity of sexualities and gender identities.

Care settings refer to adult care settings as well as adult, children and young people's health settings. In this qualification, it is adult care settings that will be our focus.

Reflect on it

1.1 Diversity

Reflect on what makes you unique and different from other people you work with and their unique differences. Do they have a disability or a visual or hearing impairment? Do they have different religious beliefs? Do these things mean that they see the world differently in any way?

What positive contributions and insights have you gained from working with these different individuals? You could make a list here of the differences and the positive contributions they have made, or the things that you have learned from them.

Remember to respect people's right to privacy by not using their real names when you produce your list.

Valuing and respecting diversity in the setting

Diversity also means recognising, valuing and respecting the differences that exist so that individuals and adult care workers can continue to be unique. Diversity and valuing is therefore very important in the work setting. It involves:

- **promoting person-centred values**. Person-centred values include things like:
  - showing **respect** for the individuals that you care for and valuing their importance
  - showing respect for people's **individuality** and showing respect towards individuals for example when communicating with them, and promoting individuality by encouraging individuals to be their own person
  - respecting their **rights**, for example to choose what they would like to eat and how they would like to dress
  - supporting their independence by encouraging them to participate in the activities they enjoy
  - respecting individuals' rights to **privacy**, for example in relation to hygiene
  - supporting people's rights to make their own choices and making sure they have the information they need to do so
  - treating people with **dignity**, which relates to the first point about treating people with respect, and valuing their beliefs
  - **working in partnership** with others including professionals outside the setting and families and carers.

Each person is different and therefore their 'person-centred values' will be different. For example, some individuals may communicate verbally, others may use signs and pictures to communicate; some individuals may choose not to eat meat while others may choose to; some individuals may enjoy going to worship in a church, others in a mosque. You can recap your knowledge of person-centred values by reading Unit 211, Implement person-centred approaches in care settings, AC 1.1.

- **developing positive working relationships**. You can do this by showing an interest in the differences that individuals and those you work with have. For example, you may ask an individual to tell you more about their culture or find out from your colleague the language

they prefer to speak. In turn, they will feel comfortable when working with you and start to build their trust in you.

- **developing yourself**. You can do this by showing your **commitment** to working together with individuals and alongside your colleagues; you will share information as well as ideas and therefore learn from one another about the different ways people live, think and behave. In this way, you can develop yourself as an individual by recognising and valuing the many different ideas and ways of life others have.

Not recognising the importance of diversity means you will not be able to provide high-quality care or support that is person-centred, build trusting working relationships that enable individuals to feel safe or develop your understanding and respect for the differences that exist in people. Remember, as an adult care worker, you are responsible for ensuring that the individuals for whom you provide care or support feel that you respect their differences and are treating them as unique individuals. In this way, individuals will develop a real sense of belonging through the good-quality care you offer and by meeting their needs (we will discuss this in LO2).

6Cs

Commitment

You will need to be committed or dedicated to promoting equality, diversity and inclusion in the setting, and working in a person-centred way in order to uphold the individuality and rights of the individuals you work with and ensure that their experiences of care and support are positive. This is important so that individuals feel valued and are able to live according to their preferences. You can show that you are committed to promoting equality, diversity and inclusion as well as person-centred values, by treating each individual with respect and showing a genuine interest in their likes and background.

How do you show that you work positively alongside individuals with care or support needs? What qualities do you show when working together with your colleagues? How can working with diverse individuals further develop your knowledge?

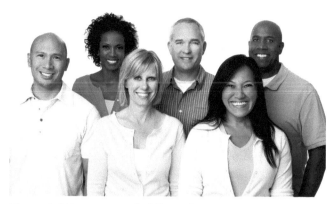

Figure 3.1 How are we all different?

What does equality mean?

First of all, it is about recognising that each person is different, understanding how they are different and then treating them in a way that respects their differences. For example, an adult care worker who provides care to three older individuals who live together would need to find out from each one how they want to be cared for. Do not assume that these

individuals all have the same preferences in their daily routine. For example, you would need to ask what time they would like to get up in the morning or whether they prefer to have a shower or bath.

As well as understanding and recognising the differences that may exist between people (this is what we mean by diversity) it is also important that you understand how to treat all the different people you come into contact with as an adult care worker fairly and respectfully. Doing so is one of the essential behaviours expected from all adult care workers. It is important to remember that treating people equally does not mean treating them all the same.

Not recognising the importance of equality means you will not be able to support people's rights and as a result they will not feel that they are being treated equally. To stop the unequal treatment of people there is legislation in place related to equality and you will learn about this later in LO2, AC 2.1 on page 98.

Dos and don'ts for treating people equally	
Do	Treat people fairly. You should treat people as individuals. This means finding out about the person they are and not making assumptions about how they want to be treated, for example ask the name they would like to be addressed by, what activities they enjoy.
Do	Respect people. You can do this by promoting a person's right to dignity and letting them make their own choices.
Do	Treat people in a way that provides them with the opportunities that are available to everyone, for example by providing them with information to access a local health service.
Don't	Ignore people's differences. Treating people equally does not mean treating everybody in the same way. First, respect their differences and then find ways to ensure that their needs are met. You can do this by asking each person about his or her differences and how they would like them to be addressed. This will also apply in your interactions with colleagues. For example, you should not make assumptions about the practices of any colleagues who follow the same culture because their beliefs and customs may vary.
Don't	Devalue people. You should support people's rights to dignity. For example, you can do this by supporting individuals to make their own mistakes and learn from them, and by supporting individuals to take risks and not let this prevent them from doing what they want to do, unless it poses a health and safety issue in which case assessing the risks of doing so must take place.
Don't	Treat people in a way that denies them access to the opportunities that are made available to everyone. For example, an individual with a visual impairment may not be able to read a leaflet, and so you should provide them with the information in a format they can read and understand. In this way, you have provided them with an equal opportunity to access the information in the leaflet. Therefore, they are not treated less fairly than anyone else.

Reflect on it

1.1 Equality

Reflect on an occasion when you or someone you know were treated unequally. This may have been because of your age, your abilities or your culture, for example. Discuss in pairs what happened, the reasons why you think you were treated unequally and how this made you feel.

What does inclusion mean?

Being included in all aspects of day-to-day life is a desire that we all have and most of us achieve. Most of us like being around friends and family, and enjoy the feeling of being part of a bigger group of people who may share our interests and hobbies. This may be in everyday life where we meet with friends and family in person, on the internet through social media such as Facebook, and group chats on our phones. Basically we like to feel included!

The term **inclusion** (see page 84 for definition) is linked closely to equality and diversity because without it you will not be able to treat people fairly and respect their differences.

As we have discussed, you will come across different people with different backgrounds, needs and preferences, and you will play a key role in making sure that they feel part of the care setting, of society as a whole and are enabled and empowered to participate in different activities. Individuals who are 'active participants' are more likely to feel and be in control of their lives because they are not having activities done for them but rather they are taking part or doing the activities they want to be involved in. (You can find out more about active participation in Unit 211, AC 4.1.) Individuals who have care or support needs may find this difficult to do on their own and so will depend on you to ensure that you either equip them with the necessary skills or provide them with the support they require.

Inclusion therefore refers not only to individuals being involved in day-to-day life but also refers to individuals:

- having a purpose or meaning to their lives, for example a paid job, being part of a group of friends
- being accepted for who they are, for example by not being left out because of their differences
- being able to play an active part in the community where they live, for example accessing any local sports facilities that are available, meeting others who live in their local community
- being valued and respected, for example being asked for their views, having their preferences taken into account
- having their differences accepted, for example by not being left out of day-to-day activities because of their differences (someone with a hearing impairment should not be left out of conversations because of their impairment)
- being included, for example by making them feel like they belong in any setting
- being empowered, for example by making them feel that their contributions are valued and that they have a role in society.

As a care worker, you will need to create a sense of inclusion. If you are not able to do this, and do not recognise the importance of inclusion, you will not be able to support individuals' well-being (a concept covered in more detail in Unit 211, Implement person-centred approaches in care settings). It also means that you will not be providing good care or support that is person-centred, which are key parts of your role.

Not supporting individuals' well-being and not being inclusive, will also impact negatively on individuals as they will not feel that they are part of a bigger group, and could lead to them feeling isolated and lonely inside or outside the setting. As a care worker, you should always make sure that you include individuals and find ways to ensure that they are involved and feel valued.

Research it

1.1 **The importance of inclusion**

Research the importance of inclusion when planning person-centred care and support.

You may like to use the **Joseph Rowntree Foundation**'s report, 'Person-centred planning in social care', as the basis of your research. You can access the report from the link below:

www.jrf.org.uk/sites/default/files/jrf/migrated/files/9781859354803.pdf

Key terms 🔑

The **Joseph Rowntree Foundation** is an independent organisation that encourages communities in the UK to work together to improve the lives of everyone.

Prejudice is a negative opinion that you may have of someone which is not based on experience or interaction.

What does discrimination mean?

Discrimination (unlike equality, diversity and inclusion that you've learned make a positive difference to individuals' lives) is a negative behaviour. It refers to treating people or groups of people unfairly or unequally. People may be 'discriminated against' and treated unfairly for many reasons including gender, sexuality, race, ethnicity and religious beliefs. It can happen when:

- people are labelled because of the characteristics they have, for example someone may be ridiculed because of their facial features, hair colour

- people are viewed as the same because of an assumption or generalisation about the group they belong to which is untrue (stereotyping), for example 'all individuals with mental health needs are dangerous'

- people are prejudged because of a preconceived opinion that is inaccurate and not true. '**Prejudice**' occurs when you make

assumptions about people that are not based on facts or reason, for example 'all older people cannot learn new skills'.

We will discuss this and the ways in which people discriminate deliberately, and discriminate without meaning to, in further detail in AC 1.2.

Labelling, stereotyping and prejudice can all lead to discrimination. Discrimination is a negative behaviour because it can:

- disadvantage people, for example an individual may not be offered a job because of the characteristics they have

- disempower people, for example an individual's confidence will be affected if they are not accepted for the person they are or the beliefs they have

- disable people, for example an individual's physical, mental, emotional and social well-being will be affected if an individual is prevented from accessing the services, care or support they require.

All those who access, live and work in adult care settings have a right not to be discriminated against; this type of positive behaviour is known as anti-discrimination. For example, some of the different types of discrimination that are currently being experienced relate to the following:

- **Gender discrimination** – people can be discriminated against in relation to characteristics associated with their masculinity or femininity. For example, transgender people who are born with a gender that they feel is not true to how they feel and are, and want to live and be treated as the opposite gender to the one they were born with.

- **Racial discrimination** – people can be discriminated against in relation to their race. For example, people that share the same culture and language, such as groups of migrants, may be viewed as having poor skills and not to be trusted and may therefore be treated unfairly by employers, who may pay them less than other employees.

- **Religious discrimination** – people may be discriminated against in relation to their religion or religious beliefs.

- **Disability discrimination** – people can be discriminated against in relation to their disability. For example, a person with a physical disability who uses a wheelchair may be refused access to a building because it does not have a lift.

- **Discrimination based on people's sexuality** – people can be discriminated against for being gay, lesbian or bisexual.

Research it

1.1 Discrimination in the news

There are many cases in the news about people suffering from discrimination for various reasons. Research some stories in the news about discrimination. Discuss why these people were discriminated against and how the reasons and views can be avoided in your role. You might like to look at this story as a starting point:

www.bbc.co.uk/news/uk-england-bristol-24584855

Evidence opportunity

1.1 Promoting diversity, equality and inclusion

Think about your job role and the day-to-day responsibilities you have in the care setting where you work. Create a poster or PowerPoint presentation explaining, with examples, how you promote individuals' diversity, equality and inclusion and ensure that they are not discriminated against.

For example, this may be in relation to how you communicate with your colleagues, provide care or support to individuals.

AC 1.2 Describe ways in which discrimination may deliberately or inadvertently occur in the work setting

As you have learned already, people can experience different types of discriminatory behaviour. You will learn more about the current legislation that protects people from discrimination in LO2, AC 2.1. The following types of discrimination are examples of the main ones that are recognised in law and can occur in the **work setting** (see page 91 for definition).

Different forms of discrimination

Direct discrimination

This is discrimination that occurs deliberately, for example excluding a young adult from a social group because they are in a wheelchair. This is unfair because they are being treated this way because of their disability which is a physical characteristic. They should have a right to participate, be part of a group and feel like they belong.

Indirect discrimination

This can occur inadvertently, for example not having access for wheelchair users in the setting. This is different to direct discrimination because it is not aimed at one particular individual but rather a way of practising that is not inclusive to individuals with diverse needs. Another example of this is when a residential care home only celebrates some religious periods such as Easter and Christmas. Again this is not direct, because these practices apply to everyone in the home but negatively impact on those that do not celebrate these religious periods or wish to celebrate others.

Harassment

This is an unwanted behaviour that does not respect an individual's dignity and makes them feel uncomfortable. For example, a visitor who uses offensive language when visiting their relative in hospital makes the individual feel uncomfortable in front of others who may overhear. Harassment can be both deliberate and inadvertent, and is sometimes done very easily in the setting. You may not even mean any harm but making jokes about someone's abilities is inappropriate as this may be at the expense of certain groups of people.

Research it

1.2 Discrimination in the work setting

Research an example of the discrimination an individual with care or support needs can experience when accessing adult care services. You may want to select an individual you know about or use the internet as the basis of your research.

You may find it useful to read the article published by **Marie Curie**, 'Healthcare professionals must address discrimination to improve care for terminally ill LGBT people', in relation to the care experiences of lesbian, gay, bisexual and trans (LGBT) people with terminal illnesses. This is available from the link below:

www.mariecurie.org.uk/media/press-releases/lgbt-research2/158806#0v1gC5xHRXPMQmyb.99

Key terms

Work settings may include one specific location or a range of locations, depending on the context of a particular work role such as in an individual's home; or in a communal setting such as a residential care home.

Marie Curie is a charity that provides care and support for individuals and their families living with any terminal illness.

Victimisation

This occurs when someone is treated unfairly because they have complained about discrimination or harassment. For example, an individual who complains about an activities worker who does not make activity sheets available in a format for individuals who cannot read so that the individual is then excluded from taking part in activities that are organised by this worker.

Reasons why discrimination can occur deliberately and unintentionally

Discrimination can occur both deliberately and inadvertently (or unintentionally) in the work setting for many reasons. The things that we discuss below are similar in many ways, but it is useful to break down some of these reasons. You will notice that similar themes run through these points. Understanding and respect for differences can overcome most of these.

Care workers who do not consider the individual needs of people

When adult care workers have not spent time getting to know the individuals they provide care or support to and are therefore unaware of their unique likes, dislikes and preferences, this could lead to discrimination, both deliberate or unintentional. Look again at the examples that are listed above. This could also happen when adult care settings have not asked a new adult care worker how they can help them become part of the team. The new team member may not feel comfortable because their colleagues have a lot more experience than they do.

People who do not respect one another's differences

In adult care settings individuals and adult care workers may be from a diverse range of backgrounds and not respecting these differences may lead to some individuals being stereotyped (see below). One example may be thinking that all those who are Muslim will want to pray at the same times every day and participate in fasting, rather than checking first with each Muslim person as to their preferences for praying and fasting. Another example might be that all young people are only interested in going out with their friends to socialise and are lazy when they have to study or work.

The stereotypes that people have

This is similar to what we have just discussed above but it is different in that your prejudices may have been produced through the stereotypes that there are in society. When you stereotype someone, you form your opinion of them based on a general idea of who they are, or who you think they are, because of the 'groups' that they belong to. You might stereotype people because of their gender, sexuality, race or religion.

People usually stereotype when they do not understand people that may be different to them and because they may not personally know people that are different to them. People who stereotype do so because they have not interacted with people from these other groups, their views (both negative and positive) may be shaped by a very limited interaction they may have had, or by the ways in which certain groups are depicted on television, in films and on the news. Stereotypes can be both positive and negative. You might expect a person to be nice and friendly because they come from a certain country, but then be suspicious of someone and have a negative opinion of them because of their background and the way they look.

It is very easy to stereotype, to see a group of people in simple terms as 'all the same'. However, you should avoid this. Viewing people in these ways can lead to positive behaviour against some people and discrimination against others, whether you do this knowingly or unknowingly. To stop this from happening, as a care worker you will need to make an effort to understand people on an individual basis, and know that while people may belong to different groups, people are not all the same. They have differing needs and preferences.

Labelling others

Stereotypes can lead one set of people to label another group of people. These labels are usually negative and are placed on people to devalue them. For example, young people may be called 'lazy', migrants may be called 'thugs', travellers 'thieves', older people 'useless'. These labels are untrue and negative and have the potential to cause even more harm if the person that has the label placed on them starts behaving like the label. For example, a young person may not see the point of applying for jobs if they believe that others view them as lazy and therefore incapable of finding a job. A traveller who is labelled a thief may decide to commit theft and live up to their reputation if they think that others view them like this anyway.

People do not have knowledge about different groups of people, and up-to-date anti-discrimination practices

It is possible that both care workers and individuals may never have worked or lived as part of a group in a care setting where they would have gained experience of other individuals and adult care workers from different cultures and backgrounds with different beliefs and values to their own. As a result, you and the individuals you work with may not be aware of your own prejudices. For adult care workers, it is important that you learn about different practices and take some time out to reflect on your own prejudices and seek feedback from others – such as your manager at work or your partner at home – who know you well and may be able to provide you with further information about your own prejudices. Just working with different individuals will help to build your knowledge of different people. You should also encourage positive interaction between individuals which will help to break down any negative assumptions, and create understanding between individuals from different backgrounds. As a care worker, you must also continue to update your knowledge about anti-discrimination practices throughout your career. You will learn more about the sources of information, advice and support that are available to you later on in this unit in LO3, AC 3.1.

Dos and don'ts for working with different people	
Do	See people as individuals with different needs and preferences.
Do	Respect people's individuality.
Do	Treat people as individuals and understand that just because people belong to a particular group they are not all the same.
Do	Value people's differences.
Don't	Treat people the same. Think about how you would feel if people focused on a certain characteristic about you, for example your race, or your religion.
Don't	Make assumptions about people.
Don't	Stereotype people.
Don't	Label people.

1.2, 1.3 Preventing discrimination in the work setting

Think about what your opinions of certain groups of people are. You may think about gender, races and religions.

- What positive opinions do you have of these groups?
- What negative opinions do you have of these groups?
- Why do you think of these people in these ways?
- What can you do to make sure you do not have any 'stereotypical' views?

Then reflect on your responsibilities as an adult care worker for ensuring that discrimination does not occur in your work setting.

Perhaps you could reflect on what you can do to fulfil your duty to provide good-quality care or support to individuals that is free from discrimination and how you are keeping your knowledge and practices up to date.

1.2 Deliberate and unintentional discrimination

Think about how discrimination can occur both deliberately and unintentionally in work settings. For three types of direct and three types of indirect discrimination that you have learned about, develop posters that detail how they can occur in the work setting. Remember to include different examples of the ways that it can occur.

AC 1.3 Explain how practices that support equality and inclusion reduce the likelihood of discrimination

Equality and inclusion

As you have learned, the UK is an increasingly diverse society:

'Nearly 1 in 10 British children is growing up in a mixed-race household. Society's age structure is changing, with a growing proportion of the population aged over 50.'

Equality and Human Rights Commission, Context of 'How fair is Britain?' review, May 2016

The Equality and Human Rights Commission (EHRC) is responsible for monitoring how equal the UK is and every three years reviews how fair Britain is as a society. The review identifies how our society has changed but also shows where the inequalities between different groups are at their largest and makes recommendations for how to address these.

The information, collated as part of the review conducted by EHRC in May 2016, suggests that some groups of people are likely to experience inequality. Some examples are included below and are represented in terms of their:

- **health** – Pakistani and Bangladeshi groups are more likely to experience poor mental health, to report a disability and find it harder to access and communicate with their GPs than other groups
- **education** – lesbian, gay, bisexual and transgender young people are treated unfairly and experiencing bullying in school and in other education establishments
- **employment** – women are much more likely to be low paid than men throughout their working lives
- **care and support** – Bangladeshi, Black African, Black Caribbean and Pakistani children under the ages of 18 are more likely to have caring responsibilities compared to White British children.

Equality and Human Rights Commission, 'How fair is Britain?', Online summary, May 2016 (www.equalityhumanrights.com/en/how-fair-britain/online-summary)

Inequalities, or people being treated as less than others, may come about because some groups of people are being disadvantaged and not being treated fairly because of the labels that other groups have placed on them. This may mean that they are being denied the rights and opportunities that everyone in the UK has.

Inclusion

In a fair and equal UK there should be nothing to stop people from participating in all aspects of society. People's differences should therefore not act as barriers that would stop them from taking part in all aspects of society. For example, a day care setting that does not allow for wheelchair access is one that is looking at individuals with physical disabilities in a negative way i.e. not having the ability or right to participate in day-to-day activities. Instead of focusing on the disability of the individual, the focus should be on the failings of the care setting to provide an environment that is inclusive of everyone and does not exclude anyone because of their individuality. It is the care setting's responsibility to provide care or support to everyone, and it is also part of anti-discriminatory practice which we will discuss shortly.

Practices that support equality and inclusion

Supporting equality and inclusion involves:

- finding out about people's backgrounds
- not making assumptions and stereotyping
- being fair and valuing individuality.

You can find out more about the practices that support equality and inclusion and reduce the likelihood of discrimination on the next page.

Figure 3.2 identifies the key practices that support equality and inclusion.

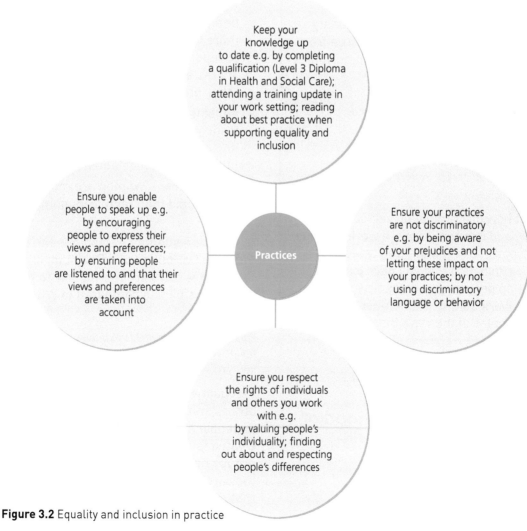

Keep your knowledge up to date e.g. by completing a qualification (Level 3 Diploma in Health and Social Care); attending a training update in your work setting; reading about best practice when supporting equality and inclusion

Ensure you enable people to speak up e.g. by encouraging people to express their views and preferences; by ensuring people are listened to and that their views and preferences are taken into account

Practices

Ensure your practices are not discriminatory e.g. by being aware of your prejudices and not letting these impact on your practices; by not using discriminatory language or behavior

Ensure you respect the rights of individuals and others you work with e.g. by valuing people's individuality; finding out about and respecting people's differences

Figure 3.2 Equality and inclusion in practice

Research it

1.3 Job-seeking discrimination

Research the inequalities that people from different cultures may face when applying for jobs. The article below, 'Is it easier to get a job if you're Adam or Mohamed?', is a useful source of information:

www.bbc.co.uk/news/uk-england-london-38751307

Explain why you think these inequalities exist. What is the impact of discriminating against job applicants on the basis of their names?

How can supporting equality and inclusion reduce the likelihood of discrimination?

Stop and think about how you would feel if you were an individual in a setting and were discriminated against because you looked different to others, or because you spoke a different language, could not speak English or could speak very little English. What if you were left out of a group activity because you could not communicate in English? How would that make you feel? Now think about what you would want the people who cared for you to do to make sure that you were not left out, that you were not discriminated against. If you were treated equally, and included in activities, would this mean that you were being respected and treated as an individual? Thinking about this will help you to understand how promoting equality and inclusion can reduce or stop discrimination from occurring.

The main way in which you can support equality and inclusion is through anti-discriminatory practice. This means being 'against discrimination' and putting practices in place to make sure that discrimination does not happen in your workplace.

Anti-discriminatory practice and how this can reduce the likelihood of discrimination

Ensuring your practices are not discriminatory means that you are leading by example and that you have the courage to challenge discrimination if it occurs, which in turn can reduce the likelihood of discrimination from occurring again and again. Having an anti-discriminatory approach is good practice, it is one of the key aspects of your job as

it will ensure that the individuals in your setting will be treated equally and fairly regardless of their differences. It will also ensure that they feel valued and respected as individuals with unique needs and preferences.

In order to make sure you and your setting have an anti-discriminatory approach, you should:

- **have up-to-date knowledge about equality and inclusion**. It is important that you understand the factors that make people different and how they may be discriminated against because of these differences. This will involve you making an effort to understand what people's rights are and what your duties are with respect to promoting equality, inclusion and diversity in the care setting where you work. This means that you will be able to understand and then follow the agreed ways of working that are required for ensuring that discrimination does not occur.

- **lead by example and challenge discrimination**. To ensure your practices and those of your colleagues are not discriminatory, you should lead by example and display good positive behaviour towards all individuals that you care for. To lead by and set a positive example means that you should also have the courage to challenge discrimination if it occurs. This in turn can reduce the likelihood of discrimination from occurring again. For example, a colleague in the setting may work in a different way with an individual by giving them less one-to-one time than they do other individuals and you may ask your manager if you could discuss their actions with them. The person or your manager may not necessarily agree with your view and that is why it can be brave to speak up about discriminatory actions and behaviour. You should not worry about the views of others if you are challenging discrimination.

- **be person-centred**. Ensure you respect the rights of individuals and others you work with, as this is part of providing person-centred care or support. You may want to refer to this concept in Unit 211, Implement person-centred approaches in care settings.

- **enable people to speak up**. You should support individuals to speak up about their rights to not be discriminated against and to be treated as unique individuals, by doing this you are empowering them to take control and to

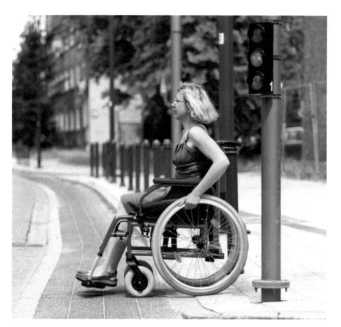

Figure 3.3 How can you support me not to be discriminated against?

be confident which in turn can reduce their vulnerability and therefore the likelihood of discrimination from occurring. It also creates a positive working environment where anti-discriminatory practices are supported and encouraged and therefore where discrimination is, again, less likely to occur.

- **make changes to the setting if and when needed**. As part of your role, you should constantly think about how to improve the lives of the individuals you care for and the changes that need to be made in order to ensure that individuals are treated equally and inclusively. For example, you may decide to ensure the weekly coffee group for individuals and their relatives who visit your work setting is held on a week day one week and at the weekend the following week. This means all individuals' relatives are given the opportunity to attend as some may only be able to visit at the weekend due to their work and family commitments.

Consequences of discriminating in the setting

Individuals who are discriminated against in care settings may experience feelings of low self-esteem, and low confidence levels. Individuals may also become withdrawn and may not want to participate. They may feel disempowered and as

6Cs   **C**

Courage

Courage refers to ensuring that you positively challenge any discriminatory practice you see and that you know may impact negatively on individuals and the people you work with. You can do this by not ignoring it and by ensuring that you report it as soon as it happens. Being courageous to support equality and inclusion will mean that you will be contributing to a discrimination-free environment. This is because you will be doing everything you can to challenge it and prevent it from occurring again.

Reflect on it   ?

1.3 Anti-discriminatory practice

Reflect on an occasion when you observed a situation that you know was unfair and discriminatory. Did you report it? Why? What impact did it have on the person's well-being?

Or you may want to think about the following questions:

- What is discrimination?
- Why does it occur?
- How can I ensure that the people and individuals I care for do not suffer discrimination from me, my colleagues and others in the setting?
- What can I do to make sure that discrimination does not occur in my setting?
- If it does occur, what can I do to make sure it doesn't happen again?

a result they may be reluctant to say or make any comments about the care they receive due to fear of having the care withdrawn or fear of upsetting their carers. All of this may in turn affect the quality of care you offer them if, for example, they then do not want to share information with you.

It is very important that your practices support equality and inclusion because as an adult care worker you are accountable for your actions. If you do discriminate, either deliberately or unintentionally, you can be disciplined for this by your employer and you could be dismissed from your job. In addition, you employer could also be held responsible for your actions.

As you will have learned, practices that support equality and inclusion and reduce the likelihood of discrimination are everyone's responsibility

in adult care settings. Read Case study 1.3 and think about the different ways the adult care workers in the residential care home are promoting people's rights to diversity, equality, inclusion and reducing the likelihood of discrimination from occurring.

Case study

1.3 Supporting equality and inclusion

Aphis care is a residential care home for older people. Every month the adult care workers in the home support the residents to meet up to discuss and share their ideas on different aspects of the home such as in relation to the activities and care services provided at the home. They discuss the things that are working well, 'what they like' and what they would like to change or improve.

Today's meeting is focused on how the residents feel about celebrating Christmas together later on in the year. They have decided to discuss this because some of the residents and their families have always celebrated Christmas and other residents have not. One of the care workers, Cindy, begins by supporting the residents to speak up about the different beliefs that are shared amongst them with respect to celebrating Christmas.

One resident explains how she has always celebrated Christmas since she was a child. Another three residents, supported by care workers Maggie and Steve, show the group photographs of them celebrating Christmas with their families while the other residents share the posters they have made to explain the different aspects involved in celebrating Christmas.

Some of the residents who have never celebrated Christmas begin to show a genuine interest in the photographs and posters being shared and ask lots of questions. Some of the residents then ask whether in the next meeting they can show the group other festivals they celebrate such as **Chinese New Year** and **Diwali**.

The residents, with support from the adult care workers, begin to put a calendar together of the different celebrations they would like to share as a group. It is agreed that the communal lounge that everyone shares will not be decorated, to show respect for the residents who decide to not be part of the festivals and celebrations. Instead, the residents decide that if they decide to celebrate any of the festivals, then they will only decorate the hallway and activities room as well as their own individual rooms for those who wish to.

Discussion points

1 How are the adult care workers supporting the residents to respect one another's differences?
2 How are equality and diversity being promoted?
3 How do you think the residents feel by being involved in these discussions?
4 How could the support provided by the adult care workers reduce the likelihood of discrimination occurring? Why?

Key terms

Chinese New Year, also known as the Spring Festival, is the most important celebration in the Chinese calendar where people share food and celebrate the year ahead together.

Diwali or Deepavali is the Hindu festival of lights celebrated every year in autumn where people share gifts and pray together.

Evidence opportunity

1.3 Supporting equality and inclusion

In pairs, take it in turns to share examples of work practices that support equality and inclusion. For each example that you share, write down how it can reduce the likelihood of discrimination occurring. Explain how as well as the reasons why.

LO1 Knowledge, skills, behaviours
Knowledge: why is equality and inclusion important in care settings?
Do you know the meanings of equality and inclusion?
Do you know how equality and inclusion link to diversity?
Did you know that you have just shown your knowledge of the importance of supporting equality and inclusion?
Skills: how can you show that you work in ways that are anti-discriminatory?
Do you know how to prevent discrimination from occurring?
Do you know what to do if discrimination does occur?
Did you know that you have just answered two questions about how your practices can reduce the likelihood of discrimination from occurring?
Behaviours: how can you show the personal qualities you have for supporting equality and inclusion?
Do you know how to show that you respect individuals' differences?
Do you know how to show your consideration when someone has been discriminated against?
Did you know that you have just answered two questions about a few of the essential behaviours that are expected for supporting equality, diversity and inclusion in care settings?

LO2 Be able to work in an inclusive way

Getting started

Think of an occasion when you were involved in an event or celebration. For example, this may be at work in relation to someone leaving the setting for a new job or at home in relation to a surprise birthday party. How did it make you feel being involved and part of these important celebrations? How do you think it would make you feel if you were not asked to be involved and only found out about the events afterwards?

Remember that working in inclusive ways also involves being considerate and putting yourself 'in other people's shoes'. This means empathising with them and showing them consideration and kindness.

AC 2.1 **Identify which legislation and codes of practice relating to equality, diversity and discrimination apply to your role**

Legislation

It is important that all adult care workers are aware of current legislation and codes of practice so that they can ensure that they are working in a fair and inclusive way and their practices in relation to equality, diversity and anti-discrimination are up to date and reflect best practice.

UK and international legislation or laws are established by governments and are in place to support our rights and protect us from being discriminated against.

The following laws are the main ones that relate to supporting equality, diversity, inclusion and preventing discrimination (it is important to note, however, that there may be changes to legislation as a result of **Brexit**, see page 100 for definition).

Table 3.1 Legislation that supports equality, diversity, inclusion and the prevention of discrimination

Legislation	
Relevant Act	**What does it say?**
Human Rights Act 1998	This establishes the human rights and freedoms that everyone in the UK has. Some examples of this include: • the human right to respect for private and family life. In a setting, this includes individuals having the right to receive their visitors in private in their rooms • the right not to be tortured or treated in an inhuman or degrading way such as individuals having the right not to be abused or harmed • the right to liberty such as the right of an individual to not be locked in a room • the right to life such as the right of an individual to live their life how they want to • the right not to be discriminated against such as the right of an individual to not be excluded from an activity because of their health condition. It also states that organisations that provide services to the public such as local councils must treat everyone fairly, with dignity and respect.
Mental Capacity Act 2005	This protects the rights of individuals who lack **mental capacity** by for example: • supporting individuals' rights to make their own decisions for as long as they are able to • supporting individuals' rights to make decisions even if these conflict with the views of others or are seen by others as unwise • supporting individuals to make preparations and decisions about their future care and support needs should they lose capacity in the future.
Equality Act 2010	This states that people must not be treated unfairly because of their individual differences. It states that there are nine individual differences that are protected in law from discrimination and these are called the 'nine protected characteristics'. These are: 1 Age – for example, it will protect an individual from being excluded from an activities group because they are considered too old. 2 Disability – for example, it will protect an individual with a physical disability from being refused access to a service because there is no wheelchair ramp. 3 Gender reassignment – for example, it will protect an individual from being **victimised** because they are friends with an individual who is transitioning from one gender to another. 4 Marriage and civil partnership – for example, it will protect two individuals in a same-sex relationship from being refused entry to a social evening. 5 Pregnancy and maternity –for example, it will protect an individual from being asked to leave a community facility because she is breastfeeding. 6 Race – for example, it will protect individuals from some racial groups from being excluded when providing information about a new care service in the local community. 7 Religion or belief – for example, it will protect an individual being discriminated against for a lack of belief (i.e. referred to as Atheism). 8 Sex – for example, it will protect an individual being discriminated against when applying for an adult care worker job because they are male. 9 Sexual orientation – for example, it will protect an individual being victimised by another individual in a care setting because they are attracted to people of both sexes.

→

Table 3.1 Legislation that supports equality, diversity, inclusion and the prevention of discrimination *continued*

Legislation	
Care Act 2014	This supports making how care and support can be provided and accessed easier to understand.
	It supports making care and support services fairer.
	It introduced the 'well-being principle', This means that individuals' well-being must be the focus when making decisions.
	It developed the concept of 'personalisation' in care. This means that care and support provided must meet individuals' unique needs and preferences and support them being in control of their lives.

Key term

Brexit is a term that has been used for the United Kingdom leaving the European Union (EU). The EU was formed by France and Germany after the end of the Second World War to ensure that they would never again go to war with each other. The European Union currently consists of 28 countries of which the UK is one. The countries in the EU trade with one another and also discuss other political issues like climate change.

In 2016, the UK voted and decided that it no longer wanted to be a member of the EU. There are a number of 'EU' laws that are in place in the UK. It is uncertain how these laws will be affected when the UK finally leaves the EU, which is likely to be in 2019.

Reflect on it

2.1 Making decisions

Reflect on an important decision you have made about how you live your life. For example, it may be in relation to where you live or what you want to do in the future. How did it feel to make your own decision? Imagine now that you lacked the capacity or the ability to make this decision because of a health condition.

- Who would you ask to make the decision on your behalf?
- Why?
- How do you think you would feel if you didn't have anyone to ask to make the decision on your behalf?

Key terms

Mental capacity refers to an individual's ability to make their own decisions.

Victimised means to single out someone, or pick on them. Here, it means when an individual is treated less fairly when they support or speak up for an individual with a protected characteristic.

codes of practice or conduct that provide guidance to help adult care workers comply with best practice and agreed ways of working that relate to promoting equality and diversity and reducing and challenging discrimination.

Organisations such as care providers usually develop their own codes of conduct that they expect their employees to comply with. Perhaps you could speak to your manager to find out if the care setting where you work has one in place and, if so, what it says?

Codes of conduct

Codes of practice are sometimes also called codes of conduct. In this section we are referring to the

Table 3.2 lists examples of codes of conduct that are in place for all those who work in care settings.

Table 3.2 Examples of codes of conduct and what they say

Code of conduct	What does it say?
Code of Conduct for Healthcare Support Workers and Adult Social Care Workers in England	This is overseen by Skills for Health and Skills for Care, and established the following principles for all those who work in health and adult care settings. It advises that workers should: • be accountable for their actions or omissions, for example by ensuring all care or support provided is documented • promote and uphold the privacy, dignity, rights, health and well-being of individuals and their carers who use care and support services at all times, for example by ensuring your day-to-day practices take into account their individual preferences and needs • work in partnership to ensure the delivery of high-quality, safe and compassionate care and support by working together with their colleagues and manager • communicate openly and effectively to promote individuals' and their carers' health, safety and well-being, for example by asking individuals and their carers how they want to be supported • respect a person's right to confidentiality, for example by supporting them to read their post in private • be committed to continuing professional development to improve the quality of care and support provided, for example attending an equality and diversity training update • promote equality, diversity and inclusion, for example by following best practice when providing care or support to individuals.
Mental Capacity Act Code of Practice	This includes guidance on how the Mental Capacity Act 2005 should be applied. It sets out what must be done when representatives act or make decisions on behalf of individuals who can't act or make those decisions for themselves. It states that the individual's best interests must always be the focus of all decisions made.

Evidence opportunity

2.1 Codes of conduct

Produce a code of conduct for an adult care worker in a care setting that relates to the principles that support the promotion of equality and diversity and anti-discriminatory practices. Write down what your code of conduct says about how to promote equality, diversity and discrimination in your day-to-day working practices.

Are you promoting all three? If so, how?

Fundamental standards

CQC has some fundamental standards which individuals' care must never fall below. The standards state that individuals have the right, for example, to expect person-centred care (care that meets their unique needs and preferences); they have the right to be treated with dignity and respect, have their privacy maintained, be treated equally and have their social inclusion promoted so that their independence is promoted.

AC 2.2 Show interaction with individuals that respects their beliefs, cultures, values and preferences

This AC requires you to demonstrate or show that you can interact with individuals in ways that respect their beliefs, cultures, values and preferences.

Before we discuss how you can show interaction with individuals that respects their beliefs, cultures, values and preferences, we should think about what beliefs, cultures, values and preferences are.

What are beliefs, cultures, values and preferences?

Beliefs

Beliefs may be strong principles that govern the way we live. They can affect how we live, the places we go and the things we eat. For example, people who do not eat meat may not do so because they believe that killing animals for food is not right.

Beliefs may also be religious or political.

Cultures

Cultures refer to particular traditions or customs that are used to describe a group of people who share those certain customs, traditions and values or people from one country or group.

Often Britain is described as a multi-cultural society, which means that it is made up of different cultures and groups of people who originate from different countries such as Africa, France, India, Italy, Poland, Romania and Russia.

Values

Values refer to those things in our lives that we value as very important and can include for example our family, friends, our health, our freedom and our rights. Review how this reflects your previous learning around the Human Rights Act; what rights and freedoms are considered as important to everyone who lives in the UK?

Preferences

Preferences refer to our likes and our own personal choices. This can for example include our preferences for food, clothes, activities and health. Our beliefs and values may affect our personal choices. How would you feel, for example, if your choices and preferences were not respected? Perhaps you prefer not to eat meat but are told that there are no vegetarian options on the menu at a restaurant. How would that make you feel? Why?

How your own beliefs, cultures, values and preferences affect you and your interactions

It is very important to be aware of your own beliefs, values and prejudices, and how they may affect your work so that you can ensure that they do not impact negatively. For example, you should be aware of the positive and negative feelings you have about different groups of people and reflect on how these may affect your work, especially if you think they could affect your role negatively. For example, if you believe that young people have a tendency to be lazy, how could this affect the way that you interact with them? What could you do to stop this affecting your interactions negatively?

It is encouraging to know that some beliefs will affect your role positively, but it can be tricky to face up to perhaps some of the more negative attitudes you have towards people, especially if they are likely to impact individuals in negative ways. Being honest with yourself, discussing this with your manager and understanding how you can address any issue will not only enhance the care that you offer individuals but it will also make you a more informed, reflective care worker who is likely to address prejudice in the setting. That is why it is important to think about this and discuss it with your manager.

Reflect on it

2.2 How your beliefs affect your interactions

Look at this list of beliefs that people may have:

- All human beings are equal and should be treated fairly.
- People with disabilities cannot do a job as well as people who do not have a disability.
- Refugees should not be allowed into Britain.
- People should not have to retire by the age of 65 and should work until they feel they are able to.

If you have or were to have these beliefs, how could they affect the way you interact with the individuals you support?

Dos and don'ts for interacting with individuals respectfully	
Do	Show that you value the individuals that you care for. You can do this through your communications with them. It would be useful to go over Unit 203 on communication and understand how you can make sure that you communicate with individuals and empower them through **communication**.
Do	Be aware of your own prejudices.
Do	Value and respect the opinions and views of individuals as well as the positive contributions that people from different backgrounds make.
Don't	Stereotype and assume that all people from a certain group are the same.
Don't	Talk down to people, or patronise them.
Don't	Use any offensive or patronising language when working with individuals. For example, by using their first name to address them when they want to be addressed by their surname or by calling them 'dear' or 'love' when the individual finds this offensive and patronising.

Reflect on it

2.2 Communication skills

Reflect on the communication skills and qualities you have. How can you use these to show interaction with individuals that respects them?

Why is it important to interact in ways that respect beliefs, cultures, values and preferences?

As you have learned earlier on in this unit, in order to be inclusive as care workers, we should support individuals to live their lives fully and respect their unique differences such as their likes, dislikes, needs, wishes, beliefs, culture, values and preferences.

Interacting with individuals in this way is:

- essential for showing best practice
- essential for providing high-quality, safe, effective care and support
- essential for respecting and supporting individuals' rights
- essential for empowering individuals and raising their self-esteem.

How can you show interaction with individuals that respects their beliefs?

- **Get to know the individual you are interacting with:** find out what their beliefs are, for example whether they follow any religious practices, how their beliefs affect how they dress, what they eat.

6Cs

Communication

Good communication involves building good working relationships with individuals that instil mutual trust and respect. This is because communicating well makes individuals feel like they are being listened to and that their thoughts and opinions are valued.

Good communication also makes individuals feel respected and involved. You can ensure that you communicate well by showing that you are aware of individuals' communication preferences and are able to show respect for these during all your communications with individuals. You may also like to refer to Unit 203, Communication in care settings.

- **Do not make assumptions about individuals' beliefs:** ask the individual how you can take into account their beliefs, do not assume you know how to and treat all individuals with the same beliefs the same.

- **Ensure you take into account individuals' beliefs:** before interacting with individuals, remember to prepare yourself for your interaction with them by checking that you've understood how they want you to take into account their beliefs.

- **Be accepting of their beliefs and reflect on any of your own prejudices that you may have:** understand that their beliefs may be different to your own. You may agree or disagree with their beliefs but they are entitled to hold those beliefs just as you are entitled to your beliefs.

How can you show interaction with individuals that respects their cultures?

- **Get to know the individual, their background and culture:** talk to them about their culture or find out about the individual's culture from those who know the individual well such as their family, friends or advocate. You may also carry out your own research about their culture.

- **Ask the individual about their culture:** ask them about any associated beliefs, ideas or customs they have and follow.

- **Ask the individual to show you how to respect their culture:** if there is anything you do not fully understand, or are unsure of, it is okay to politely ask the individual. You may for example ask them about what is seen as respectful and disrespectful when speaking to them, when providing them with care or support and the reasons why.

How can you interact with individuals to show that you respect their values?

- **Find out what the individual's values are:** support them to show you what is important to them and ask them how you can support them.

- **Do not make judgements about an individual's values, particularly if they are different to your own:** ensure your interaction has the individual and their values as the focus, not yours. The concept of person-centred care is covered in Unit 211, Implement person-centred approaches in care settings.

- **Do not allow your values to influence the interaction:** remain fair and **objective** at all times.

How can you interact with individuals to show that you respect their preferences?

- **Empower individuals to share their preferences with you:** encourage them to talk about their choices, what makes them the person they are, what good care or support looks like to them.

Key term

Objective is to be fair, and not influenced by your own feelings or beliefs.

- **Take into account individuals' preferences at all times:** ensure that you have agreed on ways to do so with individuals.

- **Do not impose your preferences on individuals:** empower individuals to speak about themselves, their preferences and how you can show respect for their preferences without influencing them with your own preferences. You may of course suggest alternatives which will benefit their care and well-being but make sure that the individual is able to communicate their preferences to you first and foremost.

In all interactions with individuals it is important to address the following.

- **Observe individuals**, for example observe the individual through your interaction to ensure that they are showing you whether they have received your interaction positively, i.e. by what they say, what they don't say, their body language. You will find it useful to refer to Unit 203, Communication in care settings, in relation to verbal and non-verbal communication.

- **Be aware of your interaction** with individuals, for example are you using non-discriminatory language when talking to individuals about their beliefs? Is your body language showing that you are genuinely interested in their beliefs?

You will find it useful to review Unit 203, Communication in care settings, in relation to SOLER on page 28.

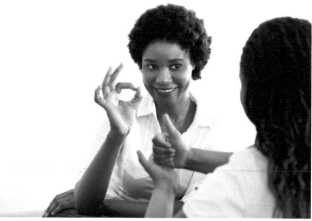

Figure 3.4 What am I communicating? Why is it important to observe individuals carefully to understand what they are communicating?

2.2 Respecting others' beliefs, cultures, values and preferences

Your practices will be observed for AC 2.2. Make arrangements for interactions with two different individuals or people you know. For example, you may arrange to be observed meeting with individuals to discuss an issue that is important to them or supporting individuals with a care or support activity. (Ensure you plan this with your assessor in advance.)

For each individual, ensure you show how you respect their unique beliefs, culture, values and preferences.

AC 2.3 Describe how to challenge discrimination in a way that encourages change

It is very important for you to work in inclusive ways and know how to challenge those not doing so constructively and positively.

Working in an inclusive way involves being able to:

- recognise practices that are discriminatory
- know what to do if you become aware of or see discrimination taking place either in or outside of the care setting where you work
- challenge discrimination positively.

Discrimination, as you have learned at the beginning of this unit, involves the unfair or unequal treatment of an individual or group. It can be deliberate or unintentional. It can occur for different reasons such as:

- a lack of clear understanding or knowledge about equality, diversity and/or inclusion
- a lack of awareness of own and others' behaviours at work and towards individuals
- fear or a lack of confidence over how to respond to an individual's needs, for example when they behave aggressively or have a condition such as dementia.

If you do not challenge discrimination in a way that encourages change then this may lead to the discrimination becoming worse and occurring more regularly. You may also be inadvertently reinforcing these negative unwanted behaviours and individuals may think that you are encouraging the discrimination to continue. It will also mean that you will be failing in your **duty of care** (see page 106 for definition) towards the individuals you provide care or support to; this concept is covered in Unit 205, Duty of care.

When challenging discrimination in a way that encourages change it is important to follow some 'dos and don'ts'.

Dos and don'ts for challenging discrimination and encouraging change	
Do	Act straight away to make it clear that it will not be tolerated.
Do	Support others to act straight away to make it clear that it is unacceptable.
Do	Record all incidents to ensure the details of the incident are documented. This includes who was affected and what actions were taken. This document can be referred to at a later stage if necessary.
Do	Report all incidents so that the necessary actions can be taken.
Do	Keep up to date with good practices so that you can constructively challenge discrimination.
Do	Ensure you know your work setting's agreed ways of working for constructively challenging discrimination.
Don't	Accept it.
Don't	Ignore it.

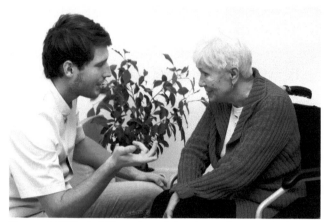

Figure 3.5 What skills and qualities do you have to challenge discrimination?

Reflect on it

2.3 Challenging discrimination

Reflect on an occasion when you challenged something that you felt was unfair. What did you say and why? What did you do and why? How did this make you feel and why?

Challenging discrimination in a way that encourages change involves being positive, supportive and constructive. You can do this by:

- having a discussion with the person responsible so that they understand why their practices are discriminatory
- suggesting self-reflection so that increasing their awareness of or insight into their behaviour reduces the likelihood of the discrimination occurring again; Unit 207, Personal development in care settings has more information about the self-reflection process and you may find it useful to refer to this
- suggesting further training so that they can update their knowledge about inclusive and anti-discriminatory practices

- suggesting shadowing more experienced colleagues so that they can observe and learn about good ways of working when supporting individuals in inclusive ways
- accessing an **advocate** and others who do not work in the setting in order to support individuals to challenge discrimination and ensure their rights and choices are upheld
- ensuring that you voice your suggestions and discuss them with your manager so that these can then become part of the setting's agreed ways of working for everyone to follow
- empowering individuals and encouraging the active participation of individuals so that they can themselves challenge discrimination and any barriers they may come across.

You can also recap all the things we have discussed with regards to diversity, equality, inclusion and anti-discriminatory practice in this unit (see page 83 onwards).

The reflective exemplar on page 107 provides you with an opportunity to explore in more detail how adult care workers in care settings must work in inclusive ways, challenge discrimination positively and the consequences if they don't.

	Reflective exemplar
Introduction	I work as an adult care worker in a day care centre that provides activities for older adults with learning and physical disabilities. I work alongside two colleagues who are very experienced and also have a very supportive manager.
What happened?	This morning my two colleagues and I were preparing the main sitting area for the planned quiz. While we were doing so, one of the individuals who participates in the quiz arrived early and asked whether he could help us with preparing the sitting area. My two colleagues both said 'No' at the same time and explained that he wasn't a staff member like they were and so for this reason couldn't help.
	The individual withdrew immediately from the area where the three of us were standing and sat in an armchair in the corner.
	A little while later when my two colleagues were busy welcoming everyone, I went over to the individual and gave him a copy of the quiz. He looked at me and threw it on the floor.
What worked well?	I think that the fact that the individual felt he was able to approach us and express his preference to help us with setting up this morning's activity was excellent.
What did not go as well?	My colleague's reactions to this individual's request were unfair.
	My reaction to their responses was not good enough; I did not do anything and because I stood by and watched, the individual then got annoyed with me too and this was why he threw the quiz I gave him on the floor.
What could I do to improve?	I think I need to speak with both my colleagues about what happened and challenge their responses by explaining why I think these were unfair; after all we should be supporting individuals' active participation.
	I think I will also need to record the incident and report what happened to my manager. I think I may also need more training on how to challenge discrimination when it occurs.
	I think the individual is owed an apology and reassurance that this will not happen again. Perhaps he can be asked whether he would like to help with preparing the next morning's activity? I think I need to show my **compassion** and evidence of good-quality **care** to this individual.
Links to unit assessment criteria	ACs 1.1, 1.2, 1.3, 2.2, 2.3

6Cs

Compassion

Compassion will involve you showing concern for the well-being of individuals if they are being discriminated against, and caring enough to challenge it. This will not only show that you are taking a stand against discrimination in the setting and saying that it will not be tolerated, but it also shows your regard and respect for the rights of the individuals for whom you provide care. You can show compassion by supporting individuals who have been discriminated against and recognising the impact this has had on them personally; allow yourself to empathise with the individual, this in turn will allow you to understand how they are feeling and find a solution that will bring about a long-term change and make a positive difference.

Care

Care, here, will involve you doing what you can to ensure that if an individual is discriminated against, then you are able to do what you can to improve the situation and have their well-being as the focus. It is about showing that you can make a positive difference to an individual's life through your role. Again, you can show this by:

- positively challenging all discrimination you may come across
- showing that you care through your communication
- making sure they know that you have their best interests at heart.

This is important for ensuring that individuals trust you to support them and promote their rights to live in a way that is free from discrimination.

Research it

2.3 Best practice when challenging discrimination

Research 'best practice' when challenging discrimination in the adult care sector.

You could speak to adult care workers who work in different care settings as the basis of your research or you could use the internet to read about good practice success stories.

Evidence opportunity

2.1, 2.3 Code of conduct for challenging discrimination

Produce a 'code of conduct' for a new adult care worker that describes how to challenge discrimination in a way that encourages change. Ensure you are clear about the worker's responsibilities under the code of conduct. You may want to recap what codes of conduct are by rereading AC 2.1, pages 100–101.

LO2 Knowledge, skills, behaviours
Knowledge: what are the principles of working in an inclusive way?
Do you know what the Equality Act 2010 says about discrimination?
Do you know why the Care Act 2014 is relevant to supporting inclusion in care settings?
Did you know that you have just showed your knowledge of the key legislation relating to equality, diversity and discrimination?
Skills: how can you show that you are able to work in an inclusive way?
Do you know how to communicate with individuals in relation to their values?
Do you know how to interact with individuals to show that you respect their beliefs?
Did you know that you have just demonstrated a few of the skills required for promoting inclusion in your day-to-day working practices?
Behaviours: how can you show the personal qualities you have in your day-to-day working practices?
Do you know how to show your personal confidence when challenging discrimination?
Do you know how to challenge discrimination using positive behaviours?
Did you know that you have just demonstrated a few of the essential behaviours required when challenging discrimination in a way that encourages change?

LO3 Know how to access information, advice and support about diversity, equality and inclusion

Getting started

Think about an occasion that arose at work that you found difficult to deal with. Why did you find it difficult? Did you get advice from someone? Who was it and why? Did this help? If yes, why? If not, why? What could you have done differently next time?

What difference does it make when you have someone to support you when you come across difficult situations at work? Why?

AC 3.1 Identify a range of sources of information, advice and support about diversity, equality and inclusion

Ensuring that your working practices promote diversity, equality and inclusion is your responsibility as well as that of the care setting where you work and your employer.

Being aware of all the different sources of information, advice and support about diversity, equality and inclusion that are available to you is essential for:

- following or complying with agreed ways of working to ensure safe and effective care
- following 'best practice' for providing person-centred care (see AC 1.1 for more information on person-centred care. You could also refer to Unit 211 on person-centred care)
- creating a positive working environment where individuals' rights are protected and supported.

Figure 3.6 includes some examples of the main sources where you could access information, advice and support about diversity, equality and inclusion.

Reflect on it

3.1 Consequences of not having access to information, advice and support

What would be the consequences of not knowing where you can access information, advice and support about diversity, equality and inclusion? How would this impact on your working practices? And on your **competence**?

6Cs

C

Competence
Competence involves being aware of how to effectively apply your knowledge and skills in your role which is essential if you want to provide high-quality care for individuals.

A part of being competent involves you continuing to learn about improving and developing your practices in relation to promoting diversity, equality and inclusion.

You can demonstrate that you are competent by showing that you know about the different sources of information, advice and support available to you, both inside and outside your setting. If you are aware of the different sources, you can seek out the best source for advice in order to improve your practice. This will also allow you to access up-to-date knowledge and working practices, without which you cannot develop professionally or practice high-quality care or support.

Also see the Competence 6Cs box in AC 3.2.

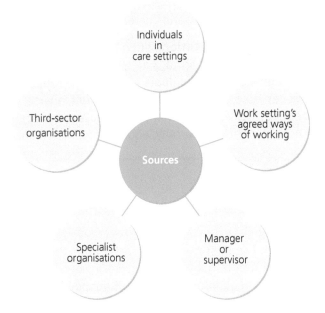

Figure 3.6 Sources of information, advice and support

As you have learned, **individuals** in care settings are the experts in what care or support they require to meet their unique needs and preferences. They should be the first people you turn to for information and advice when you want to check that your practices are inclusive.

Your **work setting**'s agreed ways of working, including the policies, procedures and working 'codes of practice' that there are can provide useful information about how diversity, equality and inclusion are supported in your day-to-day working practices and in the service as a whole. It may be useful to review your work setting's relevant policies, procedures and codes of practice now.

Your **manager** or **supervisor** is a good source of advice and support, particularly when you have had to report discriminatory practices. They can also help when you want to clarify your understanding of your role and responsibilities in relation to promoting diversity, equality and inclusion.

Specialist organisations such as the Equality and Human Rights Commission (EHRC) provide useful information, advice and support on all matters relating to promoting diversity, equality and inclusion. You can seek advice from their specialist advisors and you can also read about best practices in the adult care sector and current legislation.

Third-sector organisations such as the Alzheimer's Society, Mind, Age UK and local support groups for individuals with care or support needs can also provide useful information, advice and support for ensuring that you are able to support individuals' rights to diversity, equality and inclusion.

> **Research it**
>
> **3.1 Sources of information, advice and support**
>
> Research two charities or support groups that you know about that you can access in your local area if you need information about supporting the rights to equality, diversity and inclusion for:
>
> - individuals who have mental health needs
> - individuals who have a learning disability.
>
> For each charity, produce a leaflet to show the information it can provide.

AC 3.2 Describe how to access information, advice and support about diversity, equality and inclusion

How you access sources of information, advice and support about diversity, equality and inclusion will vary across different care settings and will depend on your current job role and responsibilities including what the expected standards are. You could access information, advice and support by:

- **Asking your line manager or supervisor** – they will be experienced and can provide you with the support you need; you may for example have a question about working practices that you think are unfair. You may want to recap the key points from the discussion you had with your manager or supervisor for Evidence opportunity 3.1.

- **Speaking to the individual** – the individual or their representative, such as their family or advocate, can provide you with some useful insight into how their care or support could be improved. This may give you ideas for the changes you can make to your working practices. For example, by speaking to the individual, you may discover that the individual wants to be asked how they feel about the care or support provided on a more regular basis or they may tell you that they would like to be asked for their ideas on improvements that could be made.

- **Accessing personal development opportunities** – access to training courses and other sources of information such as articles written about 'best practice' in care settings can provide you with useful up-to-date information. You can make arrangements for training through your manager and during the supervision process as part of the personal development plan process. You may want to review your learning of Unit 207, Personal development in care settings.

- **Accessing your work setting's agreed ways of working** – review the policies and procedures that you are required to follow in your work setting along with any guidance included about diversity, equality and inclusion on a regular basis. Make sure you know where these are and that you understand what they say so that you can carry out your job role with **competence**, applying the knowledge you've learned to various different situations that may arise. If you are in any doubt, ask your manager.

- **Accessing external organisations and/or charities** – these external organisations can provide you with some useful ways of supporting diversity, equality and inclusion. They may also be able to share with you their ideas and/or case studies that they know about that support 'best practice'.

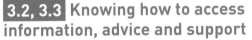

Case study

3.2, 3.3 Knowing how to access information, advice and support

Harjinder is 64 years old, has a learning disability and lives on his own. He receives support for day-to-day living tasks such as cooking, cleaning and shopping from his support worker and is also visited regularly by his daughter who lives close by.

This morning Harjinder is accompanied by his daughter to the GP's surgery so that he can collect the results of his recent blood test. On arrival, the receptionist explains to Harjinder that he will be seen by the nurse to discuss his blood test results rather than his GP as his GP has been called away to an emergency.

Harjinder and his daughter meet with the nurse who brings out Harjinder's blood test results and shows them to Harjinder's daughter. Harjinder stands up and says to the nurse, 'These are my results, talk to me face-to-face'. With immediate effect, the nurse asks Harjinder to leave and explains that his behaviour will not be tolerated. Harjinder immediately phones his support worker and tells him he's been treated unfairly.

Questions

1 How could Harjinder's daughter better support Harjinder in this situation?
2 What are Harjinder's rights in this situation?
3 What actions should Harjinder's support worker take? Why?

6Cs

C

Competence

Competence, as we have addressed in AC 3.1, refers to effectively applying the knowledge and skills you have consistently and accurately learned so that you're able to provide individuals with good-quality care or support that are in line with agreed ways of working.

It is important that you know what to do if you are unable to support equality, diversity or inclusion during your day-to-day working practices and that the individual knows that you are doing your very best to work in inclusive ways and support their rights to be included and treated fairly.

In this section, you can show that you are competent in knowing the process to follow for accessing information, advice and support from your work setting. You can do this by following the advice that is offered here, as well as discussing this with your manager and colleagues.

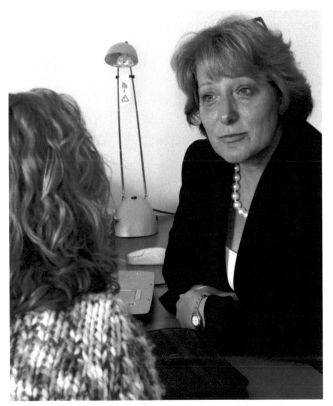

Figure 3.7 How are you supported? Who would be able to help you access information, advice and support about diversity, equality and inclusion?

3.2 Procedures to promote equality and challenge discrimination

Research the procedures in place in your work setting for:

- challenging discrimination
- supporting equality
- promoting diversity.

Discuss with your manager the key points in the procedure and how they can support you in your work role.

3.1, 3.2 Sources of information, advice and support and how to access them

Discuss with your assessor where you can access support, information and advice about keeping your knowledge and skills up to date in relation to diversity, equality and inclusion. Describe to your assessor how you go about accessing this information, advice and support.

AC 3.3 Identify when to access information, advice and support about diversity, equality and inclusion

Knowing where the sources of information, advice and support about diversity, equality and inclusion are and how you can access them is very important but only if you also know when you should do so. Remember not doing so at the correct time can mean that discriminatory practices continue to go unnoticed and ultimately could become worse.

Below are some examples of when you should access information, advice and support about diversity, equality and inclusion.

- **When you start work in the adult care sector** – this may be in your first job, in a new team or in a different service or organisation. As explained earlier on in this unit, each care

3.3 Dealing with discrimination

Research an occasion when discrimination occurred in a care setting and it was not dealt with correctly. You can use newspapers and the internet as sources of information.

Discuss the impact this had on the individuals with care or support needs and those who worked in the care setting.

setting will have its own agreed ways of working. It's important that you find out what these are for the role and responsibilities you are carrying out. If you are new to working in adult care then it is really important that you seek information, advice and support from those you work alongside as this will help to inform your knowledge in this area and ensure that you are working to the expected standards.

- **When you're unable to support diversity, equality and inclusion** – this may be because there is a conflict between your duty of care (see page 106 for definition) and individuals' rights to have their preferences respected. For example, an older individual who is prone to falling asleep when on their own in the evenings wants to smoke in their armchair; you are worried that they may fall asleep while doing so and cause a fire. You have a duty to support the individual's preferences but you also have a duty to ensure that you support the individual's safety. You should respect the individual's rights to smoke but protect them from danger, for example by suggesting they smoke before they start to feel tired in the evenings or smoke only when someone is present.

- **When you're unsure about your practices or those of others** – this may be because you have seen an experienced colleague interact with an individual in a way that you view as discriminatory but that they and the individual do not. For example, your colleague may speak to an individual using a patronising tone of voice. In these situations, you must report your concerns to your manager; you can explain to your colleague and the individual that you will seek clarification from your manager.

- **When an individual or their representative such as their family or advocate request information, advice or support about diversity, equality and inclusion** – it may be that they want to see your work setting's 'equality and diversity policy' or have heard that there have been changes to current legislation or have witnessed an individual being treated unfairly. You should seek advice from your manager or supervisor in the first instance so that they can advise you about the best course of action to take.

Reflect on it

3.3 Consequences of not seeking advice about diversity, equality and inclusion

Reflect on the consequences of not seeking advice from your manager or supervisor if an individual or their family or advocate request information, advice or support about diversity, equality and inclusion.

What may unintentionally happen if you provide them with incorrect or inaccurate information? How would they feel? How would you feel? What actions may your manager or supervisor take as a result?

Evidence opportunity

3.3 When to access information and advice about diversity, equality and inclusion

Identify two sources of information, advice and support about diversity, equality, inclusion and discrimination that are available to you in the care setting where you work. For each one, list the situations when you might need to access them.

Discuss your list with your assessor. Is the information you recorded correct? If not, why not?

LO3 Knowledge, skills, behaviours
Knowledge: what are the sources of information, advice and support that are available to you about diversity, equality and inclusion?
Do you know who to ask for support in relation to supporting individuals' diversity?
Do you know where you can access more information about supporting equality and inclusion?
Did you know that you have just shown your knowledge of different sources of information, advice and support?
Skills: how can you show that you can access information, advice and support effectively?
Do you know how to follow your work setting's policy if an individual tells you they've been treated unfairly?
Do you know when to access advice and support from your colleagues about diversity, equality and inclusion?
Did you know that you have just demonstrated some of the skills required to support diversity, equality and inclusion in your current job role?
Behaviours: how can you show the personal qualities you have when you're accessing information, advice and support?
Do you know how to actively listen when seeking advice from your manager or supervisor?
Do you know how to be thorough when reading your work setting's equality, diversity and inclusion procedures?
Did you know that you have just demonstrated a few of the essential behaviours required to support diversity, equality and inclusion?

Suggestions for using the activities

This table summarises all the activities in the unit that are relevant to each assessment criterion.

Here, we also suggest other, different methods that you may want to use to present your knowledge and skills by using the activities.

These are just suggestions, and you should refer to the Introduction section at the start of the book, and more importantly the City & Guilds specification, and your assessor who will be able to provide more guidance on how you can evidence your knowledge and skills.

When you need to be observed during your assessment, this can be done by your assessor, or your manager can provide a witness testimony.

Assessment criteria and accompanying activities	Suggested methods to show your knowledge/skills
LO1 Understand the importance of equality and inclusion	
1.1 Reflect on it (page 85) 1.1 Reflect on it (page 88)	Write a personal statement about your understanding of the four terms: diversity, equality, inclusion and discrimination. Include examples of what they mean in the context of your job role and the care setting where you work. Address the points in the activities.
1.1 Research it (page 89) 1.1 Research it (page 90)	You could provide a written account to evidence your research and discussions.
1.1 Evidence opportunity (page 90)	You could create a poster or PowerPoint presentation explaining how you promote individuals' diversity, equality and inclusion and ensure they are not discriminated against. Or you could write a reflective account and address the points. You could also tell your assessor about your understanding of the terms diversity, equality and inclusion. You could tell your manager, who will be able to provide a witness testimony.
1.2 Research it (page 91)	Read the article. Write an account addressing the points outlined in the activity. Discuss with your assessor the different ways that discrimination may deliberately or inadvertently occur in the work setting. Ensure you include examples of how both may arise. You will need to have a good understanding of what is meant by discrimination. Or you could write a reflective account about an occasion when discrimination occurred either deliberately or inadvertently.
1.2, 1.3 Reflect on it (page 93)	Write a short reflective account addressing the issues in the activity.
1.2 Evidence opportunity (page 93)	Create a poster as instructed in the activity. You could also write an account about your experience of when discrimination (deliberately or inadvertently) occurred in your own work setting.
1.3 Research it (page 95)	Read the article. Write notes detailing your findings and address the points in the activity.
1.3 Reflect on it (page 96) 1.3 Case study (page 97)	Write a reflective account addressing the points in this activity. You could also write a reflective account about an occasion when your work practices supported equality and inclusion. You will need to include examples of both, and then explain how they reduce the likelihood of discrimination occurring. The case study will help you.
1.3 Evidence opportunity (page 97) 1.3 Case study (page 97)	You could provide a written account to evidence your discussion. You could also discuss this with your assessor, and even show them how your own work practices that support equality and inclusion reduce the likelihood of discrimination in your own work. The case study will help you.
LO2 Be able to work in an inclusive way	
2.1 Reflect on it (page 100)	Write a reflective account.
2.1 Evidence opportunity (page 101)	Provide a written account to address the points in the activity. You could also tell your assessor about these.

→

Suggestions for using the activities

2.2 Reflect on it (page 102) 2.2 Reflect on it (page 103)	You could write personal statements or reflective accounts about your experience of occasions when you were able to show how you interacted well with individuals and respected their beliefs, culture, values and preferences. What communication skills and qualities helped you to do this? You could also discuss these with your assessor. Explain your experience of working in an inclusive way in your own work setting. When thinking about communication skills, you could think about topics covered in Unit 203, Communication in care settings, and why it is important to observe an individual's reactions when communicating, for example.
2.2 Evidence opportunity (page 105)	As instructed in the activity, you must arrange for your work practices to be observed so that you can show interactions with at least two different individuals that respect their unique beliefs, culture, values and preferences. To support the observation, you could also show relevant records or reports that reflect the individuals' individual needs and preferences.
2.3 Reflect on it (page 106)	Write a reflective account. Or you could produce a presentation about how to challenge discrimination in a way that encourages change in the context of your job role. Include examples of the different methods that can be used to challenge discrimination positively. You will find your work setting's agreed ways of working are a useful source of information because they will set out the process you must follow.
2.3 Research it (page 108)	Carry out some research in your work setting. Provide a short written account detailing your findings.
2.1, 2.3 Evidence opportunity (page 108)	You could produce a 'code of conduct' as instructed in the activity. You could also describe to your assessor how to challenge discrimination in ways that encourage change. You could include an example of how you coped on an occasion when you challenged discrimination in a way that encouraged change. You can revisit the reflective exemplar on page 107 for some ideas on this.
LO3 Know how to access information, advice and support about diversity, equality and inclusion	
3.1 Reflect on it (page 109)	Produce a spider diagram that includes examples of a range of different sources of information, advice and support that are available to you in relation to diversity, equality and inclusion. You may want to discuss the different sources available to you with a colleague; you could also include whether either of you has used them. You could write down the main points that came out of your discussion.
3.1 Research it (page 110)	Produce the leaflet as instructed in the activity. You could produce a poster instead or a written account. You could cover either individuals who have mental health needs or those with a learning disability, or both.
3.1, 3.2 Evidence opportunity (page 112) 3.2, 3.3 Case study (page 111)	Discuss the points in the activity with your assessor. You could also provide a written account. You could also show your assessor or manager how you access information, advice and support about diversity, equality and inclusion. The case study will help you.
3.2 Research it (page 112)	Research the procedures for promoting equality and challenging discrimination. You could discuss the points with your manager. Make notes detailing your discussion.
3.3 Research it (page 112)	Write notes to evidence your research. You could even think about a situation in the setting.
3.3 Reflect on it (page 113)	Write a reflective account about the consequences of not seeking advice about diversity, equality and inclusion. You may have been in a situation when you have been faced with one of the consequences of not doing so, so you could reflect on that.
3.3 Evidence opportunity (page 113)	Discuss the points in the activity with your assessor. You may like to detail specific example of when you have had to access information and advice about diversity, equality and inclusion. You could also write a personal statement.

Legislation	
Relevant Act	**It states that:**
Human Rights Act 1998	everyone in the UK is entitled to the same basic human rights and freedoms. This includes individuals who have care and support needs. The Act supports individuals' rights to dignity, respect and to be treated fairly when accessing care or support services.
Special Educational Needs and Disability Act 2001	schools, colleges, universities, adult education providers, statutory youth services and local education authorities are required to make reasonable adjustments for people with disabilities. This is so that they can be offered the same opportunities and choices as people who do not have disabilities, e.g. a specialist support person for an individual with a learning disability or the provision of teaching and learning materials in alternative formats such as in Braille for individuals who have sight loss.
Children and Families Act 2014 and the Special Educational Needs and Disabilities (SEND) Code of Practice 2014	the Children and Families Act 2014 introduces a range of new legislation regarding adoption and family justice. In Part 3 it includes a new Special Educational Needs and Disabilities (SEND) Code of Practice. This supersedes the Code of Practice from 2001 (but does not replace the Special Educational Needs and Disability Act 2001). You can find more information here: **www.gov.uk/government/publications/send-code-of-practice-0-to-25**
Mental Capacity Act 2005	individuals have the right to make their own decisions for as long as they are able to and to be supported to make arrangements for when they may lack the capacity to make their own decisions in the future, i.e. in relation to their care and support.
Equality Act 2010	it is unlawful to discriminate against individuals that have one of the nine protected characteristics, i.e. age, disability, gender reassignment, marriage and civil partnership, pregnancy and maternity, race, religion or belief, sex, sexual orientation.
Care Act 2014	information and services for the provision of care and support should be made fairer and clearer to understand to everyone involved. It also introduced the well-being concept as the basis of all person-centred care.

Resources for further reading and research

Books and booklets

Butt, J. (2006) 'SCIE Race equality discussion paper 03: Are we there yet? Identifying the characteristics of social care organisations that successfully promote diversity', Social Care Institute for Excellence

Care Quality Commission (2015) 'Equal measures: Equality information report for 2014', Care Quality Commission

Ferreiro Peteiro, M. (2014) *Level 2 Health and Social Care Diploma Evidence Guide*, Hodder Education

INVOLVE (2012) 'Diversity and inclusion: What's it about and why is it important for public involvement in research?', INVOLVE

Weblinks

www.equalityhumanrights.com The Equality and Human Rights Commission's (EHRC) website for information and resources about the Human Rights Act 1998 and the Equality Act 2010

www.gov.uk The UK Government's website for information about current legislation including the Human Rights Act 1998 and the Equality Act 2010

www.mind.org.uk Mind's website – resources and information about the Mental Capacity Act 2005, including useful terms to know about

www.rethink.org Rethink Mental Illness – resources and information about mental illness and mental capacity, the Mental Capacity Act 2005 and the accompanying code of practice

www.scie.org.uk Social Care Institute for Excellence (SCIE) – resources and information about the Care Act 2014 in relation to the well-being concept

www.skillsforcare.org.uk Skills for Care – resources and information on the Care Act 2014, the code of conduct for adult care workers

www.skillsforhealth.org.uk Skills for Health – resources and information on the Care Act 2014, the code of conduct for adult care workers

Duty of care (205)

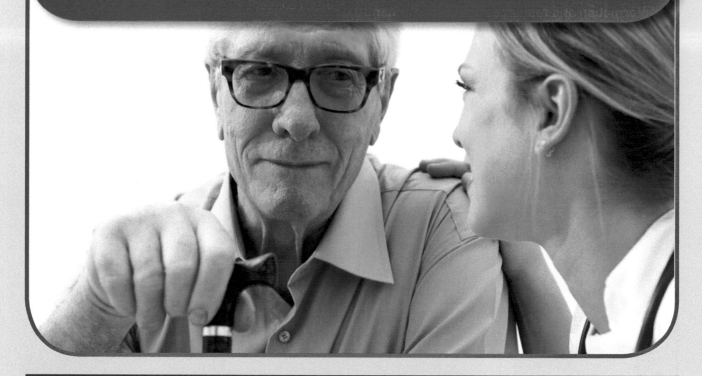

About this unit

Credit value: 1
Guided learning hours: 7

Everyone who works in an adult care setting has a duty or responsibility to care not only for the individuals that have care or support needs, but also for other people involved in the care setting (including their employer, colleagues and the individuals' families and friends) so that danger, harm or abuse is avoided. This means placing the best interests of all those people at the heart of everything you do and making sure that they are kept away from harm. In this unit, you will begin by learning more about the meanings of the term 'duty of care' including how it affects your work role. Being open and honest in the way you work must underpin your work practices and behaviours at all times and this unit will provide you with an opportunity to think about the links that exist between the duty of care and the duty of candour.

Fulfilling your duty of care and supporting an individual's rights can be difficult at times and this unit will help you to identify the dilemmas that may arise and understand where you can access support and advice to resolve such dilemmas. The ability to make improvements when care goes wrong is important and so this unit will provide you with a good insight into how to respond to and handle complaints effectively.

Learning outcomes

LO1: Understand the implications of duty of care

LO2: Understand support available for addressing dilemmas that may arise about duty of care

LO3: Know how to respond to complaints

LO1 Understand the implications of duty of care

Getting started

Think about someone you care about, for example a family member who you are close to or a good friend. How do you show that you care about this person? Do you treat them differently to other people you know? If so, how? Can you think of an occasion that you were worried about this person? Why were you worried? What did you do to show the person you cared about them? How did that make the person feel? How did that make you feel?

AC 1.1 Define the term 'duty of care'

Duty of care towards the individuals that you care for is a key part of your role and it will underpin everything that you do in your job. You will have a duty of care not only towards the individuals that you provide care and support to in the care setting where you work but also towards others such as individuals' families, visitors, your colleagues, manager, employer and other professionals who you work with.

All adult care workers are legally required to have a duty of care. Do you know what this means?

Act in the best interests of individuals and others

First, your duty of care means that you must always act in the best interests of individuals when carrying out your responsibilities and make sure that they are kept safe from any harm. This means taking into consideration what will be best for them, allowing them to make their own decisions but ensuring that you make the individual aware of the risks associated with any decisions before they make them. We will discuss this in AC 2.1. You will also need to act in the best interests of others when carrying out your job role and responsibilities and keep them safe from harm. This could include reporting that the carpet in the entrance hall is frayed so that visitors and your colleagues do not accidentally trip over on it, have a fall and harm themselves. This is discussed below.

Take action to prevent harm

Duty of care also means to take action to prevent harm. For example, if you see that the person you support is leading an inactive lifestyle and smoking, it is your responsibility to make them aware of the consequences of this (we will discuss this in more detail in AC 1.3 Describe how the duty of care affects your work role). You may also, for example, observe a colleague use unsafe practice when cleaning a spillage on the floor. Your duty of care to the individuals you support, your colleagues and visitors to the setting means that you must say something. Not reporting unsafe practices can lead to others slipping over or if the spillage contained, for example, body fluids it may lead to the spread of infection.

This also goes hand in hand with promoting individuals' safety, by ensuring individuals are kept safe not only from harm and injury but also from being abused. You can do this, for example, by ensuring you report any changes in an individual's behaviour that concern you. For example, you may notice that they become withdrawn or very tearful every time a specific family member visits them. This could possibly be a sign that the visitor is abusing them. This will not always be the case of course, but not reporting this may result in the individual continuing to be subjected to abuse.

Work within the agreed scope of your job role

Here, your duty of care means that you only carry out the tasks that you are able to, and have the knowledge and skills for. For example, if a colleague asks you to assist them with operating a hoist to move an individual from one position to another and you have not been trained in how to use moving and handling equipment then you must not do so. You should explain to them that this is because you do not have the **competence** to do so, as you do not have the necessary knowledge and skills. Saying yes to things that you have no knowledge and experience in will lead to unsafe practice, and potential harm. As a responsible care worker, you will need to ensure that you work within the scope of your role. There is more on this in Unit 202, Responsibilities of a care worker, AC 2.1.

If the individual to whom you provide care or support is also your employer, then the agreed ways of working will have been developed by the individual and/or their representative. You will be informed of this through your contract of employment, which will set out the agreed ways of working, as well as through any specific guidance that the individual and/or representative provides you with; this may be in writing and/or verbally explained.

Promote individuals' well-being

This goes hand in hand with working for the best interests of the individuals you care for. Here you can exercise your duty of care by supporting individuals' rights to for example choice, privacy, dignity and respect, by working in person-centred ways that indicate that you genuinely care about individuals and aim to always provide good-quality care. This is all part of your duty of care.

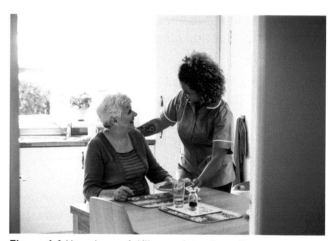

Figure 4.1 How do you fulfil your duty of care?

Remember that a duty of care is a legal requirement that you must fulfil when caring for or supporting individuals.

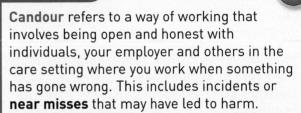

Evidence opportunity

1.1 What does 'duty of care' mean?

Produce a poster of the key aspects that underpin your duty of care to the individuals you care for or provide support to and to all those others you work with in your care setting.

AC 1.2 Describe how duty of care relates to duty of candour

What is 'duty of candour'?

The 'duty of candour' is your legal responsibility to be open and honest when care or support goes wrong.

This applies to all health and social care services, including where you work, and was introduced and recommended as a result of the Francis Inquiry report published in February 2013 into Mid Staffordshire NHS Foundation Trust. The inquiry examined the causes of serious failings in care over a period of 50 months between 2005 and 2009 at Stafford hospital (a small district general hospital in Staffordshire) where a disputed estimate of 400–1200 patients died because of poor care. The report made 290 recommendations, one of which was the statutory or legal duty of candour for all health and social care workers and services. As a result of the report and its findings, you as a care worker have a legal responsibility to ensure the following.

- Openness – this means that you must enable individuals and others to raise concerns and complaints freely without fear.
- Transparency – this means that you must only share true information about the care of individuals with for example team members and regulators such as the Care Quality Commission (CQC).
- **Candour** – this means you will need to ensure that any individual that is harmed by the care or support services is informed of this, as they may have been or be harmed without them realising it. For example, an individual may have been assisted with their personal hygiene by a care worker who is still recovering from the flu; the risk of potential infection must be explained to

Key terms

Candour refers to a way of working that involves being open and honest with individuals, your employer and others in the care setting where you work when something has gone wrong. This includes incidents or **near misses** that may have led to harm.

Near misses refer to incidents that have the potential to cause harm such as a delay to administering an individual's medication or a hoist battery that runs out just before an individual is about to be moved from one position to another. It may be that the individual is not actually harmed, but they could have been, and so it is a 'near miss'.

Research it

1.2 Mid Staffordshire NHS Foundation Trust

Research the serious failings in care discovered by the inquiries into the Mid Staffordshire NHS Foundation Trust. Find out about the causes of these failings and the impact they had. You will find the link below useful:

www.theguardian.com/society/2013/feb/06/mid-staffs-hospital-scandal-guide

Write an article about your findings.

the individual. An appropriate solution must be offered, regardless of whether the individual or someone else acting on their behalf has made a complaint or has raised any queries.

Legislation

The relevant piece of legislation that made the duty of candour into a legal duty was the Health and Social Care Act 2008 (Regulated Activities) Regulations 2014: Regulation 20. This legislation applies to all health and social care organisations that are registered with the regulator in England, which is the Care Quality Commission (CQC). The duty of candour regulations came into force in November 2014 for the NHS and in April 2015 for all other organisations.

'Duty of care' and 'duty of candour'

The legal duty of candour relates to the duty of care because under these regulations all care settings that provide care or support to individuals must:

- **tell individuals or their representatives when their care or support has gone wrong, has caused significant harm or has the potential to cause significant harm in the future.** In this way you will be promoting individuals' rights to be safe and free from harm and acting in their best interests.

- **inform individuals and their representatives what happened as fully as possible**; this must also be put in writing and include an apology. It must also include what actions will be taken next. For example, the safety measures that will be put in place and sources of support available for those affected. In this way you will be promoting individuals' and others' well-being by upholding their rights to being informed, communicated with and treated with respect, like an equal partner in the working relationship.

- **be open and honest about all incidents that appear to have caused or have the potential to cause significant harm to individuals and others.** In this way you will not be failing to act when care or support goes wrong by working in line with the agreed scope of your job role. By being honest about any mistakes you have made, you can then ensure you learn from these and ensure you try not to make those mistakes again.

If it is not just you who has made a mistake, and you have concerns that the care setting you work in is not complying with the duty of candour, you must in the first instance follow your agreed ways of working for making a complaint. (We will explore in more detail how to respond to complaints later on in LO3 of this unit.) If you are dissatisfied with the response you receive from your complaint, then you can raise your concerns directly with the regulator, the CQC, and/or seek further independent advice from an external organisation such as the charity Action against Medical Accidents (AvMA). If organisations and care settings fail to comply with the duty of candour, they can face serious consequences such as being closed down, heavy fines and even criminal prosecution.

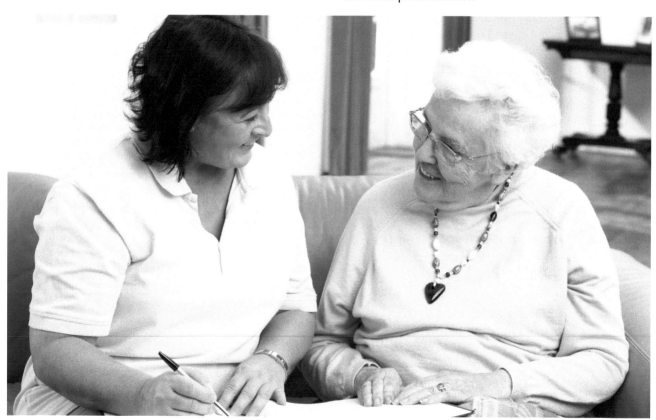

Figure 4.2 How open and honest are you when care goes wrong?

Reflect on it

1.2 Reporting

Reflect on the importance of reporting when you have a concern that your care setting has failed to comply with its duty of candour. What are the potential consequences for all those involved?

Evidence opportunity

1.2 Duty of candour

Read through your employer's agreed ways of working for complying with the duty of candour. Produce a one-page information handout about what it says about how it is going to comply with this legal duty. How does your duty of candour relate to your duty of care?

AC 1.3 Describe how the duty of care affects your work role

As you have learned, working in a setting that provides care or support means that you will have a duty of care towards the individuals and others you have working relationships with. There is more information on the different working relationships you have with individuals and others in Unit 202, Responsibilities of a care worker.

How duty of care affects your role

Duty of care affects your work role in different ways. In order to make sure that duty of care underpins and is the basis of your role you will need to ensure that you adhere to the considerations described below.

Consider the best interests of the people you provide care for

You can do this by:

- ensuring that any decisions you make are informed by the individual's best interests
- getting to know the individuals and ensuring this informs the care provided
- involving others who know the individual and have their best interests as the focus.

Consider the health and safety of individuals as well as that of the others in the care setting where you work

You can do this by:

- complying with your employer's health and safety procedures such as attending all health and safety training provided by your employer
- reporting unsafe practices immediately
- wearing personal protective equipment (PPE) when carrying out work activities that involve coming into contact with individuals' body fluids, to avoid the risk of infections and illnesses spreading.

Your work role responsibilities in relation to your duty of care towards your own health and safety and that of individuals and others can be explored in more detail in Unit 210, Health, safety and well-being in care settings.

Consider the well-being of the individuals that you provide care for

You can do this by:

- treating an individual with respect and promoting their personal dignity when providing them with care by supporting the individual's choices for daily activities
- protecting the individual from abuse and neglect by reporting all concerns immediately
- supporting individuals to maintain personal relationships with family and others by facilitating visits and positive communications.

Work to a high standard and ensure that the care and support you provide to individuals reflects best practice

You can do this by:

- reading, understanding and following your employer's agreed ways of working (if you are unsure about any aspects of your work activities you should raise this in the first instance with your manager)
- familiarising yourself with the standards expected of all adult care workers (such as the Care Certificate) and ensure you take these into account when you practise
- seeking information, guidance and support from your manager and colleagues in relation to how you can continue to further improve and develop your work practices.

Research it

1.3 Care Certificate 2015

Research Standard 3: Duty of Care. There is a useful link below:

www.skillsforcare.org.uk/Documents/
Learning-and-development/Care-Certificate/
The-Care-Certificate-Standards.pdf

Discuss with a colleague the duty of care standard and what it means for the way you work.

The duty of care will inform the agreed ways of working or the policies and procedures in your particular care setting, as well as the codes of practice that you are required to follow. It will affect all aspects of your care and your everyday duties, including everyday conversations and work activities where you will need to ensure that the best interests of the individuals are at the heart of your care. You will be accountable for the care you give to individuals, in other words it is your responsibility to ensure that you fulfil this key part of your role, as you are answerable for this.

As you will have learned, to fulfil your duty of care you must ensure that you uphold individuals' rights, respect their individuality and differences as well as work in ways that maintain individuals' safety and protection from danger, harm and abuse.

Sometimes individuals are unable to make decisions for themselves because they do not have the capacity to do so, for example due to a learning disability or a mental health condition. In these situations, decisions can be made on their

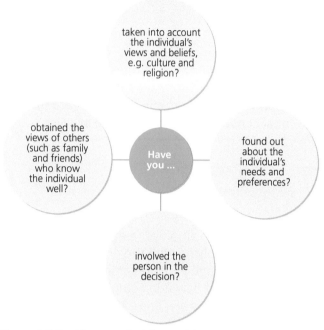

Figure 4.3 Best interest decision making

behalf and these are referred to as best interest decisions. It is still very important to record the reasons why the individual lacks capacity to make a decision and what has been done to maximise their capacity so that you can show the reasons behind your actions. It is your duty of care to work within the Mental Capacity Act (this is covered in more detail in AC 2.1). Figure 4.3 identifies some points for good practice when decision-making in the best interest of an individual who lacks capacity.

While we have covered examples of how your duty of care affects your role, Table 4.1 provides some examples that you may come across in your work setting.

Table 4.1 Scenarios you may come across in the setting

Scenario or situation you may come across in the setting	What is your duty of care and how will you carry it out in your role?	How might you address this situation?
An individual you care for is obese. They eat a lot of sugary food and consume sugary drinks. You find leaflets on healthy eating that you could give to them but they are only available in English and the individual has difficulty reading English.	Your duty of care is to ensure that the individual is aware of the dangers that their diet poses to their health. You cannot force them to change their diet. However, you should make them aware of the information that is available about healthy eating and the dangers	Speak to the individual about the dangers and risks that their lifestyle poses. Ensure you give them information on healthy eating and the dangers of eating too much sugar.

Table 4.1 Scenarios you may come across in the setting *continued*

Scenario or situation you may come across in the setting	What is your duty of care and how will you carry it out in your role?	How might you address this situation?
	to their health of eating too much sugar and by speaking to them about this.	If the leaflets are only available in English, then you should access leaflets available in the language they are able to read. If their eating habits are severely affecting their health, then you should also consult your manager who will advise you if you should speak to the individual's GP for further advice.
You need to assist an older individual (for whom you have cared for 6 months) to have bath.	First, your duty of care is to make sure that you check that the individual would like to have a bath. If they are happy with this, you will need to ensure you assist them to walk to the bathroom safely, for example with the use of a wheelchair or by walking alongside them if they are a little frail. You should check with them upon arrival at the bathroom if they are happy to proceed with having a bath.	This situation is straightforward because you have worked with the individual and you understand their needs and preferences. However, it is important that you continue to ask the individual about their needs and preferences each time you carry this out, even if it is an activity you support them with on a regular basis. Do not assume that they will be happy to have a bath at a set time. It may be that they are feeling unwell and may not necessarily want to bathe or they may decide that they want to have a shower instead.
Your colleague asks you to assist them with moving an individual from their bed to their chair but you have no skills and previous experience in this.	As you have no experience with the moving procedure, the best course of action is to speak up and say so. If you decided to go ahead, just because you have been put on the spot, you risk the safety of the individual being compromised. By speaking up, you have fulfilled your duty of care to the individual by ensuring they are not at risk and shown that you have their best interests at heart. You have also fulfilled your duty of care to the setting where you work as you could have potentially breached your job role and responsibilities and the agreed ways of working.	Speak up and say you cannot carry out the moving and handling procedure. Inform another colleague and ask someone that has the skills to complete the task. Inform your manager of what has happened and explain your reasons for not wanting to complete the task. Ask for training in moving and handling so that you are able to gain the knowledge and skills in order to complete these tasks.

Consequences of not maintaining your duty of care

Not maintaining your duty of care to individuals and others can have serious consequences.

- If you do not support individuals' rights to make their own decisions, then this could mean that individuals feel that they are being discriminated against and your practices will also negatively impact on the working relationships you have with them to provide them with good-quality care. The benefits of working in partnership with individuals and others are covered in more detail in Unit 202, Responsibilities of a care worker.

- Neglecting your duty to follow your employer's agreed ways of working for maintaining the health and safety of individuals and others during your day-to-day work activities will mean that you will be placing individuals and others in danger of harm or abuse.

- If you do not maintain your duty of care to report harm or a potentially harmful situation, your actions or lack of action could result in you being held responsible for a fatality, a serious injury or the cause of harm, and being prosecuted. Your actions or lack of action could result in you being dismissed from your job as well as the care setting where you work being deemed unsafe and closed.

Don't spend your day worrying about the consequences. However, it is important to be aware of them, so that they inform your day-to-day practice so that you continually think about how to prevent harm, maintain a safe environment and ultimately maintain your duty of care.

Case study 1.1, 1.2, 1.3 provides you with an opportunity to review the learning you have undertaken in LO1 and think about why duty of care is important.

Case study

1.1, 1.2, 1.3 Duty of care

Jennie has been a care worker for many years and now works weekends in a residential care home that only provides care to older people. Jennie is very hard working and takes her responsibilities as a care worker very seriously.

Today, Thursday, Jennie has come into work because it is the monthly staff meeting and all staff must attend. As Jennie has arrived a little early, she has time to have a coffee break in the staff room where she meets with some of the other members in her team. As discussions amongst the staff ensue, some of the team members comment that as Jennie is only a weekend worker she doesn't really have a duty of care towards the individuals she supports (or the others she works with) – because duty of care only applies to those team members who work full time (as they are the ones who see the individuals who live in the home regularly and know them best).

Jennie joins in the discussion and begins by saying that she thinks that everyone who works in the home has a duty of care towards the individuals as well as others they work with. Jennie adds that having a duty of care has nothing to do with how often you work with an individual or how many hours you do. Having a duty of care, Jennie states, is about working in a way that does not put individuals' or others' health and safety at risk. It also means being responsible and supporting individuals to take the lead and be in control of their lives. Sometimes, Jennie explains, this may also mean recognising when the care provided is not effective and being honest about this with individuals and others involved in their lives.

Questions

1. How would you have felt if you were Jennie in this situation? Why would you feel this way?
2. Would you have acted in a different way? Why might you act in a different way?
3. Is there anything else that Jennie could have included about the meaning of duty of care?
4. Does Jennie say anything about the duty of candour?

Evidence opportunity

1.3 **How duty of care affects your role**

Discuss with your manager how your duty of care affects your job role. You can think about how it affects the way you carry out your role and responsibilities, how it affects how you work with individuals, how it affects the care and support you provide to individuals. (This can be evidenced through a witness testimony from your manager.)

LO1 Knowledge, skills, behaviours
Knowledge: what is the meaning of the term 'duty of care'?
Do you know three key aspects of the term duty of care in relation to your care setting?
Do you know how duty of care relates to duty of candour?
Can you describe three ways in which the duty of care affects your role?
Did you know that you have just answered three questions about what the term 'duty of care' means?
Skills: how can you show your duty of care in the care setting where you work?
Do you know how to uphold individuals' rights to privacy, dignity and respect?
Do you know how to protect individuals from danger, harm and abuse?
Do you know how to use your body language to show you are listening to an individual?
Did you know that you have just answered three questions about how duty of care affects your work role?
Behaviours: how can you show the personal qualities you have in your duty of care?
Do you know how to show your professionalism when working with others to support individuals to live the lives they want to?
Do you know how to be open and honest with individuals and their families when you have made a mistake?
Did you know that you have just answered two questions about a few of the essential behaviours that are expected of all adult care workers and their duty of care?

LO2 Understand support available for addressing dilemmas that may arise about duty of care

Getting started

Think about an occasion when you faced a dilemma that meant you felt compromised. For example, this may be in relation to a friend asking you to keep something private about them secret.

It might be something that is unsafe or dangerous to their health, and they may have asked you not to tell anyone, not even your parents. Or you may have been asked to do something by a member of your family that you do not believe in or approve of.

How did you feel? Why do you think you felt this way? Did the dilemma get resolved? If so, how did it get resolved? Reflecting again on what happened, do you think anything else could have been done?

AC 2.1 Describe dilemmas that may arise between the duty of care and an individual's rights

Your duty of care, although an integral part of your job role and responsibilities, may also conflict at times with an individual's rights, views or wishes. As you know, you have a duty to empower individuals to take control of their lives as much as possible, and a duty of care to ensure you do what is in their best interest, but individuals are still entitled to make their own choices! You cannot force them to follow an action just because it is in their best interests. This is where conflicts between your duty of care and making sure you uphold the rights and decisions of individuals are balanced.

If this is not handled well it could lead to a situation or problem where a difficult choice has to be made and your working relationship with the individual may suffer.

Dilemmas

In your role, you may face various dilemmas between the duty of care and an individual's rights. Here are some examples.

- The agreed ways of working that you follow may support some but not all individuals' rights. For example, you may be required to support an individual to learn the guitar in his room; it is the individual's right to do so. However, the individual is disturbing the other two individuals who share the same house. This means that supporting the individual's right to play the guitar is denying the rights of the other individuals to live peacefully and not to be disturbed.
- You are bound by the agreed scope of your job role and its associated duty of care. For example, an individual may ask you not to wear gloves when supporting them to change a dressing on their hand because this is their preference; they do not like the feel of the glove on their hand. However, you are required by your duty of care to wear gloves because

of the risk of infection that may result (if you come into contact with the individual's blood).

- Your duty of care may be in direct conflict with an individual's rights. For example, you may have a duty of care to an individual with respect to their safety when going out late at night – this is in direct conflict with an individual's right to be independent, to be treated like an adult and take risks if they want to.
- An individual may not understand the duty of care you have towards them and others. For example, an individual may feel that you are talking to them about the risks of smoking because you want to prevent them from exercising their right to smoke rather than because you want them to make an informed choice and think about the safety issues that this involves when smoking in the house where others are present.

Figure 4.4 includes more examples of dilemmas that may arise between the duty of care and an individual's rights. Can you think of any that have arisen in the care setting where you work?

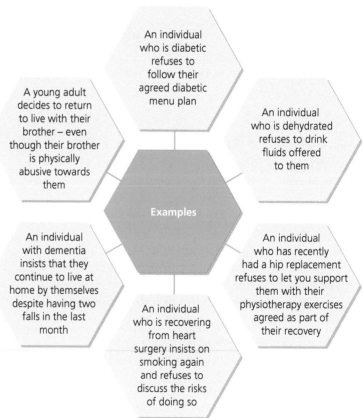

Figure 4.4 Dilemmas between duty of care and an individual's rights

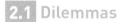

Reflect on it

2.1 Dilemmas

Reflect on the examples of dilemmas included in Figure 4.4 and think about how these can conflict with the duty of care? Now put yourself in the individual's shoes in each case. How do you think they may feel about being denied their rights? How may they view your duty of care? How may this be different to your view?

How to overcome dilemmas and support individuals

Supporting an individual's rights while maintaining your duty of care requires you to be knowledgeable about the individual you are working with as well as what is expected from you by your employer. It also involves you showing compassion when providing care or support to individuals and treating them with dignity and respect.

The dilemmas that arise between duty of care and an individual's rights do not mean that you cannot support the rights of the individual. In order to support individuals, there are measures you can take and these are discussed in detail below.

Make sure individuals have all the necessary information to make informed decisions

A key part of your role is to encourage individuals to make their own choices and live as independently as possible. However, individuals' choices may not necessarily be what you think is right for them. The individual is entitled to their choice but it is your responsibility to make sure that you inform them of what their choice means and what the consequences of their decision may be. Perhaps an individual you care for would like to stop taking vitamin tablets that the doctor has suggested, because of the side effects. However, you know that the tablets are beneficial to their health because they do not eat the vegetables that they are given at mealtimes. You could give them leaflets about the benefits of taking the vitamins and explain the consequences of not doing so, or explain that they will need to eat more vegetables if they decide not to take the vitamins. You could ask that they speak to a doctor, who would be

able to advise them further. In all instances, you should think about the things covered in Unit 203, Communication in care settings, making sure that you effectively communicate information to the individual in ways that they can understand and in a manner that allows you to check they understand what is being communicated.

Ensure that individuals understand what duty of care means

You should ensure that you and everyone you work with support individuals to understand the meaning of your duty of care, the reasons why it is important and why this doesn't mean that their rights will not be upheld. You can do this by ensuring you explain your duty in a way that individuals understand, for example in a format they can understand such as by using pictures, photographs or signs or by using a representative such as their advocate.

Ensure that individuals are at the centre

You should ensure that you, and others you work with, ensure the individual is at the centre of all discussions you have about any dilemmas that occur. You can do this by showing that you respect that every individual is unique, has a right to make their own choices and decisions and is always consulted.

Use positive ways of working to maintain rights

You should ensure that you and others use positive ways of working when supporting individuals to maintain their rights. You can do this by supporting individuals' rights to complain if they are unhappy about any aspect of their care or support and by ensuring that you remain open and honest with individuals about your duty of care and their rights.

Follow agreed ways or working to support rights

You should ensure that you and others follow your work setting's agreed ways of working relating to your duty of care and supporting individuals' rights. You can do this by following what your employer has agreed for you to do as part of your job role when supporting individuals' rights and by asking questions if there is any aspect of your role and responsibilities that you do not understand.

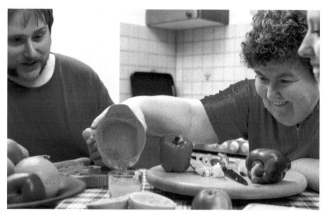

Figure 4.5 How do you support the rights of the individuals you care for?

Research it

2.1 Supporting individuals' rights

Carry out some research in the care setting where you work and find out your work setting's agreed ways of working for supporting individuals' rights. Share your findings and discuss these with a colleague. What are the main points for supporting individuals' rights?

6Cs

C

Compassion

Compassion refers to taking a genuine interest in how the individual you care for may be feeling, or putting yourself in their place. Here it refers to you trying to understand the reason why individuals may make certain choices and decisions. Being compassionate is important because without it you will not be able to see things from the perspective of others and thus build effective working relationships with individuals and others involved in their lives. You can show your compassion when dilemmas arise between your duty of care and an individual's rights by listening carefully to what they are saying and observing what they are expressing so that you can then respond with kindness and consideration to their beliefs and preferences. You will need to think carefully about things from their perspective to try and understand why their views, preferences and decisions may be different to your own.

Evidence opportunity

2.1 Dilemmas between duty of care and individuals' rights

Think about two dilemmas that have arisen in the care setting where you work. For each one describe what the conflict was and how it caused difficulties between your duty of care and supporting individuals' rights.

Instances where you may need to go against the wishes of the individual

A key part of your role is to empower individuals to make their own decisions and decide what is best for them. However, there will be times when you will need to take the best course of action even though this may not be what the individual has asked for. This can happen for many reasons and we discuss these below, as well as how you may want to tackle these issues.

The individual does not have capacity to make decisions

Having the 'capacity' to make decisions refers to the ability to make decisions. In the setting where you work, you will come across individuals that may not have the capacity to make their own decisions and this may be for various reasons. This may be due to health issues, although you should never assume that just because someone is suffering from depression, for example, that they do not have the capacity to make their own decisions. You, your colleagues and the others that care for the individual will have an idea of whether they have the ability to make their own decisions by understanding their medical history and from working with and caring for them. You should also take into account the particular situation and the type of decision that needs to be made. For example, an individual with mental health needs will at times be able to make their own choices about going out and participating in activities.

In order to help individuals to make their own decisions, you can make sure that you give them all the information that they need. This includes telling them about the positives as well

Table 4.2 Example of how to make sure individuals have the relevant information to make informed decisions about their care

Situation	Explain the positives	Explain the negatives, the consequences and the risks that they face
An older individual has been prescribed a course of antibiotics by their GP for a chest infection. However the individual is unwilling to continue taking them as they think the antibiotics are not making them feel better.	You cannot force an individual to take medication; you must respect their right to refuse and record their refusal. You could explain to the individual that the course of antibiotics they are taking will prevent their chest infection from developing into anything worse but that the whole course has to be taken for this not to happen. You could also explain that the course of antibiotics they are taking has a proven track record and will mean that if taken they will make the individual feel better and therefore restore their health and sense of well-being.	If there are any side effects to the medication, then you could explain what these are. You should explain the risks if they do not take the medication, which may mean reiterating the benefits of taking the medication. You could explain to the individual that antibiotics will only be effective if the whole course is taken. Not completing the course will mean that the individual will not experience the full benefits. You could also explain to the individual that a chest infection if not treated can make the individual deteriorate quickly; the individual's life may be at risk as a result. An emergency hospital admission may result. If the individual pulls through, a long recovery period may follow before the individual's health and well-being are restored.

as the negatives of the decision they are about to make, and then any risks and consequences they may face as a result. If you do not have the knowledge, or are unsure about anything, then you should ask for advice from your manager or others who may have a better understanding of the area. The example in Table 4.2 explains how you might go about doing this.

In 2005 the Mental Capacity Act was introduced and aimed to protect and give some power back to individuals who lacked capacity. It was also designed so that those working in health and social care could assess whether individuals have capacity. It outlined ways in which care workers could support individuals to make decisions. The Act outlined five principles which are important for you to know and understand in your role as you have a duty to comply with this.

The five principles state that:

1 You must presume capacity: you must assume that a person has the capacity to make their own decisions unless you can prove that they do not.

2 Individuals have the right to be supported to make their own decisions: you cannot treat them as if they are unable to make their own decisions. You must support them to do so, unless you have taken all necessary steps and you then decide they are unable to make their own decisions.

3 Individuals have the right to make unwise decisions: you may disagree with a decision and feel it is unwise but individuals have the right to make such decisions.

4 Best interests: any decision made on behalf of the individual who lacks capacity must be made in their best interests.

5 Least restrictive option: before you make the decision for the individual who does not have capacity, you must make sure that this will be the least restrictive when it comes to their rights and freedoms.

There is also the two-stage functional test of capacity that you should undertake to decide whether an individual has the capacity to make a decision:

Stage 1 Is there an impairment of or disturbance in the functioning of a person's mind or brain?

Stage 2 Is the impairment or disturbance sufficient that the person lacks the capacity to make a particular decision?

These two questions are taken from SCIE's 'Mental Capacity Act 2005 at a glance' (www.scie.org.uk/mca/introduction/mental-capacity-act-2005-at-a-glance)

The MCA also introduced new bodies such as the Lasting Power of Attorney (LPA) which means people over the age of 18 can formally choose people that they want to make decisions for them if they are unable to make decisions in the future. The MCA also introduced a Public Guardian to ensure that people who lack capacity are not abused and it also states that it is a criminal offence to neglect or ill-treat someone who lacks capacity. The Act is accompanied by a code of practice that provides guidance to people who act or make decisions on another person's behalf.

All of this stresses the importance of maintaining your duty of care to individuals and to do all you can to ensure that you empower individuals to make decisions but also follow best practice when they are unable to.

Research it

2.1 Mental Capacity Act 2005

Find out more about the Mental Capacity Act here:

www.scie.org.uk/mca/introduction/mental-capacity-act-2005-at-a-glance

The individual's decision will harm them or put others at risk of harm

There might be times when an individual's decision not to follow what you have advised may put them at serious risk of harm. It may be that they do not want to follow your advice about their eating habits and they are endangering their health as a result. At times like this, it is important that you tell your manager about the situation. If you decide that you cannot allow the individual to ignore your advice, then you will need to explain to your manager your reasons for doing so. You manager will be able to advise you of the best course of action with regard to the agreed ways of working in your setting.

Another example may be where the individual's actions may harm others, and you cannot allow this to happen. It may be that the individual ignores your advice about the dangers of smoking, and they decide that they would like to smoke inside the communal living area even when you suggest that you can take them outside. This means that others in the living area will be exposed to the smoke fumes which could be harmful to their health, and so you cannot follow the individual's request. Similarly, you should seek your manager's advice and discuss how to tackle the situation based on the agreed ways of working in your setting. In both situations, you should communicate clearly the reasons you cannot allow the individual to follow their own decisions.

Just think for a second about how you would feel if someone made a decision for you and did not explain why they did not follow what you had asked for, just because it was in your best interests. Would you want to know the reasons behind their decision? You should follow the advice on pages 128–31 about how you can support individuals (even when you do not agree with them).

The individual's decision means that they will be taking part in something that goes against the setting's agreed ways of working

There may be times when the individual makes a request or makes a decision that goes against the policies and procedures of the setting in which you work. Think about the example above. It may be that your setting simply does not allow individuals to smoke in the living area and here you would need to take action. First, you should tell your manager. However, an appropriate response would be to politely tell the individual: 'I understand that you would like to smoke in the living area so you do not miss the group activity, but I can't allow you to smoke here because it is not safe for the other individuals in the room and the policies in our setting won't allow me to let you do this. I can however, take you outside, or to another quite room if you prefer?' That way you are explaining your reasons to the individual, still allowing them the chance to smoke and giving them a choice of alternative places to smoke.

The individual's decision means that they will be taking part in something that is morally wrong, illegal or criminal

It may be that you discover that an individual you provide care for is partaking in something that is illegal or a criminal activity; you cannot ignore this and must report your concerns to your manager first and foremost who will advise on the best course of action.

AC 2.2 Explain where to get additional support and advice about how to resolve such dilemmas

At times, because the dilemmas that arise between your duty of care and an individual's rights can be quite difficult to resolve it will be necessary for you to ask for additional support and advice about how these can be resolved satisfactorily.

Getting additional support and advice is a must because doing so means that any dilemmas that arise can be dealt with quickly which means that the conflicts they could potentially cause will be limited and this will therefore protect individuals' and others' safety. Getting additional support and advice will also show individuals that you genuinely **care** about respecting and promoting their rights and consider how the care you provide impacts them as you have gone to the effort to seek advice.

6Cs

Care

Care is not just about meeting an individual's needs and preferences. Care is about showing your genuine interest in ensuring that the support you provide improves and makes a positive difference to an individual's life. This is important because without good support you will not be able to support an individual's rights and preferences. In this section in particular, you can show you care by seeking advice from others when you are trying to resolve dilemmas. It is only if you genuinely care for the well-being of individuals that you will seek advice to efficiently and effectively resolve the dilemma.

A range of sources of support and advice about how to resolve dilemmas is available both within and outside of the care setting where you work. If faced with a dilemma, the first person you should speak to should be someone senior to you (such as your manager, team leader or supervisor) so that you can discuss what you feel is in the best interests of the individual. They should be able to offer you advice on how to address the dilemma and may also be able to tell you about their experiences of dilemmas they have faced. However, there will be other sources of support that you can approach for support and advice, including colleagues, bodies outside your setting including trade unions that you may be part of, or charities that may have more expertise in areas that you do not. We explore some of these sources of advice and support below.

Reporting your concerns to external organisations, if necessary, is part of your legal duty of care and you have a legal right to do this knowing that you will not be penalised by your work setting for doing so; this concept is known as **whistle-blowing** (see page 134 for definition); it is important you always follow your agreed ways of working for whistle-blowing.

> ### Key term
>
> **Whistle-blowing** is when you reveal or expose a serious fault or something that is seriously wrong in your setting. This might be something that is unethical or illegal, or a way of working that is not best practice and is having a negative impact on the individual or others.

The additional support and advice you seek will depend on a range of circumstances.

- **The nature of the dilemma** – for example, if the dilemma involves the rights of an individual with dementia, you may require additional support from the individual's partner about their preferences as well as advice from a professional such as a dementia nurse about how you can promote their choices safely.
- **What your role is** – for example, if you are a care worker then your agreed ways of working may require you to seek additional support and advice about resolving dilemmas from your supervisor in the first instance. Or, if you are a supervisor, your agreed ways of working may require you to seek additional support from the manager in the first instance.
- **The setting where you work** – for example, if you are a personal assistant (see page 2 for definition), the individual you care for may also be your employer and so you may be required to seek additional support and advice from an independent person such as from a staff member who works for the organisation supporting the individual. Or if you are a residential care worker who cares for individuals with support needs, dilemmas that arise may be resolved by seeking additional support and advice from the individuals themselves, their families and friends, your colleagues, other team members, your manager, other professionals who visit, such as GPs, nurses and social workers, and external organisations.
- **Any expert advice you may need** – there may be times when you require some expert advice in areas that you are not knowledgeable in. For example, you may need to contact charities such as Mind for advice on how to support an individual who lacks capacity. You may need to consult the Alzheimer's Society for advice on how to promote the choices of an individual with dementia. You may need to consult the Care Quality Commission (CQC) for more specific advice on how to promote your duty of care while maintaining good standards of care or the Health and Safety Executive (HSE) for advice on how to carry out risk assessments effectively.

Although there is a wide range of different people and organisations and services that can provide you with additional support and advice, it is worth remembering that it may or may not be appropriate to involve an individual and/or their family or friends in resolving dilemmas that arise. If an individual does not have the capacity to make their own decisions, they may not be able to understand and make sense of the information they are given to help with resolving the dilemma. Similarly, if an individual's previous experiences and current relationships with their family or friends are not positive then it may not be in the individual's best interests to involve their family or friends. An independent representative such as an advocate can be one effective way of ensuring an individual's best interests and preferences are being put forward when resolving such dilemmas.

Importance of effective working relationships when resolving dilemmas

How effective you are in resolving dilemmas that arise depends on the working relationships you have with individuals and others. If you have positive working relationships built on mutual trust and respect then it will be more likely that a solution everyone is happy with will be found. Positive working relationships as well as the ability to resolve such dilemmas are underpinned by good communication. It is important that when you seek additional support and advice you are able to communicate clearly what the dilemma is, what action you have taken and the reasons why so that you are able to obtain the support and advice you need and so that the dilemma can be resolved as quickly as possible.

6Cs

C

Communication

Communication is crucial to getting additional support and advice about how to resolve dilemmas that may arise between your duty of care and an individual's rights. It is important because communicating effectively and clearly explaining the details around the dilemma will mean that you are able to source relevant advice and support enabling you to resolve the dilemma. In other words, if you seek advice from your manager, you will need to ensure you know and communicate:

- the details around the dilemma
- what you would like the individual to do and your reasons
- what the individual would like to do and their reasons
- why these conflict.

All of this is so that your manager has a clear understanding of the situation, the 'different sides' or viewpoints, and can advise you.

Communicating clearly and being clear, open and honest with an individual means that you can maintain good working relationships with them in order to resolve dilemmas. Good communication will avoid misunderstandings and any delays in resolving such dilemmas. You can show good communication by:

- explaining clearly to the individual why there is a dilemma
- outlining what action you are going to take to resolve it
- reporting and recording information about the dilemma fully and accurately.

Reflect on it

2.2 Resolving conflict in the setting

Reflect on an occasion when you were involved in a conflict and tried to resolve it. What techniques did you use to resolve it? Were these techniques successful? Why do you think they were successful? Did you use effective communication skills? What personal qualities did you show and did you think were essential for resolving the situation? Were you patient? Were you honest? Were you sensitive?

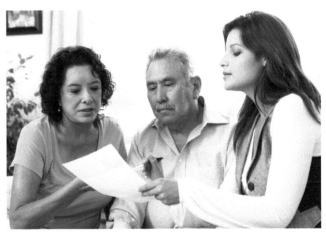

Figure 4.6 Are you an effective communicator?

The reflective exemplar below provides you with some additional information about the benefits of getting additional support and advice regarding how to resolve such dilemmas.

Reflective exemplar	
Introduction	I work as a senior care worker in a nursing home and part of my job role involves, supporting care workers carrying out their work duties by monitoring their work practices and providing them with additional support and advice when they require it.
What happened?	Last week, during an afternoon shift I was approached by one of the care workers, who expressed her concerns over one of her colleagues not supporting an individual's rights because this was in conflict with her duty of care. The care worker explained that her colleague had observed an individual behaving very rudely to another individual over lunch and how the care worker had challenged the individual immediately because the individual's behaviour had been discriminatory. The care worker went on to explain that she did not think her colleague should have challenged the individual so publicly in front of everyone at lunchtime because this upset the individual and the others having their lunch. I thanked the care worker for her concern and explained that she had done the right thing reporting this to me. I then sought advice from my manager and discussed the situation with her in full.
What worked well?	I received the care worker's concerns in a positive manner and sought advice from my manager immediately.
What did not go as well?	I should have explained to the care worker the actions I was going to take to resolve the dilemma, i.e. seek advice from my manager. I should have approached all those involved after discussing the situation with my manager to ensure that everyone could participate in resolving the dilemma that had arisen over lunchtime and to reinforce with everyone how the care setting is in support of all individuals' rights.
What could I do to improve?	I think I will need to reflect on my actions today and think about how I could improve my practice if a situation like this were to arise again. Also, I plan to discuss this with my manager at my next supervision meeting.
Links to unit assessment criteria	ACs 2.1, 2.2

Evidence opportunity

2.2 Additional support and advice about resolving dilemmas

Produce an information handout that explains where to get additional support and advice on how to manage dilemmas that involve duty of care and an individual's rights.

You might like to carry out some research in the care setting where you work to find out about the different people and organisations you can access for additional support and advice to resolve dilemmas that may arise between the duty of care and an individual's rights.

LO2 Knowledge, skills, behaviours
Knowledge: why do dilemmas arise about duty of care, the importance of addressing these and where to seek additional advice and support?
Do you know the reasons why duty of care may conflict with an individual's rights and the dilemmas that may arise?
Do you know what dilemmas could arise between the duty of care and an individual's rights?
Do you know why it is important to seek additional support and advice about resolving such dilemmas?
Did you know that you have just answered three questions about the dilemmas that may arise in care settings and why it is important you take action to address these?
Skills: how can you show that you understand the support available for addressing dilemmas?
Do you know how to access additional support and advice on how to resolve these dilemmas?
Do you know how to ensure your work practices comply with fulfilling your duty of care and supporting individuals' rights?
Did you know that you have just answered two questions about a few of the skills you have in relation to addressing dilemmas that may arise about duty of care?
Behaviours: how can you show the personal qualities you have when addressing dilemmas about duty of care?
Do you know how to be understanding and patient when your duty of care conflicts with an individual's rights?
Do you know how to be assertive when asking for support and advice about how to resolve dilemmas?
Did you know that you have just answered two questions about a few of the essential behaviours that are expected for addressing dilemmas that may arise about duty of care?

LO3 Know how to respond to complaints

Getting started

Think of an occasion when you were dissatisfied or unhappy about a service you received. This may be in relation to waiting too long for an appointment at your GP surgery or about the food you were served at a restaurant (perhaps the food was too cold or not what you ordered). Perhaps you have been unhappy about the quality of customer service you received when buying a new mobile phone.

Did you take any action? If so, what did you do? If not, why not? How did it make you feel afterwards? Why do you think you felt this way?

AC 3.1 Describe the process to follow when responding to complaints

All organisations that provide health and social care services are required by law to have a process in place to respond to complaints. We will look in more detail at what the law says about the main points that should be included in agreed procedures for complaints

in AC 3.2, but first we will look at the process that you should follow when responding to complaints.

Who might complain and why?

Complaints are made when a person is not satisfied with an action, or lack of action, taken by an employee or organisation and seeks to express their unhappiness. Complaints in adult care settings may be made by the following people:

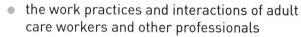
Reflect on it

3.1 Complaints

Reflect on any occasion you have experienced in the care setting where you work when an individual or another person told you they were unhappy with an aspect of the service they received. What were they unhappy about? Did you consider this to be a complaint or did you think they were just sharing their concern with you? What did you do? Why?

Why does having a process for responding to complaints lead to the provision of (providing) good-quality care and support services? You may want to discuss your thoughts with your manager.

- **an individual who requires care or support** may complain about a care worker who always arrives late to assist them with having breakfast

- **an individual's family or friends** may complain about the time made available to their relative by the care team when supporting them to access facilities in their local area

- **a team member** may complain about how an individual, being provided with support, has been treated unfairly by one of their colleagues

- **a visitor** might complain about how the care setting has failed to respond to their concerns about not keeping the main fire escape routes in the building clear

- **a professional from another organisation** may complain about a care worker who has failed to respond to their communications in relation to an individual's agreed plan of care or support.

The nature of complaints can therefore vary significantly in adult care settings and may be in relation to a number of different aspects, including:

- the quality or amount of care or support provided
- the type of services provided

- the work practices and interactions of adult care workers and other professionals
- the lack of information provided
- concerns over the health, safety and well-being of individuals and others.

Responding to complaints

Making a complaint can be a scary prospect for many people. Often, we worry that we will offend someone by making a complaint and this may stop us from making one. Individuals in your setting may feel the same way when they make complaints. However, you should remember that complaints can lead to improved practice and so it is crucial that you make individuals feel that their concerns and complaints are welcome and taken seriously.

Every health and social care organisation will have developed their own process for responding to complaints and this must be followed *every time* a complaint is made. It is important that all complaints are responded to fairly; so that the **complainant** feels that their complaint has being treated seriously and quickly so that any issues or concerns can be resolved and improvements made.

Responding to complaints in this way will encourage mutual trust and respect between the complainant and the care setting. It will also inspire confidence in the other people who use the service including the families of individuals as it will show them that the care setting is doing its very best to promote best practice.

You can promote best practice when you deal with complaints by following some simple guidance outlined in the 'dos and don'ts' table on page 140. There is some overlap here between responding to complaints and handling complaints in AC 2.2. However, this is useful for you to know in both situations.

There may be circumstances when the individual does not want to make a complaint, but simply to know how to make one. Here, you should support them by making them aware of your setting's procedure.

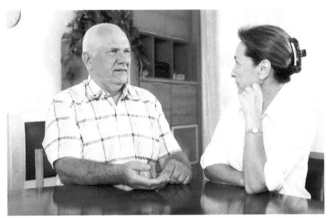

Figure 4.7 Do you have the skills to respond to complaints?

The process

Any process for responding to complaints must include the following key stages.

1. **Acknowledge the complaint when you receive it**. For example, the complainant may make an **informal complaint** verbally to a care worker or a **formal complaint** in writing to the manager of the service or organisation. Both types of complaint must be acknowledged; this is usually done by writing to the complainant. In this way, the complainant will know that you are taking their complaint seriously.

2. **Acknowledge the complaint in writing and within the agreed timescale**, for example within three days of the complaint being received. In this way, you can act upon the complaint quickly.

3. **Make a decision over how to handle the complaint**. For example, you could arrange for the complainant to meet with the manager of the adult care service to discuss the issues

raised or you could arrange for a formal investigation to take place.

4. **Reach a decision on how to handle the complaint** and discuss this with the person making the complaint. You may need to discuss the reasons why a meeting or a formal investigation is required as well as how long it will then take to reach an outcome. You can do this verbally first but you should then document it in writing. Again, this must be communicated within the agreed timescales, for example, within ten days of the complaint being acknowledged.

5. **Contact the complainant and any others involved for further information**. For example, you may need to tell them if a formal investigation will take place and inform them that the person conducting the investigation will be impartial (neutral) and that they may request to interview the complainant and any others involved.

6. **After reaching a final outcome**, make sure you put together a formal response and send this document to the complainant. This might be in the form of a full report into the investigation that has taken place, its findings and any suggestions for improvements that will be made as a result.

7. **If the complainant thinks that their complaint has not been responded to fairly** or has not been dealt with by following the correct process then you will need to inform them that they have a right to contact an external organisation which will investigate their concerns further. This may be the **ombudsman** (see page 140 for definition) if you are complaining about the council or the Care Quality Commission (CQC) if you are complaining about an independent provider of adult care services.

All of the stages will of course depend on how serious the complaint is, but these stages will be in most settings' complaints procedures. You should, however, check your setting's policies and procedures for responding to complaints or discuss with your manager for more information.

Key term

Ombudsman is a free independent service that investigates complaints against an organisation.

Evidence opportunity

3.1 The process for responding to complaints

Produce a diagram that describes the process you must follow when responding to complaints in the care setting where you work. This can be in the form of a flow diagram.

	Dos and don'ts for responding to and handling complaints
Do	Remain calm and listen to the person who makes the complaint; find out the facts around what happened to ensure that you fully understand the complaint.
Do	Find out what outcome the person making the complaint would like (what they would like to happen) to make sure that this is something you are able to do and do seek advice from a senior colleague or your manager about how best to deal with it.
Do	Reassure the individual, understand that it may be hard for them to make the complaint, and continue to support them as they make the complaint so they understand that their complaint is important to you and that you are 'on their side'.
Do	Think of complaints positively so that any complaints that have been made informally (maybe just 'I didn't like the way you spoke to me earlier') can be addressed and do not become bigger issues.
Do	Act quickly on the complaint.
Do	Follow your setting's policies and procedures for handling complaints.
Do	Keep your manager informed about all complaints made, no matter how big or small. This will allow them to keep informed about practice and address any issues. They may also decide that they should handle the complaint and the process.
Do	Keep the complaint confidential.
Do	Keep the complainant informed of the progress made with their complaint. Inform the complainant that if they are not happy with the outcome, then they can refer the complaint to the ombudsman (see AC 2.2).
Do	Learn from the mistakes and complaints made. Share this information afterwards. Produce a summary at the end of the year detailing any complaints and show how you have addressed the complaints and improved the service as a result of them.
Don't	Rush to try and resolve the issue before you have understood the situation. Take some time to give the individual your full attention and understand all the details.
Don't	Just think about what you feel is the best way to deal with the complaint. It is important that you understand what they would like to see and discuss this with a senior member of staff to see if this is possible and decide how best to deal with the complaint.
Don't	Be defensive. Complaints can be a criticism of your work, but remember that complaints and criticism can help to inform and better your ways of working. It can be hard to take criticism but don't let this demotivate you! Use it as a way to learn, and be an even better care worker.
Don't	Think of complaints as 'one-offs' or 'that won't happen again'. Make a note of it, and know not to make the same error again. That way, you can stop an informal complaint from becoming a formal complaint.
Don't	Just file the complaint away, however minor it may be. It is important that you find a solution to the issue. You may not feel it is an urgent issue but it might be to the person making the complaint. This is all part of being a compassionate and considerate care worker.

→

Dos and don'ts for responding to and handling complaints	
Don't	Tell the individual how you will deal with the complaint if you are unsure of how it will be addressed and before you have spoken to your manager.
Don't	Tell all your colleagues about the complaint. You may need to tell your manager, but ensuring confidentiality is part of your duty of care and the last thing you want to happen is for the individual to find out that the complaint they made is common knowledge, especially if they struggled to complain in the first place.
Don't	Overload your manager with information when you tell them about the complaint. Communicate accurately and clearly the details of the complaint made, and stick to the facts, so that you deal with the complaint exactly as it has been made.
Don't	Forget to inform them or think that just because it will take time to resolve that you should not contact the complainant. Make sure that you tell them how the situation is progressing.
	You do not have to say whom the complaint was made against but it is important that others learn from it too.

AC 3.2 Identify the main points of agreed procedures for handling complaints

Agreed procedures refer to the agreed ways of working in your setting, or the policies and procedures of your setting, and here these refer to your work setting's procedures for handling complaints. Every work setting will have a complaints procedure and one to follow for handling complaints. This will not only be made available to you, but it should also be made available to everyone else who uses the setting's services so that they too know how to make a complaint should they need to.

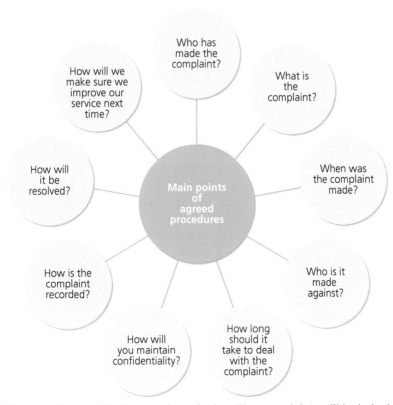

Figure 4.8 Your setting's procedures for handling complaints will include these points

How to make sure people are aware of the complaints procedure

In your role, you will be dealing with complaints and supporting people when they make them, but you may also need to advise individuals to make complaints and simply tell them about the procedure for doing so. A good way to make sure that this information is readily available to everyone is to make sure it is on display on your notice board and in leaflets in your setting – as well as on your setting's website. This information should be clearly displayed in reception areas so that visitors can see it and even included in any mail-outs to service users and their families. You will also need to ensure it is accessible and so should be available in different languages including Braille. Remember that complaints can ultimately lead to improvements so should be welcomed.

As you have learned, following a process when responding to complaints aims to ensure that complaints are dealt with fairly and resolved as quickly as possible.

Handling complaints can be difficult particularly if they are in relation to a conflict between for example the duty of care and an individual's rights. Therefore, it is important that all complaints are handled professionally, sensitively and with **courage**.

When you handle a complaint it is important that you:

- **remain impartial** – you should remain non-judgemental and non-discriminatory (this means you should treat every complaint seriously and not make judgements about the complainants)
- **remain professional** – be polite, calm and assertive when receiving a complaint, following your agreed ways of working
- **listen attentively** – do not interrupt, listen to what is being communicated so you can understand the complaint
- **pay attention to both verbal and non-verbal communication** – you will find it useful to refer to Unit 203, Communication in care settings, in relation to the messages that are expressed from verbal and non-verbal communication

- **be open** – be honest, including when you record information, by making sure you complete full and accurate records (refer to Unit 206, Handle information in care settings, to find out how to complete records fully and accurately)
- **act in individuals' best interests only** – taking into account their needs and showing respect for their rights will show your **commitment** to ensuring that needs are met and rights upheld.

Also see the table on pages 140–1 for 'dos and don'ts' on responding to and handling complaints.

6Cs

C

Courage

Courage here relates to doing the right thing when you are handling complaints. This is important because you need to comply not only with your employer's agreed ways of working but also with all the current legislation. You can show courage by not ignoring any complaint, however small, and by ensuring you always handle and respond to all complaints respectfully.

Commitment

Your determination to ensure that your way of working makes a positive difference to individuals' lives is important when handling complaints. It means that complainants are more likely feel that they can approach you with any concerns they have (i.e. they will not be deterred from complaining about any aspect of their care or support that they are unhappy about). You can show your commitment by following the agreed ways of working for your setting – showing an interest in what the complainant has to say and keeping them informed about how their complaint is being handled. Look at the list above and the 'dos and don'ts' table on pages 140–1 for more advice on how to respond to and handle complaints.

Reflect on it

3.2 Your skills in handling complaints

Reflect on the skills and personal qualities you have in relation to handling complaints. Which ones do you think are the most important and why? What are the consequences of not having these personal qualities when responding to complainants?

Research it

3.2 Handling complaints and the Care Act 2014

Research what the Care Act 2014 says about handling complaints about care or support. You will find Skills for Care's and gov.uk's websites useful sources of information; both have produced factsheets and resources about the Care Act.

Produce your own factsheet with the key points about handling complaints.

Legislation

The main points of agreed procedures for handling complaints about adult care settings are set out in regulations and legislation and these will inform the policies and procedures in your setting. The main regulations and legislation are as follows.

Health and Social Care Act 2008 (Regulated Activities) Regulations 2014: Regulation 16

This states that:

- all complaints received must be investigated
- all complaints must be acted on, i.e. when there are serious failures
- there must be an effective system in place for identifying, receiving, recording, handling and responding to complaints by individuals and others, i.e. this must be managed by the person with overall responsibility for the adult care setting such as the registered person
- the registered person must provide to the regulator, i.e. Care Quality Commission (CQC) Commission, when requested, a summary of all the complaints made as well as the registered person's response to these and all related correspondence in relation to the complaints made.

The Care Act 2014

This makes it clear that individuals have a right to complain about any decisions the local council makes about their care or support, for example how much care or support they need, what they have to pay for, what services they can access. It also requires the council to have clear information in place for handling complaints.

Data Protection Act 1998

This sets out rules for how personal information about individuals must be handled and this also applies to personal information that may be shared by complainants, for example how its security will be maintained when recorded, used, stored and shared during the complaints process. You can find more information about the Data Protection Act in Unit 206, Handle information in care settings.

The regulator for health and social care services, the Care Quality Commission (CQC), also produced in 2014 the guidance document 'How to complain about a health or social care service'. It includes the following main points of agreed procedures for handling complaints in adult care services.

- All complaints must be investigated and responded to promptly and fully.
- All services must make available a copy of their complaints procedure and this must include information about who to contact, how complaints will be handled and the improvements that will be made as a result of the complaint made.
- Complaints can be received in person, over the telephone, by letter or email, and if a complaint is made in person or over the telephone then the service must provide the complainant with a written copy of their complaint.
- The service must let you know how long they think it will take to investigate the complaint and must provide you with a response.

Some people may find it difficult or overwhelming to complain about adult care services and settings. Some specific organisations that can provide support and advice when making complaints are:

- the Relatives and Residents Association (R&RA) – a national charity for older individuals in residential care, their families and friends

- Citizens Advice – a national service that provides free, confidential and independent advice.

Case study 3.1, 3.2 provides you with an opportunity to review your learning about best practice points of agreed procedures for handling complaints.

Case study

3.1, 3.2 Handling complaints

Geoff is a care worker in a residential care home and this afternoon he sat down to speak with one of the residents, Derek, who was having a coffee in the lounge and who had recently moved in to the home. Derek tells Geoff that he is enjoying staying at the home because he has found that now he is no longer living on his own he does not have to worry about anything any more such as bills and shopping. Derek also tells Geoff about how much he enjoys the food at the home and his surroundings, particularly his view from his bedroom window as it overlooks the garden.

Just as Geoff is about to get up Derek mentions that he doesn't like coming down to the lounge because it is very noisy, also at the same time, Derek's sister arrives to see him. Geoff tells Derek that as his sister has arrived he will leave them alone and say goodbye to them both.

The next day Geoff's manager calls Geoff to the office and tells him that there's been a complaint made by Derek's sister who has been told by Derek that he had complained to Geoff that he found the lounge too noisy but how Geoff did nothing about his complaint. Geoff apologises and tells his manager he didn't realise that Geoff was making a complaint and because his sister had arrived at the same time he wanted to give them some privacy.

Questions

1 What action should Geoff have taken?
2 Why should Geoff have taken action?
3 What are the consequences of not responding to complaints?

Evidence opportunity

3.2 Handling complaints – the main points for agreed procedures

Develop a poster showing the main points of agreed procedures for handling complaints about the quality of care or support provided in the care setting where you work.

LO3 Knowledge, skills, behaviours
Knowledge: do you know how to respond to complaints?
Do you know why all complaints must be responded to promptly?
Do you know the consequences of not responding to an individual's informal complaint?
Do you know the process to follow when responding to complaints?
Did you know that you have just answered three questions about the importance of responding to complaints?
Skills: how can you show that you can follow the process and procedures for handling and responding to complaints?
Do you know how to listen attentively to a complainant?
Do you know how to record all complaints received fully?
Do you understand your employer's agreed ways of working for handling complaints and the main points they include?
Did you know that you have just answered three questions about some of the skills you have in relation to handling complaints?
Behaviours: how can you show the personal qualities you have when responding to and handling complaints?
Do you know how to be sensitive towards a complainant?
Do you know how to remain focused and calm when handling a complaint?
Did you know that you have just answered two questions about some of the essential behaviours that are expected of you to be able to respond to and handle complaints in your care setting?

Suggestions for using the activities

This table summarises all the activities in the unit that are relevant to each assessment criterion.

Here, we also suggest other, different methods that you may want to use to present your knowledge and skills by using the activities.

These are just suggestions, and you should refer to the Introduction section at the start of the book, and more importantly the City & Guilds specification, and your assessor who will be able to provide more guidance on how you can evidence your knowledge and skills.

When you need to be observed during your assessment, this can be done by your assessor, or your manager can provide a witness testimony.

Assessment criteria and accompanying activities	Suggested methods to show your knowledge/skills
LO1 Understand the implications of duty of care	
1.1 Research it (page 120)	Discuss your findings with your manager. Write a personal statement that provides a definition of the term 'duty of care'. Ensure you have related the meaning of this term to your job role and to the care setting where you work.
1.1 Reflect on it (page 120)	You could write a short reflective account. You can also base the account on experience.
1.1 Evidence opportunity (page 121) 1.1, 1.2, 1.3 Case study (page 126)	You could produce a poster. Or you could discuss the meaning of 'duty of care' with your assessor. Agree on a definition of the term. The case study will help you to think about the meaning of 'duty of care'.
1.2 Research it (page 121)	You could write an article as instructed, or tell a colleague about your findings and provide a written account to detail your findings.

➡

Suggestions for using the activities	
1.2 Reflect on it (page 123)	You could tell your assessor about the importance of reporting when you have a concern that your setting has failed to comply with duty of candour, and the consequences. You could also write a reflective account.
1.2 Evidence opportunity (page 123)	You could produce a handout as instructed in the activity.
	Or you could write a personal statement that describes how duty of care relates to duty of candour. You will need to ensure that you show your understanding of the term 'duty of candour'. You will then need to detail how the two are linked. You could use examples from your care setting. Discuss the links between both terms with your work colleagues. Detail the main links between both and how each one influences the other.
1.1, 1.2, 1.3 Case study (page 126)	The case study will help you to think about the meaning of duty of candour and how it relates to duty of care.
1.3 Research it (page 124)	Discuss with a colleague the duty of care standard and what it means for the way you work.
	Produce a presentation that describes how the duty of care affects your job role in the care setting where you work.
1.3 Evidence opportunity (page 127) 1.1, 1.2, 1.3 Case study (page 126)	You can discuss this with your manager or write a short account answering the questions in the activity. This can be evidenced through a witness testimony from your manager.
	The case study will help you to think about how your own work role is affected by your duty of care.
LO2 Understand support available for addressing dilemmas that may arise about duty of care	
2.1 Reflect on it (page 129)	Think about the issues in the first reflective activity. This will help you to relate to the issues in this section. You could write a reflective account addressing the points in the activity.
2.1 Research it (page 130) 2.1 Research it (page 132)	You may wish to discuss your findings with a colleague or tell your manager about these and write a short piece detailing your findings.
2.1 Evidence opportunity (page 130)	Write a personal statement that describes different dilemmas that may arise between the duty of care and an individual's rights. Remember to include in your description the conflict that exists and the reasons why, and how it caused any difficulties between your duty of care and supporting individuals' rights.
2.2 Reflect on it (page 135)	Write a short reflective account and address the points in the activity.
2.1, 2.2 Reflective exemplar (page 136)	The reflective exemplar is a useful source of information as it will help you with thinking about the conflicts that may arise when carrying out your duty of care and supporting individuals' rights.
2.2 Evidence opportunity (page 136)	Produce an information handout as instructed in the activity.
	For the research part, you could produce a presentation explaining where to get additional support and advice about how to resolve different dilemmas. Include sources of support and advice both within and outside the care setting where you work.
	Or you could write a personal statement to explain the process you must follow to get additional support and advice about how to resolve dilemmas that arise.
	Ensure that the details you include are in line with your employer's agreed ways of working. You could also discuss this with your assessor.

→

Suggestions for using the activities	
LO3 Know how to respond to complaints	
3.1 Reflect on it (page 138)	Write a personal statement that describes the process to follow when responding to complaints. You could discuss some of the questions with your assessor, especially how having a process for responding to complaints leads to improved care and support.
3.1 Evidence opportunity (page 140)	You could produce a diagram, or discuss the importance of responding to complaints and the process to follow with your manager, who can provide a witness testimony, or your assessor.
3.2 Reflect on it (page 143)	You could discuss your thoughts with a colleague and write a reflective account.
3.2 Research it (page 143)	Produce a factsheet that identifies the main points of the agreed procedures for handling complaints. Or you could create a presentation to explain your findings.
3.2 Evidence opportunity (page 144)	You could produce a poster or a presentation to discuss the main points of the agreed procedures for handling complaints in the care setting where you work.
3.1, 3.2 Case study (page 144)	You will find your agreed ways of working, as well as the case study, useful sources of information and guidance about the main points for handling complaints.

Legislation	
Relevant Act	**It states that:**
Human Rights Act 1998	everyone in the UK is entitled to the same basic human rights and freedoms. This includes individuals who have care and support needs. The Act supports individuals' rights to dignity, respect, to be treated fairly when accessing care or support services and to live safely and free from harm or abuse.
Mental Capacity Act 2005	individuals who lack the capacity to make their own decisions have a right to be empowered and supported to do so. It states that everyone has the right to make their own decisions and be supported to do so when they are unable to themselves. The Act also enables individuals to decide who they would like to act in their best interests should they lack capacity in the future.
Care Act 2014	individuals have a right to make a complaint about their care and treatment if they are unhappy. It requires the local council to provide clear information about how to complain about its services.
Health and Social Care Act 2008 (Regulated Activities) Regulations 2014: Regulation 16	individuals have a right to make a complaint about their care and treatment if they are unhappy. It requires health and social care providers to have an effective system in place for identifying, receiving, handling and responding to complaints from individuals using the service and others. It requires that all complaints are investigated thoroughly and action taken in response to any failures identified. It also requires providers to make available to the CQC a summary of the complaints made along with all relevant correspondence.
Health and Social Care Act 2008 (Regulated Activities) Regulations 2014: Regulation 20	health and social care providers must be open and transparent with individuals and others such as their families and advocates in relation to individuals' care and treatment. It also requires providers to act when things go wrong with care and treatment, including informing those involved about the incident, providing support, true and accurate information and an apology when things go wrong.

Legislation	
Relevant Act	**It states that:**
Data Protection Act 1998	all individuals' personal information, including that shared during the complaints process, must be kept secure and handled lawfully when recorded, used, stored and shared.
General Data Protection Regulation (GDPR) 2018	In May 2018, the General Data Protection Regulation (GDPR) came into force. It provides detailed guidance to organisations on how to govern and manage people's personal information and this will need to be included in care settings' policies, procedures, guidelines and agreed ways of working.

Resources for further reading and research

Books

Ferreiro Peteiro, M. (2014) *Level 2 Health and Social Care Diploma Evidence Guide*, Hodder Education

Hawkins, R. and Ashurst, A. (2006) *How to be a Great Care Assistant*, Hawker Publications

Weblinks

www.avma.org.uk Action against Medical Accidents (AvMA) – information from the charity for patient safety and justice, and leaflets about the duty of candour

www.citizensadvice.org.uk Citizens Advice – a service that provides free, independent and impartial advice on a range of issues

www.cqc.org.uk Care Quality Commission (CQC) – information from the regulator of all health and social care services about the standards expected from care settings and workers providing care and support to individuals, information and guidance on the duty of candour

www.gov.uk The UK Government's website for information about current and relevant legislation for the duty of care such as the Care Act 2014

www.relres.org The Relatives and Residents Association – the national charity for older people in or needing care and for their relatives and friends; provides advice on care and what to do when things go wrong

www.skillsforcare.org.uk Skills for Care – information about the knowledge, skills and behaviours expected from adult care workers, including information about the Care Certificate

Safeguarding and protection in care settings (201)

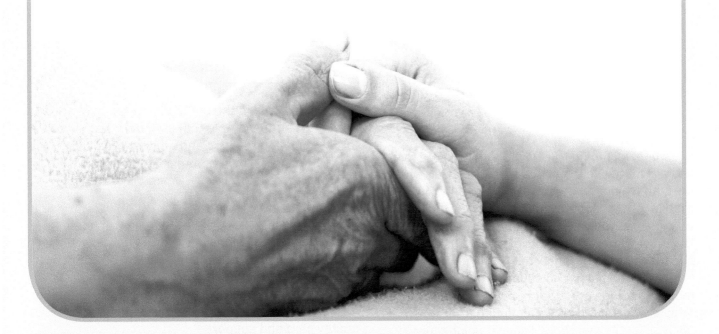

About this unit

Credit value: 3
Guided learning hours: 26

One of the most important aspects of your role as an adult care worker is to protect individuals with care or support needs. This unit will equip you with the principles that underpin safeguarding including understanding the different types of abuse, their associated **signs** and **symptoms** as well as the factors that may make an individual more vulnerable to abuse.

You will explore your safeguarding role and responsibilities for responding to **suspicions** and **allegations of abuse** including how to ensure that evidence of abuse is preserved. Understanding the legislation, national policies and **local systems** that underpin your working practices for reducing the likelihood of abuse will enable you to understand how the likelihood of individuals being abused can be reduced by managing risks and focusing on prevention. Recognising and reporting unsafe practices and understanding the principles of online safety will ensure you carry out your duty of care.

Learning outcomes

LO1: Understand principles of safeguarding adults

LO2: Know how to recognise signs of abuse

LO3: Know how to respond to suspected or alleged abuse

LO4: Understand the national and local context of safeguarding and protection from abuse

LO5: Understand ways to reduce the likelihood of abuse

LO6: Know how to recognise and report unsafe practices

LO7: Understand principles for online safety

LO1 Understand principles of safeguarding adults

Getting started

Think about a story you have heard or read about in the media that involved adults being abused and not being kept safe. For example, you may have read or heard about care homes where individuals were neglected by staff or other care homes where older individuals died as a result of poor-quality care.

How did these news stories make you feel? Why?

AC 1.1 Explain the term 'safeguarding'

Everyone, including the **individuals** you care for, has a right to live their lives safely and free from hurt, **abuse** and **neglect**. To safeguard individuals means to protect them from **harm** and abuse. In your role, you will be working with some of the most vulnerable people in society, not only because of health issues, but because they may have suffered harm and abuse. It may be that the individuals you care for are being abused by the people who should be protecting them from abuse such as family members, friends, neighbours, other individuals in the setting and even care workers – all the people that are supposed to care for the individual. Abuse and neglect can occur in the individual's own home, at work, in care settings, medical settings – again places where individuals should feel safe!

In order to safeguard individuals, you will need to know about the signs to look for, identify when someone is being abused and know the actions to take. Safeguarding also means promoting individuals' rights to good health and **well-being**. This involves providing individuals with good-quality care and support.

Key terms

Individuals refer to the people you care for and support.

Abuse occurs when someone is mistreated in a way that causes them pain and hurt. This does not just mean physical abuse but can also mean sexual or psychological or mental abuse. Neglecting someone and not caring for their needs is also a form of abuse. It is important to be aware of the different types of abuse because you will be working with vulnerable people. See AC 1.3 for more information on the different terms used to describe abuse.

Neglect means failing to care for someone so that their needs are not met. See Table 5.1 for more information on neglect. Also see AC 1.3, page 155, for a description of the term 'self-neglect'.

Harm is caused as a result of abuse. Someone may have come to harm physically (they may be bruised or injured) or emotionally (they may be frightened or worried). This may not be intentional. For example, someone may hurt themselves at home because of a tear in the carpet which went unnoticed; in which case the harm caused is accidental.

Well-being is how a person thinks and feels about themselves, physically, mentally and emotionally. More generally, it can also mean being healthy and in a positive state.

duty of care. (You may want to refer to this concept in Unit 205.)
As we mentioned earlier, as a care worker, you will need to know about the signs to look for and what to do if you think that someone you care for is being abused. It is important to follow the agreed ways of working in your care setting as these will set out what is expected from you in the safeguarding process.

However, there are some important ways of working that you must follow to support individuals to remain safe from abuse and neglect.

Understand different situations where abuse may be occurring and stay alert

This will mean knowing the different signs to looks for, which we will discuss in LO2. You should constantly be mindful of these. Individuals you care for may be vulnerable and may not disclose or tell you about abuse that they are suffering. It may be that they fear what may happen if they do. It may even be that they do not realise they are being abused or think that they are the problem and so deserve what is happening to them. It may also be that they cannot communicate abuse to you as they are either too weak given health issues or because of their age.

Therefore, you should constantly look for signs or clues that may suggest they are being abused. That is not to say you should be suspicious of everyone the individual comes into contact with. However, you will need to consider it as a possibility if individuals you care for have an injury that they cannot explain to you, or are behaving differently to how they normally do or behave differently around different people.

If you are aware of the signs, dangers and risks that individuals face, whether they are physical dangers in the setting (such as a spillage on the floor) or abuse from people (such as family members), then you will be well placed to identify abuse and can act immediately to investigate the situation and to protect the individual.

Your first port of call should be to consult your agreed ways of working in your setting. Your manager will also be able to advise you on what to do.

Research it

1.1 The Care Act 2014 and Safeguarding

Research what the Care Act 2014 says about the meaning of safeguarding adults who have care or support needs. Produce a poster with your findings.

You will find it useful to access Skills for Care's resource about the Care Act and its role in safeguarding adults:

www.skillsforcare.org.uk/Document-library/Standards/Care-Act/learning-and-development/care-act-implications-for-safeguarding-adults-briefing.pdf

---

Evidence opportunity

1.1 What does 'safeguarding' mean?

Identify an individual who has care or support needs. Write down a definition of the term 'safeguarding'. How can this individual be safeguarded and protected from harm and abuse? Think about all the different aspects of safeguarding.

AC 1.2 Explain your role and responsibilities in safeguarding individuals

Everyone involved in the lives of individuals who have care or support needs has a responsibility to safeguard them from abuse and neglect. This includes you and your colleagues, their families, friends and neighbours and other professionals such as GPs and social workers.

Your role and responsibilities

Discovering that an individual you care for is being abused can be one of the most challenging situations you face in your role, but you must remember that protecting and safeguarding individuals is your responsibility and part of your

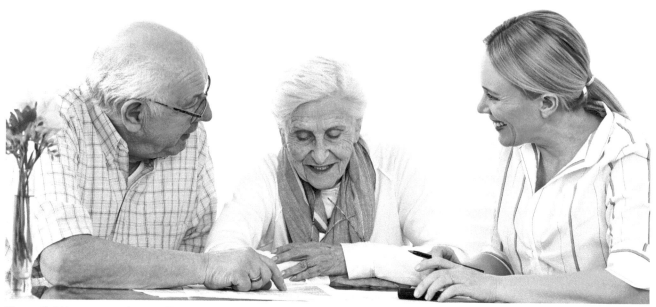

Figure 5.1 How can you be an effective partner in care?

Make sure that you accurately record details of why you suspect abuse, or if someone has disclosed it to you, then accurately record this so that you can clearly communicate this to your manager.

Prevent individuals from being subjected to any danger, abuse or neglect

You can do this by developing an individual's knowledge and understanding about the meaning of danger, abuse or neglect and what they must do if this happens to them. Reassure them that they will always be supported if they are being abused or neglected or if they report that they are being abused or neglected. You may need to seek support from the individual's advocate and adapt the information you provide so that it can be understood – by using pictures or signs if needed. This is to make sure the information is accessible. This is important, because in this way you will supporting the individuals to learn how to safeguard themselves and as a result make them less likely to be abused by others, or if they are already being abused, then you will be able to stop it from happening. There is more on the ways to reduce the likelihood of abuse in LO5.

> ### Evidence opportunity
>
> **1.2** Safeguarding roles and responsibilities
>
> Carry out some research in the care setting where you work to find out what your roles and responsibilities are for safeguarding individuals. For example, they may include your reporting and recording responsibilities as well as how you must support individuals. Discuss this with your manager, decide on the key points and make detailed notes.

AC 1.3 Define the different terms of abuse

To safeguard adults with care or support needs it is important that you are aware of and understand the different forms that abuse can take. Individuals may experience one or several types of abuse at the same time – or at different times. Therefore, being aware of all the different types of abuse that there are will be important.

As we discussed right at the start, abuse can take place by people who are supposed to

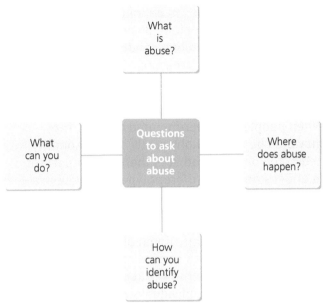

Figure 5.2 Questions to ask about abuse

care for the individuals. Abuse can happen in all sorts of places (including places that are supposed to provide care); not only in their own homes and care settings, but also at the home of someone they know, outside in a public area or in an office or place of work. Therefore, abuse can happen anywhere, by anyone and at any time.

When you think about abuse, consider the questions outlined in Figure 5.2.

The Care Act 2014 defines abuse as falling into ten different categories. You will have an opportunity to learn more about this in LO4.

Different types of abuse and what they mean

Physical abuse

Physical abuse is unwanted contact leading to injuries or pain. This can include hitting, hair pulling, scalding, slapping, pinching and other physical actions that can cause harm.

However, some other forms of physical abuse are less obvious. Physical abuse can also include overuse of medication, withholding food, unlawful isolation such as locking an individual in their room, unlawful restraint such as not allowing an individual to get up from their bed by keeping the bed rails up.

Domestic abuse

Domestic abuse can include controlling and coercive or bullying behaviour between family members and partners. This can include threats, humiliation, isolation (such as from their friends), **honour-based violence** and **female genital mutilation (FGM)**.

Sexual abuse

This includes individuals being subjected to unwanted sexual contact and involvement in sexual activities and relationships. This can include rape, sexual assault, sexual harassment, making an individual watch pornography or sexual acts, and indecent exposure.

There will be situations where individuals you care for will be in sexual relationships, ones they have consented to, but you will need to recognise the difference between this and ones where individuals are being abused by partners, family members or even care staff. (See AC 2.1 Identify the signs and symptoms associated with each type of abuse.)

Basically, any sexual activity that the individual has not consented to, was forced to consent to, unable to consent to or tricked into consenting to can be defined as sexual abuse.

The issue of consent is a very important one here as many of the vulnerable individuals you work with will not have the capacity to consent or make informed decisions.

Emotional and psychological abuse

These are abusive actions that make an individual feel worthless and humiliated. This can include bullying, threatening harm or intimidation, controlling and denying an individual's right to privacy, dignity and choice. It can also include isolating people from others or from accessing services, or being verbally abusive by swearing or shouting at them. This type of abuse underpins all the others because individuals will of course experience emotional pain when they are being abused in other ways. It is hard not to be emotionally hurt when you are physically abused.

Remember that not all abuse may be so obvious or it may not be actual abuse but it still causes distress. Often behaviour that is harsh and unacceptable can be offensive and cause emotional hurt. This can include belittling someone, treating them like a child, patronising them or bullying them. You should also be aware of this and the potential for this to cause harm. It could also lead to further and different types of abuse.

Financial and material abuse

This is the unauthorised use (without permission from the individual) of a person's finances. This can include theft, fraud, misuse of benefits or direct payments, threats or manipulation in relation to wills and inheritance. It can include abusing and exploiting them to benefit financially.

It may result in vulnerable individuals who are not able to look after their finances becoming victims of theft and fraud and losing their homes in extreme cases. For example, think about the news stories you have either heard about or read in relation to people being the victims of fraud. It is happening more and more now as technology is being used to exploit people.

Modern slavery

This means the exploitation of a person in order to serve others (domestic servitude) without being paid. This includes slavery – human trafficking where individuals are exploited by others and sold as slaves. Slaves do not have a choice, they are forced to work. It is forced and compulsory labour.

You will have learned that slavery has occurred throughout history. However, this is something that still occurs today, not just in other countries, but also in the UK. The Modern Day Slavery Act 2015 is in place to prevent the enslavement and trafficking of people. See AC 4.1 for more information on legislation.

Discriminatory abuse

This is the unequal treatment or denial of a person's rights based on a protected characteristic (that is, as defined in the Equality Act 2010). This can include discrimination because of age, disability, gender reassignment, marriage and civil partnership, pregnancy and maternity, race, religion and belief, sex or sexual orientation.

When people are discriminated against, they may also be harmed physically or emotionally, neglected or harassed. It is therefore important to understand how different types of abuse are connected and linked to others.

Institutional and organisational abuse

Institutional or organisational abuse occurs when the setting focuses its service on the needs of the organisation and the workers rather than on the needs of the individuals who access the service. This might include rigid routines and systems such as specific times for individuals to get up, go to bed, isolating individuals from families and friends, disrespectful behaviours towards individuals such as swearing and being patronising.

You may not even realise that you and the setting are being abusive in this way. It may be that you think your setting is being efficient by specifying routines and times for meals and bed, or think that it is in the best interest of the individual. However, in this way, the individuals' needs are *not* at the centre – yours are! Individuals are being forced into routines to suit you. This may be because of budgeting restraints or staff shortages, or not having the right training but the fact remains that this is still abuse. Not having the right training is not an excuse!

This type of abuse can also include neglecting the care needs of individuals to suit yourself. For example, you may decide that you do not want to take food to the individual because they have requested it after your shift ends – so you leave the individual in a situation where they are forced to eat food at a time that is convenient for you.

Sometimes institutional abuse is more obvious. Think about some of stories you may have read about individuals being ill-treated in care settings, where they have been neglected or handled in an aggressive way. This is a serious breach of duty of care and abuse not only of the individuals but abuse of the care worker's responsibility. Also see AC 1.5 on restrictive practice.

Self-neglect

This is the failure of individuals to care for themselves and meet their own needs. This can result in them causing harm to themselves. Self-neglect can include showing no care for one's own personal hygiene, not eating or drinking healthily, or perhaps not taking prescribed medication, not accessing care and support services available. They may do this because of health reasons, disabilities or simply because it is their choice to follow a certain lifestyle. You should also read about self-harm, covered below in AC 1.4.

Neglect by others

This is a failure by others to care for and meet an individual's needs which results in harm being caused to the individual. This can include not providing support for or access to food, water, heating, clothes, physical activity or moving/mobility, medical or personal care, or not taking into account an individual's cultural and religious needs. It can also mean leaving individuals in unsafe environments, generally not supporting them with their needs and simply leaving them to be alone.

You should refer to the section on institutional abuse, but remember that families and friends and others who are supposed to care about individuals can also be guilty of neglect. This may be because they are finding it difficult to care for the individual alongside other things in their life, or it may be a very deliberate and even cruel type of neglect.

Many of the types of abuse that we have discussed are criminal offences, which means those committing the acts can be prosecuted by the police. Whatever form of abuse you suspect is happening, do not ignore it. Follow your agreed ways of working so that you can stop any abuse that may be happening and safeguard and protect the individual.

You should also remember that a lot of abuse spans several of the categories we have discussed, and so often the category is less important than actually identifying that abuse is taking place.

Research it

1.3 Abuse reported in the media

Research two cases of abuse that have recently been reported in the media. You can, for example, choose cases in relation to domestic abuse such as honour-based violence and modern slavery. You will find newspapers, the television and the internet useful sources of information. Produce an information handout about each case. You may find it useful to look at the following stories as a starting point:

www.bbc.co.uk/programmes/p05bdb3d

www.bbc.co.uk/news/uk-england-northamptonshire-41935223

Case study

1.3 Different types of abuse

Wood Green is an established supported living scheme where three men with autism and other complex needs live together. One afternoon, all three individuals are sitting in the lounge. A care worker asks Jonas, one of the individuals with care needs, whether he is ready to cook his evening meal. Jonas kicks the care worker hard on the leg and runs upstairs. The care worker runs up after Jonas and shouts at him angrily, telling him that she will not tolerate him abusing her and for that reason instructs him to remain in his room for the rest of the evening. The care worker goes back downstairs and tells the two other individuals in the lounge that Jonas will not be eating this evening and will remain in isolation until he apologises to her.

Discussion points

1 What types of abuse are taking place in this care setting?
2 Why do you think these types of abuse occurred?
3 How could these types of abuse have been prevented?

AC 1.4 Describe harm

The ten types of abuse that you learned about in AC 1.3 and that are identified in the Care Act 2014 are the ones that cause harm through abuse and neglect. An individual who has care or support needs may be at risk of harm if they are or have experienced one or more of these types of abuse and neglect.

Therefore, the term 'harm' refers to any type of abuse or neglect that can have a negative effect on an individual's physical, emotional or social health and well-being.

Self-harm

Harm may not always be caused by others but by the individuals themselves. Others involved in the care of the individual, such as GPs and their family, will be able to tell you if they have a history of, or are currently self-harming and are a risk to themselves, or are likely to self-harm. Self-harming may include individuals physically abusing themselves by cutting for example. Whatever the form the self-harm takes, you should follow the policies and procedures in your setting for working with someone who self-harms and make sure that their care plan and your practice is informed by this. You may also need to

seek advice from organisations and charities that have specialist knowledge in this area.

AC 1.5 Describe restrictive practice

Restrictive practice includes actions that deliberately limit an individual's movement or freedom. As we will discuss, there are times when you may need to use restrictive practice. However, there are times when restrictive practice may cause abuse, harm and neglect if it is used inappropriately or unlawfully. This might include physically restraining an individual for no reason by tying them to a chair so that they are unable to move or using medication to make an individual drowsy. It could also include locking an individual in the house so that they are unable to leave their home on their own.

Restrictive practice denies an individual their basic human right of freedom and movement and can have serious consequences including pain, harm, suffering and even fatalities if not used correctly.

When restrictive practice may be needed

Restrictive practice must only be used legally and when necessary. It is used only as the last resort and when there are no other options. This point cannot be stressed enough. For example, it may be that other more proactive practices that encourage discussion and reassurance to diffuse situations that may arise have broken down.

It may only be legal and necessary for restrictive practice to be used by trained professionals in the following situations (although all settings will be different and you should check with your manager about the policies and procedures in your setting).

- In an emergency, for example when an individual with mental health needs is self-harming by biting his arms. In this situation, it may be necessary for trained professionals to physically restrain him so that he does not continue to harm himself.

- When an individual requires life-saving treatment, for example when an individual with dementia is having a heart attack and prevents hospital staff from administering medical treatment because they are very anxious and physically hitting out. It may be necessary for trained professionals to use medication to calm the individual down so that their condition does not deteriorate.

- When escaping violence, for example this might be when an individual who is dependent on alcohol and drugs physically abuses another individual or adult care worker and causes damage to the setting, or displays threatening behaviour. Here, it may be necessary for trained professionals to use physical restraint to prevent the individual causing further harm to others and further damage to the environment.

Restrictive practice can also include deprivation of an individual's liberty. See Unit 211, Case study 3.3.

Reflect on it

1.5 Consequences of not using restrictive practice

Reflect on the importance of restrictive practice only being used when it is absolutely necessary and legal to do so. What are the consequences of you not doing so? What are the consequences for *you*? What are the consequences for the *individual*? What are the consequences for the care setting where you work? What about the individual's setting?

Evidence opportunity

1.5 Restrictive practice

List two examples of appropriate restrictive practice and two examples of inappropriate restrictive practice. Describe how the appropriate practices can be used to safeguard individuals. Explain why the inappropriate practices are inappropriate. Keep a copy of your list and make notes to evidence this.

LO1 Knowledge, skills, behaviours
Knowledge: what is the meaning of safeguarding?
Do you know your safeguarding responsibilities and how you can promote the safety of individuals with care or support needs?
Do you know how safeguarding links to promoting individuals' health and well-being?
Do you know the meaning of these two types of abuse: emotional/psychological abuse and self-neglect?
Do you know what harm is?
Do you know what restrictive practice is and why it can and cannot be used?
Did you know that you have just answered five questions about the meaning of safeguarding adults?
Skills: how can you show your understanding of how to safeguard adults?
Do you know how to empower an individual in relation to safeguarding?
Do you know how to protect individuals from harm?
Do you know what your role and responsibilities are in relation to restrictive practices?
Did you know that you have just answered three questions about the principles of safeguarding adults?

→

LO1 Knowledge, skills, behaviours
Behaviours: how can you show the personal qualities you have when safeguarding adults?
Do you know how to work in partnership with others to provide good care and support?
Do you know how to show your awareness and understanding of the different types of abuse that exist?
Did you know that you have just answered two questions about a few of the essential behaviours that are expected of all adult care workers when safeguarding adults?

LO2 Know how to recognise signs of abuse

Getting started

Think about someone you know well. How can you tell if this person is not being their usual self? For example, do they act differently – perhaps they are unusually quiet when usually they are very chatty? Perhaps they appear different, they may look unwell or unhappy? Perhaps they tell you how they are feeling. Are they anxious, worried, angry? Perhaps you notice changes in their personality. Do they suddenly become very irritable or withdrawn?

Recognising these signs means that you know when there is something wrong. Knowing there is something wrong means you can take action to put it right.

AC 2.1 Identify the signs and symptoms associated with each type of abuse

You can only carry out your role and responsibilities to safeguard individuals from abuse, harm and neglect fully if you are able to recognise the **signs** and **symptoms** that may suggest an individual is being abused.

Table 5.1 lists the different signs and symptoms of abuse. You should remember, however, that these signs are not evidence of abuse. It may be that there are other reasons for a visible injury that the individual cannot explain.

The most effective way that you can safeguard individuals and protect them from harm or abuse is by getting to know every individual so that you notice and act upon any unusual changes that they do show, however small.

Working with colleagues and other professionals will also help you to understand any wider context, for example the individual's medical history will inform you of any bruising and injury in the past. Therefore, you will need to look at the signs in the wider context of the individual's life and care. You may also need to observe and communicate with the individual to understand any injuries better.

It is important to remember that because all individuals are unique, the way they may experience abuse or harm will also be unique. This means that individuals will not necessarily show the same signs and symptoms associated with each type of abuse.

Nonetheless, Table 5.1 will provide you with a good understanding of common signs and symptoms that may indicate abuse and ones that you should look out for and be mindful of. You will see that that there is overlap in some of the signs and symptoms for the different types of abuse and although the table does not cover all the possible signs and symptoms, it will give you an idea of the major ones to look out for.

Key terms

Signs are outwardly visible to others – you can see them. Signs of abuse can include unexplained or unusual bruises, sores and malnutrition. Signs can also present as changes in behaviour and moods.

Symptoms are experienced by individuals. They are an indication of something, for example feeling upset, angry, scared or alone. Symptoms could be the result of an illness, or abuse.

Table 5.1 Signs and symptoms of abuse

Type of abuse	Examples of signs	Examples of symptoms
Physical abuse	Unexplained or unusual bruises, cuts, scratches, burns, frequent unexplained injuries, fractures, rashes or pressure ulcers, weight loss, general worsening of their health and mood. There may be some signs in their behaviour like flinching in the presence of the abuser, wearing long sleeves in hot weather to cover up bruises, or they may not want to see visitors. Some more obvious ones might include cigarette burns, black eyes that indicate violence, repeatedly falling or repeated overdosing. Individuals may also be unable to explain the injuries.	Being in pain and discomfort, showing fear, being withdrawn particularly in the presence of another person.
Domestic abuse	Unexplained or unusual bruises, cuts, burns, broken bones (see signs of physical abuse above), being humiliated in front of others. Others showing controlling or aggressive behaviour can also be an indicator. Other signs can include those associated with physical, emotional/psychological, sexual and financial abuse.	Low self-esteem, fear of socialising with others or reluctant to let others come to the house, increased isolation from family and friends. Other symptoms can include those associated with physical, emotional/psychological, sexual and financial abuse.
Sexual abuse	Physical signs include unexplained or unusual bruises around the thighs, buttocks, breasts and genital area. There may also be burns or scratches and even bite marks, unexplained bleeding, stained or torn underclothing, difficulty in walking or sitting. The individual may have (repeated) urinary infections or genital infections, they may be pregnant. There may be some signs in their behaviour, they may seem more withdrawn, they may attempt suicide, they may be unable to explain where they have been. Others showing aggression or suggestive sexual behaviour may also be an indicator.	Poor concentration, inability to sleep, withdrawn, fear of relationships with others, fear of being alone in the presence of the other person/people, aggression, anxiety, withdrawal of care and support services, they may for example refuse assistance with personal hygiene.

→

Table 5.1 Signs and symptoms of abuse *continued*

Type of abuse	Examples of signs	Examples of symptoms
Emotional/ psychological abuse	A change in eating habits, i.e. leading to weight loss or weight gain, being uncooperative, becoming aggressive towards others. Remember that being teased or humiliated, belittled, treated like a child with no regard for them as an individual with their own opinion is also a sign that someone may be abused or that this could lead to abuse. If you care for someone in their home, it may be that neighbours have reported shouting or you may see that people living in the area are continually parking outside their home so that the individual is unable to park. It may even be that someone is using language that is not obviously racist, but still stereotypical. Often people experience emotional distress from things that may not be obviously abuse, but is still hurtful and could lead to abuse.	Disturbed sleep, low self-esteem, very under-confident, distressed, becoming upset easily, withdrawn particularly in the presence of the other person, feeling unwell, feeling anxious.
Financial/material abuse	Unexplained lack of money and withdrawals of money, unexplained living conditions, i.e. personal possessions disappearing or insufficient food. The individual may not be kept informed of what is happening with their finances, or not be allowed to manage this aspect of their life. Their property may be sold without their knowledge. They may be unable to pay for their care or relatives may be reluctant to pay. Their will may be changed.	Feeling anxious about paying bills, not wishing to pay for essential food shopping items, fear of not being able to manage financially.
Modern slavery	Appearing malnourished, looking unkempt, i.e. appearing dirty, not wearing clean clothes. Other signs can include those associated with physical, emotional/psychological abuse.	Becoming isolated from others, fear of speaking to others, appearing fearful or withdrawn in the presence of the other person/abuser. Other symptoms can include those associated with physical, emotional/psychological abuse.
Discriminatory abuse	Becoming aggressive towards others, not being supported, or being offered support or services that do not meet the individual's needs. Individuals may be denied access to care, places, people and activities. They may not be given information on how they can be supported to tackle discriminatory behaviour. See signs of emotional abuse as well.	Becoming isolated, feeling fearful, frustrated, anxious, withdrawal from services. They may also have low self-esteem.

Table 5.1 Signs and symptoms of abuse *continued*

Type of abuse	Examples of signs	Examples of symptoms
Institutional/ organisational abuse	Poor care standards, for example individuals being hungry, dehydrated, lack of management, inadequate staffing, rigid routines, lack of choices and individuality, e.g. lack of access to personal possessions, lack of individual care plans, denial of individuals' rights, e.g. dignity, privacy, independence, absence of visitors. Individuals may not be allowed to go outside; medication is not properly or appropriately administered.	Low self-esteem, feeling frustrated, anxious, angry, upset.
Self-neglect	Malnutrition, dehydration, weight loss, poor personal hygiene, looking unkempt, living in dirty or unsafe conditions, failure to access care or support services, or ignoring their health and medical needs. They may need emergency medical treatment for an injury or illness. General apathy for their own well-being.	Feeling confused, low in mood, anxious. Becoming withdrawn and isolated from others.
Neglect by others	Malnutrition, dehydration, living in dirty or unsafe conditions, pressure sores, wearing inappropriate clothing, for example items that are worn, inappropriate for the weather conditions, untreated injuries and illnesses. There may be general worsening of health and the individual may be deprived of access to medical and healthcare needs. Some of the physical signs of abuse will also apply here.	Feeling confused, low in mood, fear of involvement from others such as professionals, services, withdrawal from socialising with others such as family and friends.

You have a duty of care to inform individuals of any dangers, but not to make decisions for them, unless they lack the capacity to do so. However, make sure you consider the different factors you have learned about with regard to consent and capacity. You will find it useful to refer to Unit 205, ACs 1.3 and 2.1, as well as Unit 211, AC 3.3.

Feelings that individuals may experience

Individuals may experience a range of feelings and emotions when they have suffered from abuse. This can include a range of emotions including anger, frustration, depression and sadness and suicidal feelings. These feelings can arise whether the abuse is fairly recent and has only occurred once or if the abuse has been going on for a long period of time. Abuse can change a person significantly, it can change the way they view others and the world generally. You will need to ensure that you try to understand what the

individual may be going through. Learn from them, learn from the experience you may have had, learn from the experiences of people you know and the experiences of your colleagues so that you can empathise with individuals, and provide appropriate and long-lasting care. You may need to draw on the expertise of others such as therapists where this is beyond your experience.

Taking care of yourself

While it is important to look for signs of abuse, you must also remember to be aware of your own feelings when you are dealing with someone who has been abused. This is a tricky situation to go through as a care worker, one that may cause you upset and distress. The situation may cause you to become angry for the individual. However, remember to take care of yourself and ask for support from others. Speak to your manager, speak to others in the setting or others you know,

Evidence opportunity

2.1 Signs and symptoms of abuse

Produce a written account detailing the signs and symptoms associated with each of the following types of abuse: physical, domestic, sexual, emotional/psychological, financial/material, modern slavery, discriminatory, institutional/organisational, self-neglect and neglect by others.

remembering not to be too specific when it comes to the individual's personal and confidential details. It is normal to want to tell others, and remember that you are not alone in dealing with this situation. Your setting will be able to provide you with appropriate support and you should make use of this. There are also support organisations that will be able to help you, such as the Care Workers Charity.

Taking care of the person committing abuse

Remember to always remain professional. Do not confront the person committing the abuse, remain calm and try to keep the safety of the individual as your priority. Confronting the individual will not help matters. At the same time, the person who has committed the abuse may also require help and, if this is the case, you should discuss this with your manager and find out if it is appropriate to suggest support for them. Of course, this will depend on the nature of the situation but you should be considerate of their situation too.

AC 2.2 Describe factors that may contribute to an individual being more vulnerable to abuse

The individual

Some of the factors that may contribute to an individual being more vulnerable to abuse are associated with the individual. For example:

- **individuals who depend on others for their care or support** may be reluctant to report an abuser because they may fear they will

lose their care or that the abuser may lose their job

- **individuals who have specific communication difficulties** because of a disability such as a learning disability or an illness such as a stroke may not be able to express what is happening or communicate any abuse that may be happening to them to others

- **individuals who have specific conditions such as dementia**, poor mobility, mental health needs or a history of substance misuse may have memory difficulties for example and therefore may not be able to recall what has happened. An individual with poor mobility may be frail and physically unable to defend themselves from others who may try to harm them.

An individual with mental health needs may have experienced (as part of their illness) hallucinations and false beliefs and therefore may not be believed by others about what has happened. An individual with a history of substance misuse may be targeted by an abuser particularly if they have a history of violent behaviour as they may not be believed about what is happening to them and could also be taken advantage of while they are abusing substances.

The carer

Some of the factors that may contribute to an individual being more vulnerable to abuse are associated with the carer. These can include families, the care worker and others involved in the care of the individual. For example:

Other priorities: the carer may have a family, children and others that they care for, or need to be home at certain times for. They may have a job which they need to manage alongside caring for the individual. Such strains can be a contributing factor for abuse. Not always, but significant stress can affect the care given and abuse and neglect can occur.

The individual may be seen as a 'burden': the carer may experience difficulties in terms of financing the care of the individual; they may have issues around space and accommodating the individual in their home. Job pressures mean that their time is also limited and they may have their own health issues to deal with. They may also find that their social life is affected as a result of caring for the individual.

Difficulties in relationship with the individual: the carer and the individual may already have a difficult relationship and the individual may even be aggressive or violent towards the carer. It may be that the carer has a history of violent behaviour, or is easily agitated or angered.

Lack of support: the individual may feel unsupported, or they may be inexperienced because of their age. This may lead to inadequate care and abuse of the individual even though it may not be intended.

Remember carers can experience abuse too

Remember that carers can also be victims of abuse. It may be that they suffer verbal abuse from the individual that they provide support for. They could be suffering physical and emotional abuse, for example the individual may refuse support and lash out. There is legislation such as the guidance in the Care Act 2014 to protect carers. Go to LO5, AC 5.2, for more information on this.

Case study

2.2 Vulnerable individuals

Carlos is 28, has learning disabilities and lives with his brother Pepe. Carlos goes out every day with his brother to the local shops and to visit other family members and family friends. When Pepe works at night, he is worried about Carlos going out and being taken advantage of or coming to harm by others, and so he locks him in his room to keep him safe until Pepe returns home in the morning. Yesterday, Carlos tried to leave his room by trying to kick the door down, and now Pepe has threatened that he will no longer let Carlos see his friends and family if he does not do as his brother says.

Discussion points

1 Is abuse taking place?
2 If so, what type and in what way?

The environment or setting

Other factors that may contribute to an individual being more vulnerable to abuse are associated with the environment the individual lives, works or socialises in. For example, individuals may:

- **live in a remote location** such as at the end of a quiet road, on the top floor of a building (where few visitors are received) and may become separated from the people who know them well such as family and friends. Families may be unable to visit regularly and individuals are isolated. This may make them a target for abuse because there is less likelihood that anyone will recognise the signs or symptoms that they are being abused.

- **receive care or support in settings that are poorly managed** and may be abused because there will be a lack of monitoring of care workers to check that they are following the procedures for keeping individuals safe. The abuse may be intentional, or it may be accidental if care workers follow poor practice as a result of a lack of support or training.

- **receive care or support in settings that lack resources**. Care workers who have large and stressful workloads may feel under-valued and over-worked. This may leave them feeling frustrated and stressed with the individuals they provide care and support to. There may be a shortage of staff and emphasis may be placed on the needs of the setting rather than those of

Research it

2.2 Legislation

Research legislation that is in place to support carers, such as the Care Act 2014. How does the Work and Families Act for example support individuals? What does it say about the protection that is available for carers?

the individual, all resulting in poor-quality care, lack of time made for the individual and general disregard for the individual's needs.

As before, with the signs and symptoms, these factors are not evidence of abuse. For example, just because a family member is under stress,

does not mean that they are abusing the person they care for.

Case study 2.1, 2.2 provides you with an opportunity to consider how to recognise the signs and symptoms of abuse in an individual as well as know the factors that may make them more vulnerable to abuse.

Evidence opportunity

2.2 Factors

Read through the research report produced in November 2015 by Age UK, 'Financial abuse evidence review', which explores why older people are more likely to experience financial abuse. It can be accessed here:

www.ageuk.org.uk/Documents/EN-GB/For-professionals/Research/Financial_Abuse_Evidence_Review-Nov_2015.pdf?dtrk=true

Discuss the findings with a colleague and outline your findings by producing a written account that describes the factors that may make older people and individuals more vulnerable to financial abuse. Ensure you summarise in your own words.

Case study

2.1, 2.2 Recognising abuse

Elsie is 70, has a learning disability and lives in a residential care home; you work there as an adult care worker. Elsie's family and friends have spent all Sunday afternoon with her as it was her birthday. As soon as everyone leaves, Elsie appears unhappy and tells you she is going to stay in her room this evening. Later, you go up to Elsie's room and ask her how she's feeling; she shakes her head and in a tearful voice tells you she has a stomach ache and doesn't want anything to eat this evening. You respect Elsie's wishes and leave. At the end of your shift, you record your observations of Elsie, including what she told you.

The next morning when you arrive at work Elsie appears her usual happy self. You ask her how she is and she tells you she is fine and is about to watch a film with the others in the lounge. A half hour or so later the doorbell rings. It is Elsie's brother, who says he just thought he'd visit Elsie again to ask her about whether she enjoyed her birthday yesterday. You ask Elsie's brother to come in and at the same time, notice that Elsie (looks up from the lounge) sees him, looks shocked and shouts out that she's got another stomach ache, is going to her room and doesn't want to be disturbed.

Questions

1 What are your immediate thoughts after reading this case study about Elsie's behaviour? Why?
2 Identify any potential signs and symptoms that may indicate that Elsie is being abused.
3 What factors do you think make Elsie more vulnerable to abuse?
4 Have you come across a situation like this in your setting? How did you respond? Were the signs different? Was the individual vulnerable in other ways?

LO2 Knowledge, skills, behaviours
Knowledge: what are the signs and symptoms of abuse?
Do you know three signs that you may notice of physical abuse and domestic abuse?
Do you know three symptoms that an individual may experience of sexual abuse and institutional/organisational abuse?
What factors may contribute to an individual being more vulnerable to abuse? Can you describe three of these?
Did you know that you have just answered three questions about identifying the signs and symptoms of different types of abuse and the factors that mean an individual is vulnerable to abuse?
Skills: how can you show your understanding of how to prevent individuals from being abused?
How can you work in ways that take the three factors you described above into account when providing care or support?
Do you know three environmental factors that may make an individual more vulnerable to abuse? How can you work in ways that consider these factors when providing care or support?
Did you know that you have just answered two questions about how to work in ways that prevent individuals from being abused?
Behaviours: how can you show the personal qualities you have when recognising signs of abuse?
Do you know how to respond sensitively to any changes in individuals that you notice?
Do you know how to protect individuals' privacy when you recognise signs and symptoms of abuse?
Did you know that you have just answered two questions about a few of the essential behaviours that are expected of all adult care workers in relation to recognising signs of abuse?

LO3 Know how to respond to suspected or alleged abuse

Getting started

Think about how you would feel if you were verbally abused by someone in a busy place such as in a high street and no one did anything to help you. Why do you think you would feel this way?

Now imagine you witnessed someone you did not know being verbally abused out in public. Would you intervene or not? Explain why.

AC 3.1 Explain the actions to take if there are suspicions that an individual is being abused

Recognising the signs and symptoms of abuse is not enough on its own to protect individuals from abuse because you will also need to know what to do when you suspect an individual is being abused. In addition, it could be that someone else shares their **suspicions** with you, or an individual tells you that they are being abused.

Key term

Suspicion of abuse is when you notice signs or are told by someone about signs that make you think or suspect abuse is happening.

It can often be difficult to accept that abuse may be happening, because you may worry that you could be incorrect or raise concerns unnecessarily and it may be the first time that you have come across it. However, if you have any suspicions that an individual is being abused you must always act on it; doing nothing is not an option. You must show **courage** because it is your legal duty of care to protect the individuals that you care for.

Your agreed ways of working will detail the actions you will be expected to take in line with the agreed scope of your job role if there are suspicions that an individual is being abused.

When the individual is the employer

Not all workers are employed by organisations. Sometimes individuals and/or their representatives directly employ their own personal assistant and therefore the individual is also the employer. Where this is the case, you will need to familiarise yourself with the roles and responsibilities that are set out in your contract of employment, as well as the local authority's procedures that are in place for where you work.

Actions to take

Figure 5.3 explains the key actions to take if you suspect that an individual is being abused, and each of the points are explained in a bit more detail below.

1 Do not ignore any signs that an individual may be at risk of abuse as this may place them in danger and prolong their pain and distress. Even if it is a suspicion and the individual has not made an **allegation**, you should still act immediately and follow the next step.

> **Key term**
>
> **Allegations of abuse** are when an individual tells you that they are being abused. Other people may also allege that abuse is happening to individuals.

> **6Cs**
>
> **Courage**
>
> Courage means standing up for what you believe in when you know it is the right thing to do. When you suspect that abuse is happening, you can be courageous by showing that abuse will not be tolerated and any suspicions that an individual may be at risk of being abused or harmed will be acted on straight away. You can show your courage by ensuring you discuss your suspicions, however small, with your manager as soon as you have them so that individuals will be kept safe and protected from being abused or harmed.

Do not ignore the signs that an individual may be at risk of abuse as this may place them in danger and prolong their pain and distress

↓

Ensure the individual is safe by reporting your or others' concerns to the named person in your workplace so that others can take the necessary actions; follow your agreed ways of working to ensure you safeguard individuals

↓

Keep secure any evidence you have of your or others' suspicions; follow your agreed ways of working to ensure any evidence is preserved

↓

Record with full details the facts of what you have noticed or seen or what others have told you and in the words they have used; follow your agreed ways of working for reporting accurately and preserving evidence

↓

Refer your suspicions to another organisation (i.e. police, adult social care services, CQC) if required to do so or if your suspicions are not dealt with seriously; this is so that they can be acted on and the individual's safety and well-being promoted

Figure 5.3 Actions to take for suspicions of abuse

2 Ensure the individual is safe by reporting your concerns to your manager or the named person in your setting so that others can take the necessary actions and safeguard individuals. They will be able to advise on what action to take and whether you will need support and further advice from anyone else, such as the individual's family, or medical assistance from a GP.

3 Keep evidence secure – if you or others have suspicions, follow your agreed ways of working to ensure any evidence is preserved (see AC 3.3 for more information).

4 Record in full the facts with details of what you have seen (or what others have told you) and in the words they have used – follow your agreed ways of working for reporting accurately and preserving evidence. This may take the form of a written report, or if you need to, make an audio recording ensuring you back this up with a written report afterwards. Make sure that you record what your suspicions are, with clear reasons for these. Suspicions should not be your opinions – they should be based on evidence and observation. Suspicions that others have told you about should also be clearly and accurately recorded. Detail is very important – remember do not confuse other people's opinions with facts. Record other people's suspicions at the earliest opportunity so you do not forget the exact details.

5 Refer all your suspicions to another organisation (that is, the police, adult social care services or the CQC) if your manager suggests that you should do so, or if your suspicions are not treated seriously. This is so that they can be acted on and the individual's safety and well-being is promoted.

Make sure that all safeguarding decisions are proportionate. You can do this by weighing up how low or high the risk is that an individual may be abused or neglected. In this way, all safeguarding decisions made will be relative to the risk posed to the individual.

Capacity

You may come across issues around consent here. For example, your suspicions may be based on signs of serious abuse, but the individual may not actually allege abuse, or refuse to make any sort of statement against the abuser. This poses a dilemma for you and the setting.

As we discussed earlier, your role here will be to provide as much information as possible or simply be there for the individual. For example, if you see a bruise or notice bleeding, you could help the individual by asking them if they would like any treatment: 'I notice a bruise on your arm, is it sore? Would you like a bandage for it?' Avoid asking too many questions at this point, however. Remember that if the injury is of a more serious nature, you must report this to a doctor so that they can decide on the best course of action.

	Dos and don'ts when taking actions if there are suspicions that an individual is being abused
Do	Ensure that the individual is safe if they are at risk of immediate danger, harm or abuse.
Do	Ensure you report your suspicions in private to maintain individuals' confidentiality and privacy.
Do	Raise your concerns immediately – avoid delay because it may prolong an individual's distress and pain.
Do	Follow your agreed ways of working – this will ensure you are safeguarding individuals in line with your job role and responsibilities.
Do	Make sure that medical assistance is provided if there are signs of injury and abuse.
Don't	Confront the person you or others have suspicions about because it is not your role to do so – if you do you may place the individual at further risk of abuse.
Don't	Destroy any evidence of abuse – this will be needed if an investigation takes place. (You will learn more about this later on in this unit in AC 3.3.)
Don't	Complete your records in a rush or inaccurately – doing so may mean that individuals are not safeguarded from further abuse and harm.

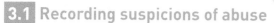
You will also need to consider issues around capacity and whether the individual has the ability to make their own decisions. Much of your actions and intervention and those of your manager will depend on whether the individual has the capacity to make decisions and refuse treatment. See pages 169–70 for more information on confidentiality and consent.

Also see page 171 for more information on working in partnership.

People you may suspect

The actions you will take when you have suspicions will generally be the same whoever you suspect is committing the abuse against the individual. However, there may be subtle differences when someone you know or work alongside commits the abuse.

A colleague: it is important you do not confront your colleague or talk about your concerns with another colleague. You must report this to your manager.

Someone in the individual's personal network: the information discussed above relates to the people that may be in their 'network'. In other words, they may be family and friends. You must report this to your manager.

Your line manager: it is important that you do not ignore your suspicions or worry about reporting this simply because it is your manager that you suspect; you must follow your organisation's whistle-blowing procedures. (See AC 4.4 for more information about whistle-blowing.)

Others: others may refer to other professionals such as an individual's tutor or physiotherapist.

Again, you must report your suspicions immediately to your manager and you could follow their organisation's whistle-blowing procedures. (See AC 4.4 for more information on whistle-blowing.)

AC 3.2 Explain the actions to take if an individual alleges that they are being abused

When working with individuals, you will get to know them and develop good working relationships with them and their families over time. This means that their trust and confidence in you will grow which may in turn lead to them to confiding in you when things go wrong. For example, an individual may disclose to you that they are being abused or someone they know, such as a family member, may allege that another person is abusing their relative. When this happens it is very important that you are compassionate towards them because the individual may be concerned that they are not going to be taken seriously or believed, or will be blamed for what has happened, and so making a **disclosure** or an allegation has taken a lot of courage and determination on their part.

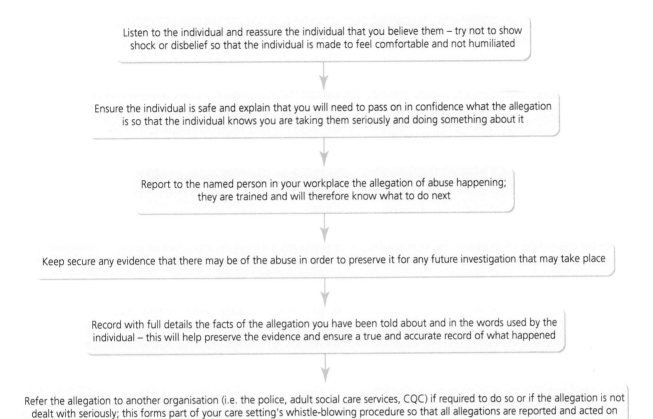

Listen to the individual and reassure the individual that you believe them – try not to show shock or disbelief so that the individual is made to feel comfortable and not humiliated

Ensure the individual is safe and explain that you will need to pass on in confidence what the allegation is so that the individual knows you are taking them seriously and doing something about it

Report to the named person in your workplace the allegation of abuse happening; they are trained and will therefore know what to do next

Keep secure any evidence that there may be of the abuse in order to preserve it for any future investigation that may take place

Record with full details the facts of the allegation you have been told about and in the words used by the individual – this will help preserve the evidence and ensure a true and accurate record of what happened

Refer the allegation to another organisation (i.e. the police, adult social care services, CQC) if required to do so or if the allegation is not dealt with seriously; this forms part of your care setting's whistle-blowing procedure so that all allegations are reported and acted on

Figure 5.4 Actions to take when there are allegations of abuse

The care setting where you work will have in place procedures and agreed ways of working for the actions to take if an individual alleges they are being abused. It is also important, as well as knowing what actions to take, that you understand the reasons why it is important to take these actions and the consequences of not doing so. Figure 5.4 will help you with developing your understanding of the key actions to take and why these are important.

Believe them if they report abuse

Individuals may not report abuse because they worry about what will happen, or worry that no one will believe them. It is important that you listen carefully when someone tells you about any abuse they are suffering. Reassure them, be compassionate and make sure that they know you believe them. If they do not want you to tell anybody else, then remember that this is one area where you may not be able to keep information confidential. You should politely and calmly explain that you will need to speak to and tell your

manager first and foremost about what they have told you, but reassure them that they will be kept informed, they will be asked before information is shared with anyone else and will be kept part of the process for safeguarding them.

Explain that you will need to pass on in confidence what the allegation is

By doing this, you can show that the individual knows you are taking them seriously and doing something about it. As we discussed above, you should explain that you will need to tell your manager. Reassure them that you will all help to protect them.

Confidentiality may be an issue here as the individual may have shared some very private information and it has taken a long time to report the abuse to just one person and so sharing information beyond telling you may be asking a lot of them. The basic rules to remember around confidentiality when someone has alleged abuse are as follows:

1 Always tell the individual who you will need to share allegations of abuse with – you should do this before you share the information.

2 Share the information only with your manager in the first instance.

3 Check with the individual first that it is okay for you to tell others who will be able to provide support and advice. Remember what you learned in Unit 206 about sharing information on 'need-to-know' terms.

4 If the individual does not consent or give you permission to share information with anyone besides your manager, tell your manager, who will advise on the next course of action.

  - Sometimes there is simply nothing you can do if the individual has said 'no' to sharing information.

  - Or, it may be that you need to breach confidentiality if the individual's life is in danger, or if a serious crime has taken place that puts the lives of others in danger. However, you must tell the individual who you will need to tell and why.

Also see Unit 203, AC 1.1 on the Data Protection Act 1998/General Data Protection Regulation 2018.

There may also be issues around capacity that you will face here, for example if an individual lacks capacity to make decisions. Also see Unit 205 for more information on capacity.

Consent

As mentioned above, consent may be another issue that you will face if the individual refuses to allow you to share information. However, it may not just be that the individual does not allow you to share information but that they refuse any action that will prevent further abuse. This can happen even if they have alleged abuse – they may have wanted to tell you about the abuse, which may have relieved some of the stress they feel, but are just too frightened about any further action and treatment. For example, they may not want police protection or their home searched, they may fear the abuser, or they may not want to be examined.

Effective communication of information about the next steps and the reasons for these will be key. Remember to provide lots of reassurance, remind the individual that they are not at fault and that you will all do everything you can to help and protect them. You will have to explain procedures carefully if individuals need to be medically examined, or you could ask medically trained colleagues to speak to the individuals as they may be best placed to provide advice here.

Also, as we discussed in the section on suspicions, there will be questions around capacity and you should refer to page 167 again here.

Empower individuals in the safeguarding process

If abuse is identified, you can empower individuals in the safeguarding process by discussing the different options for tackling the issue, including the benefits and potential risks. This is important because in this way individuals can make their own informed choices and remain in control.

Protect individuals during the safeguarding process

You can do this by ensuring that individuals have access to support and representation during the safeguarding process when they require it. For example, this may include an independent advocate and can be before or after they have reported abuse or neglect. This is important because in this way individuals will feel supported during the safeguarding process and are less likely to withdraw from the process or feel anxious.

Report the allegation of abuse

First, you will need to tell your manager or the named person in your workplace who is trained and therefore knows what to do next. Your setting will have its own policies and procedures for the recording and reporting of information. Normally there will be a report form you need to complete which will include very precise information about the allegation, such as who made the allegation, when, how and to whom. It will also require details of any actions taken such as a medical examination and whether anyone else has been consulted, for example a GP. You will also need to include any information or actions that may not have been taken and still need to be taken.

Keep any evidence secure

This is in order to preserve it for any future investigation that may take place. See AC 3.3 for more information on this.

Record with full details the facts of the allegation

As we discussed in AC 3.1, make sure you record what you have been told about and in the words used by the individual – again this will help preserve the evidence and ensure a true and accurate record of what happened.

As with suspicions, remember to record with full details the facts of the allegation – what you have been told, in the words they have used. You can record the details in written form or make an audio recording. If recorded verbally, then make a written report afterwards. Remember not to confuse the facts of what you have been told with any opinion. Accuracy and detail are key. It may be that you cannot get all the facts and information when the individual first makes the allegation, but either way you will need to accurately record what you have been told and then follow up these points once you have more information. Make sure you record information at the earliest opportunity so that you do not forget the exact details. This will be especially important if you need to make a statement to the police or in court later on.

Refer the allegation to another organisation

If required to do so, you may need to refer an allegation to the police, adult social care services or the CQC. You may need to do this if the allegation is not dealt with seriously by the care setting. This forms part of your care setting's whistle-blowing procedure so that all allegations are reported and acted on. When referring the allegation, you should make sure that you provide as much information as possible. Your setting may have its own referral form but usually this will include details of the alleged abuse, actions that have been taken, information around consent and capacity, whether the individual knows you have referred them and background information. You should, however, refer to your own setting's referral form for a better idea of what one looks like.

Work in partnership

You can do this by ensuring that you work together in partnership with individuals and others. This will include the individual's family, friends and advocates, as well as your colleagues, manager and other professionals. For example, you can ensure that you share information so that you can all work to protect the individual in the most efficient way and only use ways of working that are person-centred. This concept is covered in Unit 211. This is important because in this way you will all be working together to **care** for and support the individual and therefore make it less likely for the individual to be abused or neglected. As you get to know the individual, you will also be more likely to notice any unusual changes that may indicate that something is wrong. Working in partnership will also help with this as you will be able to learn more about the individual from others who know them well.

Be willing to account for your actions

You will need to take your role and responsibilities in safeguarding individuals seriously; this means accepting that you must account for all your actions. You can do this by ensuring that you attend safeguarding training and apply what you have learned in your day-to-day practices when working alongside individuals and others as well as by spending time and making the effort to get to know the individuals that you care for and support. This is important because in this way you are ensuring that you are maintaining your expertise in safeguarding and recognising its importance as part of your role.

When handling allegations of abuse it is really important that you know how to do this both professionally and sensitively as doing so will make an enormous difference to the experience that the individual has sharing this personal information with you. Showing good practice when an individual alleges that they are being abused is very important.

6Cs

Compassion

Compassion is essential when an individual alleges that they are being abused because without it the individual will be left feeling devalued, humiliated and at worst may even feel that what has happened to them is all their fault. Compassion involves putting yourself in the place of the individual and considering how you would feel if you shared a very intimate detail about something that happened to you with someone you trust and you were not believed or taken seriously. You can show your compassion when an individual alleges they are being abused by acknowledging what they tell you, giving them reassurance that they have done the right thing and telling them what you are going to do next so that they know that they have been listened to and taken seriously.

Care

Good care involves working in ways that are consistently positive and supportive. In relation to safeguarding individuals, working together with others to provide good care ensures that individuals' rights and safety are promoted in a consistent way by everyone. Care also promotes the well-being of individuals. Telling them about what safeguarding means, and what abuse is, can even help to prevent abuse or neglect as well as create awareness of the actions that can be taken if their rights to live safely are violated or disrespected.

	Dos and don'ts for when an individual alleges abuse
Do	Show that you believe what an individual is saying.
Do	Listen to what the individual is telling you without interrupting or questioning them. Give the individual time to talk to you and share with you how they are feeling and make sure they can see that you are listening. Refer to Unit 203, Communication in care settings.
Do	Let the individual lead the conversation.
Do	Reassure the individual that they have done the right thing by telling you. Sit with them and explain what actions you are going to take next.
Do	Inform the individual why you must report the allegations of abuse and to whom. Reassure them that all information shared will be in strictest confidence. It is also important that you ask your care setting to keep you informed of what actions have been taken and decisions reached so that you know it has been dealt with appropriately and the individual is protected.
Do	Encourage the individual to allow you to share information if they say they do not want you to. Calmly explain the reasons and benefits of sharing information.
Do	Ensure the individual is not left alone with the person they are alleging they have been abused by. This will usually involve the person accused of the abuse not being able to visit the individual until the investigation into the allegations of abuse is complete.
Do	Record all allegations of abuse made to you fully and accurately. The care setting where you work will have a form that you will be required to complete; it is important that you do so and that you keep it confidential so that the correct information is provided on which actions can be taken quickly to ensure the safety of the individual. The information you record must also be documented legibly and only contain the facts of what was disclosed to you; again, this will help with establishing what happened to the individual.
Don't	Look shocked as this may be misinterpreted by the individual as you not believing them.
Don't	Ask lots of questions.
Don't	Tell the individual that you will not share information when you know you have to. Be honest in your interactions to maintain trust in your relationship.
Don't	Move the individual from the person because this may make the individual feel that they are to blame.

3.2 Recording abuse

Carry out some research in the care setting where you work to find out about the records that you are required to complete when an individual makes an allegation of abuse.

Discuss with your manager the information that you are required to document as well as the reasons why and how you should do this in line with your care setting's agreed ways of working.

Evidence opportunity

3.2 Actions to take when abuse is alleged

Discuss with your assessor the actions to take if an individual in your care setting alleges that they are being abused. Remember to explain the reasons for your actions.

AC 3.3 Identify ways to ensure that evidence of abuse is preserved

You will also have a role to play in ensuring all evidence related to a suspicion and an allegation of abuse is preserved.

Why is preserving evidence of abuse important?

Preserving evidence is important:

- so that an investigation into what happened can take place (you may need this for further investigation in the setting or you may need to pass this on to the police)
- because evidence can support any suspicions you have and allegations that have been made
- so that the person carrying out the abuse can be prosecuted and brought to justice.

What evidence of abuse can be preserved and how?

- **Body fluids**: in the case of sexual abuse, bodily fluids that can be used as evidence include blood and semen left on the individual, on

Evidence opportunity

3.3 Preserving evidence

Discuss with your assessor your role and responsibilities when preserving evidence of suspicions and allegations of abuse. What are your employer's expectations of you when putting these into practice? Why?

clothing and bed linen. You can ensure the individual does not have a bath or shower, have contact with other people and ensure that the affected items are not touched or washed. It may even be that the individual should not remove the clothing if the abuse has just taken place. In this way, this evidence can be preserved. If possible, others should not be allowed to enter the area where the abuse has taken place.

- **Broken items or personal possessions** can be used as evidence. You should make sure that there is no attempt to clean or remove these. They should be left exactly as you found them and you should not allow anyone else to clean or remove these items.

- **Photographs**: photos of people's living environments can be used as evidence of neglect.

- **Witness testimonies**: these may be used as evidence for physical abuse that may not necessarily have left a visible injury.

- **Records**: previous records that you have made about suspicions or allegations can also be shared as evidence. This is why it is very important to record, sign and date any details of this nature straight away – as you will be less likely to forget what you have been told, the record will be more accurate and it cannot be altered later.

- **Prints**: in the case of financial abuse (fraud or theft), financial documents such as bank statements, or statements of transfer can be used. Fingerprints and footprints on items can also be preserved by ensuring that people are not allowed to touch anything or to enter the area where the abuse is suspected or alleged to have taken place.

LO3 Knowledge, skills, behaviours
Knowledge: do you know what to do if you suspect or an individual alleges they are being abused?
Do you know why it is important to take all suspicions of abuse seriously?
Do you know the first thing to do after an individual makes a disclosure of abuse to you?
Do you know why it is important to preserve all evidence of abuse?
Did you know that you have just answered three questions about the importance of responding to abuse?
Skills: how can you show that you are able to respond to suspicions and allegations of abuse?
Do you know how to record suspicions and allegations of abuse accurately?
Do you know how to ensure you follow your agreed ways of working for preserving evidence of abuse?
Did you know that you have just answered two questions about a few of the skills you need in relation to responding to suspicions and allegations of abuse?
Behaviours: how can you show the personal qualities you have when responding to abuse?
Do you know how to listen attentively when an individual tells you they have been abused?
Do you know how to remain calm when reporting abuse?
Do you know how to act professionally when preserving evidence of abuse?
Did you know that you have just answered three questions about some of the essential behaviours that are expected for responding to suspected and alleged abuse?

LO4 Understand the national and local context of safeguarding and protection from abuse

Getting started

Think about a case of abuse you have heard about in the media. You may have read about a case in the newspaper or heard about it on television. What happened? Which organisations were involved in safeguarding the individual? For example, adult social care services or the police?

Now think about the care setting where you work; who safeguards the individuals you provide care or support to in your care setting? What is your role?

AC 4.1 Identify relevant legislation, national policies and local systems that relate to safeguarding and protection from abuse

Safeguarding the individuals you work with also involves learning about the key legislation, national policies and local systems that are in place for safeguarding adults. Legislation, policies and systems change and are updated and so it is important that you keep your knowledge up to date so that you can ensure your knowledge and work practices in relation to safeguarding

individuals is up to date. You can do this by, for example attending training updates and reading through any information updates provided by your employer and referring to the Government's website (www.gov.uk) on a regular basis. You should also refer to Unit 207 on personal development and keeping up to date with your knowledge and work practices.

Legislation

Table 5.2 provides some useful information about the current legislation that exists in relation to safeguarding adults.

Table 5.2 Legislation and how it safeguards individuals

Legislation	How it safeguards adults
Modern Slavery Act 2015	• Aimed at tackling slavery, servitude and forced or compulsory labour in the UK • Addresses issues such as human trafficking and the exploitation of people
Care Act 2014	• Identifies the ten types of abuse and neglect that individuals may experience • States that individuals' safety and well-being must be promoted to safeguard them from abuse and neglect • States that organisations must work in partnership to keep individuals safe • States that effective safeguarding policies and procedures must be developed • Established the role of **Safeguarding Adults Boards** • States that individuals must have access to representation during the safeguarding process, for example access to an **advocate**. The right to an advocate is one of the areas specifically covered in the legislation
Health and Social Care Act 2012	• States that services such as health and social services (now adult social care services) must work in partnership to improve the care provided to individuals • Established the role of **clinical commissioning groups (CCGs)** to safeguard individuals who access health and social care services, for example by responding to abuse and neglect that takes place, undertaking inquiries or reviews of services where abuse or neglect has taken place • Established the role of **health and well-being boards** to oversee the provision of services in each local area
Equality Act 2010	• Safeguards individuals from unfair treatment and discrimination • Makes it unlawful to discriminate against individuals based on one of the following protected characteristics: age, disability, gender reassignment, marriage and civil partnership, pregnancy and maternity, race, religion or belief, sex and sexual orientation
Safeguarding Vulnerable Groups Act 2006	• Established the **vetting and barring scheme** that prevents people who are not suitable to work with individuals with care or support needs from doing so • Established the Independent Safeguarding Authority (ISA) which later merged with the Criminal Records Bureau (CRB) to become the **Disclosure and Barring Service (DBS)**

Mental Capacity Act 2005	• Safeguards individuals who are unable to make choices and decisions for themselves because they lack the capacity to do so, i.e. due to an illness or a disability
	• Based on five key principles:
	  1 Always assume that individuals are able to make their own decisions; never assume that they do not have the capacity to do so
	  2 Support individuals so that they can make their own choices and decisions
	  3 Respect individuals' rights to make decisions that others may not agree with
	  4 All decisions made on an individual's behalf, i.e. when they lack capacity, must always be in their best interests
	  5 Decisions made on an individual's behalf must be the least restrictive option, i.e. the option that promotes the individual's rights as much as possible

Mental Health Act 1983/2007	• Gives rights to individuals with mental health needs • Promotes individuals' rights when being assessed and treated in hospital, for example consent to medical treatment • Promotes individuals' rights when being treated in the community, for example receiving aftercare
Human Rights Act 1998	• Gives rights to every individual who lives in the UK • Promotes individuals' rights to respect, freedom, privacy, equality, dignity and fairness • Includes individuals' rights to live safely, independently and not to be harmed or treated cruelly
Female Genital Mutilation Act 2003	• Made it illegal to perform female genital mutilation (FGM), including assisting a girl to mutilate her own genitalia • Extended the previous legislation by making it an illegal act for UK nationals to perform FGM outside the UK

➜

Table 5.2 Legislation and how it safeguards individuals *continued*

Legislation	How it safeguards adults
Data Protection Act 1998	• Promotes individuals' rights to security over the use of their personal information by others, for example restricts who can access their data, how long it can be kept for • Promotes individuals' rights to privacy over the use of their personal information by others, for example gives individuals' rights to access their own data and ensure it is accurate and up to date • Replaced by the GDPR (mentioned below) in 2018
General Data Protection Regulation 2018	• Replaces the Data Protection Act 1998 • See Unit 206, Handle information in care settings, AC 1.1, for more information
Public Interest Disclosure Act 1998	• Protects workers who disclose information about malpractice including abuse at their current or former workplace for example by ensuring organisations have **whistle-blowing** procedures in place • Promotes individuals' rights to be protected from abuse or harm by ensuring any suspicions or allegations of abuse can be reported by workers free from fear of repercussions from their employers

Key terms

Safeguarding Adults Boards safeguard adults with care or support needs by overseeing local adult safeguarding systems and ensuring all organisations work in partnership. See AC 4.2 for more information on these.

An **advocate** is an independent person who supports an individual to express their views and interests when they are unable to do so themselves.

Clinical commissioning groups (CCGs) are organisations that are responsible for the provision of NHS services in England.

Health and well-being boards are health and social care organisations that work together to improve the health and well-being of the people living in the local area they are responsible for.

The **vetting and barring scheme** ensures that anyone who is not fit or appropriate to work with adults and children does not do so.

The **Disclosure and Barring Service (DBS)** is a government service that makes background checks for organisations, on people who want to work with children and adults with care or support needs.

Whistle-blowing refers to when a person exposes any kind of information or activity that is deemed illegal, unethical or not correct, for example unsafe practices, abuse, harm.

Research it

4.1 Legislation

There are various other pieces of legislation that protect people from abuse. These include the Sexual Offences Act 2003, the Health and Safety at Work Act 1974, Mental Health Act 1983, Family Law Act 1996, Criminal Justice Act 1998, Care Standards Act 2000, Protection of Vulnerable Groups 2007, Protection from Harassment 1997, Fraud Act 2006 and Office of the Public Guardian.

Research three pieces of legislation that are relevant to safeguarding and protecting adults from abuse. For each one, identify the reasons why they are relevant. Produce a poster with your findings.

You will find the UK Government's website a useful source of information:

www.gov.uk

You may wish to do some research into how health and social care policy has evolved over the years. You may like to read 'Our Health, Our Care, Our Say'.

National policies and local systems

As well as legislation there are also policies that apply nationally across England. There are also **local systems** (see page 178 for more information) in place for safeguarding adults who have care or support needs. Table 5.3 gives you some examples of both.

Table 5.3 National policies and local systems, and how they safeguard adults

National safeguarding policies	How they safeguard adults
Safeguarding Adults: A National Framework of Standards for Good Practice and Outcomes in Adult Protection Work 2011	Published by the **Association of Directors of Adult Social Services (ADASS)** (see page 178 for more information). It safeguards individuals by providing best practice guidance to those in leadership roles in services. This is so that individuals who have care or support needs can have access to (care and support) services that are more effective in terms of safeguarding them from abuse and neglect.
A Vision for Adult Social Care: Capable Communities and Active Citizens 2010	Published by the Department of Health (DoH). Promotes individuals' rights to take control of their care by ensuring information about care services is made available to individuals, therefore making them less likely to be abused or harmed. Promotes working in partnership between individuals and other agencies to ensure individuals are active partners in their care, for example in care services, housing services, the NHS. This is to reduce individuals' risk of being abused or neglected.
Think Personal: Act Local 2010	Established as a national initiative that ensures individuals who have care or support needs are the focus in their care or support, for example by promoting person-centred ways of working. Promotes individuals and other agencies working in partnership to provide effective care and support services that are person-centred.
Deprivation of Liberty Safeguards (DOLS) 2008	Safeguards individuals from having their liberty deprived unlawfully. For example, a setting such as a care home is required to seek authorisation to deprive an individual of their liberty because they feel it is in the individual's best interests.
Dignity in Care 2006	An ongoing campaign that aims to improve the quality of care or support individuals receive in adult care services. Promotes person-centred ways of working that include showing respect for individuals' rights to make their own choices and decisions thus reducing their risk of being abused or harmed.
Professional Registration and Standards	Requires professionals, for example doctors, nurses and social workers, to register with a professional body so that they can ensure they are practising to the current standards and continuing their professional development. Organisations such as **Skills for Care** (see page 178 for more information) publish codes of conduct and standards for adult care workers so that they can comply with best practice standards when carrying out their job role. For example, the Code of Conduct for Healthcare Support Workers and Adult Social Care Workers in England, The Care Certificate Standard 10 Safeguarding Adults. The Care Quality Commission regulates adult care services and sets the fundamental standards of quality and safety for all those organisations registered with it who provide care services. These fundamental standards are essential for preventing abuse, harm and neglect of adults.

→

Table 5.3 National policies and local systems, and how they safeguard adults *continued*

Local safeguarding systems	How it safeguards adults
Safeguarding Adults Boards	Local authorities are responsible for setting up a Safeguarding Adults Board (SAB).
	Provides strategies to safeguard individuals but also to deal with issues that affect specific individuals. For example, they can decide that they need to increase awareness of abuse in the local area through publicity or they may deal with complaints around abuse against a care worker in a setting.
	Made up, for example, of different agencies including the police, housing, transport, all of whom can bring their expertise to a situation. This is what is meant by multi-agency working which we discussed earlier in AC 4.2.
	A SAB is responsible for arranging a Safeguarding Adults Review (SAR) when an adult in its locality dies as a result of being abused or neglected or if there are suspicions that an adult may have experienced abuse or neglect because agencies such as care services or health services could have worked together more effectively.
Organisations' policies and procedures	All adult care services are required to have safeguarding policies and procedures in place – ones that define the different types of abuse and neglect, set out how individuals will be safeguarded, how to report concerns and arrangements for whistle-blowing.

Key terms

Local systems may include employers' safeguarding policies and procedures as well as multi-agency protection arrangements for your local area, for example a Safeguarding Adults Board.

The **Association of Directors of Adult Social Services (ADASS)** is a charity whose members are active directors of social care services and whose aim is to promote high standards of social care services.

Skills for Care is the sector skills council for people working in social work and social care for adults and children in the UK as well as for workers in early years, children and young people's services. It sets standards and develops qualifications for those working in the sector.

Evidence opportunity

4.1 Legislation

Research and reflect on the national policies and systems that are in place that influence the safeguarding arrangements at the care setting where you work. Why are these important? How do they impact on your ability to safeguard and protect the individuals you provide care for?

Make some notes on your thoughts and then produce a one-page information handout that identifies examples of relevant legislation, national policies and local systems that are in place to safeguard and protect adults from abuse.

AC 4.2 Explain the roles of different agencies in safeguarding and protecting individuals from abuse

As you will know, safeguarding and protecting individuals from abuse is achieved by agencies working together in partnership. The important work of these agencies recognises that:

- all individuals must be supported to be in control of their lives; this includes also being in control of their care or support
- all individuals have a right to live their lives in safety and free from abuse or being at risk of abuse
- everyone has a role to play in preventing abuse from happening and responding to abuse when it occurs.

Below are some examples of the roles of different agencies that have an important role to play in safeguarding and protecting individuals from abuse.

Local authorities (adult social care services) are responsible for overseeing and co-ordinating how different agencies work in partnership to safeguard and protect individuals from abuse. Local authorities are responsible for setting up Safeguarding Adults Boards so that they can ensure that all agencies are working together in partnership. One of the reasons local authorities manage how agencies are working together is to ensure individuals are being safeguarded and protected from abuse. They will ensure that all the agencies are working to the same consistent standards and ensuring positive outcomes for all individuals with care or support needs.

Safeguarding Adults Boards are responsible for working with agencies in each local authority to ensure they develop effective systems for safeguarding and protecting individuals from abuse. Safeguarding Adults Boards can safeguard and protect individuals from abuse by ensuring that agencies work in consistent ways, for example by sharing information about individuals who may be at risk of abuse. They can respond to abuse quickly and ensure they work in partnership to ensure individuals' rights, safety and well-being are protected by all agencies working with them. Safeguarding Adults Boards also promote agencies working together to share good practice so that they can learn from one another.

Health and social care settings are responsible for developing policies, procedures and agreed ways of working to ensure individuals are safeguarded and protected from abuse. Each service has a responsibility to ensure, for example, that their care workers are fully trained in safeguarding and the protection of individuals from abuse. In addition, they ensure that care workers have effective agreed ways of working in place, for example to inform the individuals they care for about what abuse is so that the individuals can be in control of their care and support and therefore less likely to be abused.

The Care Quality Commission is responsible for regulating the provision of health and care services by monitoring care and support services to ensure they safeguard and protect individuals from abuse. The Care Quality Commission also helps to safeguard and protect individuals from abuse by ensuring that best practice is highlighted and shared with, for example, organisations and Safeguarding Adults Boards. They can also raise their concerns with Safeguarding Adults Boards if they find a service is placing individuals at risk of being abused.

Voluntary agencies are responsible for providing independent advice and support to individuals, their families and workers in relation to safeguarding and protection from abuse. These can include Action on Elder Abuse, ADASS, and whistle-blowing helplines. Voluntary agencies can provide useful information and much needed support; for example, when an individual is being abused or an individual's family is worried that they may be at risk of being abused.

The police are responsible for responding to reported actual abuse, to individuals at risk of abuse or investigating incidents of abuse or alleged abuse. The police are also a useful source of information on what action to take if you think an individual is at risk of abuse or how to minimise the risk of an individual being abused. For example, the police can raise awareness about fraudulent scams that are operating in their area or provide advice on how individuals can make their homes more secure.

Evidence opportunity

4.2 Roles of different agencies

Research the safeguarding procedures in place for the local authority where your care setting is located. Find out about the different agencies that your local authority works in partnership with to safeguard adults from abuse. You will find your local authority's website a useful source of information. Discuss the roles of each agency with your manager and obtain a witness testimony.

Produce a leaflet that explains the roles of these different agencies, the professionals who work for them and how the different agencies work together. Include the key responsibilities for safeguarding and protecting the individuals for who you provide care.

AC 4.3 Identify factors which have featured in reports into serious cases of abuse and neglect

When safeguarding systems and the agencies who work together to safeguard adults from abuse and neglect are not as effective as they should be then this has very serious consequences that can result in serious failures to safeguard and protect individuals from abuse. It is these serious failures that are reported in the media and through which the public becomes aware of how care and support services for individuals can fail them. You may have heard of some of the following examples where care has gone wrong and where settings failed to protect individuals from abuse:

- Wyton Abbey Residential Home – where an individual with dementia who was on a two-week stay at the care home did not receive the care and treatment he required, which resulted in his death
- Winterbourne View Hospital – where individuals with learning disabilities were abused and neglected by the staff who worked there
- Purbeck Care Home – where individuals at a care home were abused by staff.

After a serious failure in safeguarding to protect individuals from abuse has occurred a Safeguarding Adults Review will take place. It is a detailed process that reviews:

- the abuse that happened
- how it happened
- what allowed it to happen
- how it could have been prevented
- what needs to be changed in order to prevent it from happening again
- the key lessons learned.

Safeguarding Adults Reviews also review the services provided by each organisation.

Once the Safeguarding Adults Review (previously known as a Serious Case Review) is completed, a report into its findings is published and made public so that everyone can learn from its key findings and prevent abuse from occurring again.

For example:

- The Serious Case Review report published for the abuse of people with learning difficulties at Winterbourne View Hospital found that the abuse that happened was in the main due to professionals and others not responding to incidents of abuse that took place, not challenging poor working practices as well as not understanding their own and one another's roles and responsibilities.
- The Serious Case Review report published for the abuse of Stephen Hoskin found that the abuse that happened was mainly due to the agencies supporting Stephen not sharing information they had received about the concerns that there were about Stephen's safety. In addition, the professionals supporting Stephen did not recognise the signs that he was being abused and therefore did not respond to his cries for help, which included repeatedly phoning emergency services.

Responding to abuse is everyone's responsibility and although we can all learn lessons from reports published into serious failures to protect individuals from abuse, it is important that you are able to recognise and respond to individuals at risk from abuse so that you can safeguard and protect them from being abused and neglected.

Reflect on it

4.3 Abuse reported in the media

Reflect on a case of abuse and neglect you have heard about in the media. For example, this may be one of the care settings listed above, or perhaps another example reported in your local area. How did the news report make you feel?

Now imagine you were the individual or a member of this individual's family – how do you think this made them feel?

4.3 Factors that have featured in reports

Research a Safeguarding Adults Review that has been published following a case of an individual or individuals who have been abused.

Read through this and then produce an information leaflet on the different factors that featured in the abuse and neglect.

You will find the internet a useful source of information; each local authority will also publish all the reports that it has completed on its website.

AC 4.4 Identify sources of information and advice about your role in safeguarding and protecting individuals from abuse, including whistle-blowing

To understand your role and responsibilities in safeguarding and protecting individuals from abuse you may need to seek further information and advice from the care setting where you work. This can include:

- **Your manager** will be able to guide you on how carry out the job you are employed to do in ways that safeguard individuals and protect them from abuse. Your manager can guide you with any aspect you are unsure about or arrange extra training around safeguarding. (Your manager can also advise you on how your job role fits in with other professionals and the agencies you work with.)

- **Your colleagues** will be able to inform you of the procedures to follow if you have concerns about an individual or if you witness unsafe practices that may lead to an individual being abused or placed at risk of abuse. More experienced colleagues may also be able to provide you with advice about your responsibilities for safeguarding and protecting individuals from abuse.

- **Safeguarding policies and procedures** will provide you with information about the agreed ways of working that you must follow in your care setting. They will detail the process to follow if you have concerns that an individual is being abused or is at risk of being abused. They will also include information about the whistle-blowing procedures in place including the external organisations you can seek support from if your concerns are not taken seriously.

- **Safeguarding training** provided to you will ensure that you keep yourself up to date with how to ensure that your working practices reflect best practice and current legislation for safeguarding and protecting individuals.

Other sources of information and advice can also be accessed through external organisations, such as the Care Quality Commission, who will be able to respond to any concerns you have relating to an individual being abused or at risk of being abused. Similarly, if you believe that there are failures within the care setting where you work and they are *not* being taken seriously or *not* being responded to effectively, then you can report your concerns to them. They also issue guidance on how to be a **whistle-blower**. The Care Quality Commission's website frequently publishes reports of both good practices and serious failures in the provision of care and support services to individuals.

- **The police** will be able to provide you with information and advice about what to do if an individual is being abused or is at risk of being abused, including whether a criminal act has been committed and whether any unsafe practices you may have concerns about are unlawful.

- **The local authority** adult care services department will be able to provide you with information and advice about what to do if you have concerns that an individual is being abused or is at risk of being abused. Each local authority will also have information on its website about the role and purpose of its

Safeguarding Adults Board, good practice guidance for safeguarding individuals from abuse to be shared with all agencies as well as reports based on the findings from Safeguarding Adults Reviews completed within the local area.

- **Independent organisations** whose role is to provide information and advice on best practice when safeguarding individuals from abuse, including the most effective ways of working for achieving positive outcomes for individuals. For example, the Social Care Institute for Excellence (SCIE), the Carers Direct Helpline, and whistle-blowing helplines.

Whistle-blowing

To whistle-blow means to report any unsafe or illegal working practices used in your setting. One of the key concepts of whistle-blowing is that you must have reasonable belief that disclosure is in the interest of the public. Remember, sources of information and advice about whistle-blowing can be obtained – from both your place of work and sources outside of work as mentioned above.

Whistle-blowers receive protection. For example, the employment rights or career of a whistle-blower will not be affected as a result of them reporting unsafe practice. Legislation is also in place to protect a whistle-blower (see the legislation section at the end of this unit). Your care setting will have a whistle-blowing policy and procedures in place for advice on what to do.

Remember that you have a duty of care to report any unsafe and illegal practice, even though it may seem scary to report the people you work with. If you feel you are unable to speak to the manager in your care setting then you can report your concerns to someone more senior or go directly to the Care Quality Commission. You can do this by telephoning them or emailing them with your concern(s). All information you share will be treated as confidential – and if you prefer you can do this anonymously, (this means that you do not have to leave your name or contact details when you email or telephone).

Anything you suspect that is of a criminal nature should still be discussed with your manager first, but you must then contact the police about this.

If your report is about the setting where you work and not just a colleague, then you may need to go directly to the CQC. Obviously, if there are minor concerns that you feel you are able to speak to your manager about, then you should discuss these with them first. If however, the concerns are of a more serious nature such as failures to care for individuals on the part of the setting, you may need to go directly to the CQC. You should also refer to the section on institutional abuse in AC 1.3.

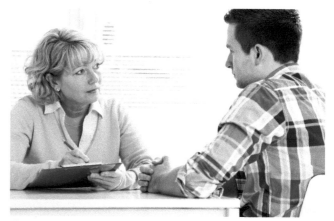

Figure 5.5 How can you raise your concerns about unsafe practices at work?

Research it

4.4 Whistle-blowing guidance

Research the guidance: 'Whistleblowing: Quick guide to raising a concern with the CQC', which can be accessed from the CQC's website:

www.cqc.org.uk/contact-us/report-concern/report-concern-if-you-are-member-staff

Discuss the key points from this document with a colleague.

Evidence opportunity

4.4 Sources of information

Develop a poster that identifies your role in safeguarding and how to source information and advice when protecting individuals from abuse. Use examples of both internal (in the work setting) and external (an organisation separate to your work setting) sources of information.

AC 4.5 Identify when to seek support in situations beyond your experience and expertise

Safeguarding and protecting individuals from abuse is part of your duty of care and responsibility as an adult care worker. At the same time, you cannot expect to know everything about abuse. Doing nothing is not an option,

therefore should a situation arise where you have no experience (or it is outside your area of expertise) it is important to seek help.

There may be times when you do not have experience and the expertise in something and you just do not know how to respond to a situation. Table 5.4 provides you with examples of situations when you will need to seek further support from either or both internal and external sources.

Table 5.4 Situations where you may need to seek support

When to seek support	The reasons for seeking support
You are dealing with a situation where a crime has been committed.	You will need to seek support from police when a crime is committed, for example when an individual has been burgled and has had their property damaged. You may not have expertise in how to handle this situation and how to preserve evidence.
You are dealing with a situation which requires a medical procedure which you have no knowledge of or skills in.	You may need to contact a medical professional when you do not know how to carry out a procedure or administer medication, for example when an individual is bleeding from the head. This will ensure the individual receives appropriate medical care and is not placed in danger.
You are dealing with an individual with an illness you have no medical expertise in, such as dementia.	You may need to contact a medical professional, or a charity such as the Alzheimer's Society for more information on supporting an individual with dementia.
You witness an individual's family member shouting at their relative during one of their visits.	Seeking support from your manager will ensure the appropriate actions can be taken and the individual can be protected from any further abuse. By doing this, you are practising your duty of care to safeguard this individual. You can ensure that your safety is also maintained by seeking the support of your manager.
You report your concerns of an individual in your care setting being at risk of abuse from a colleague and your manager is too busy to deal with this.	Seeking support from an external organisation such as the CQC will ensure that the individual is no longer at risk of abuse. By doing this, you will be protecting this individual's safety as well as others who may be at risk in the care setting where you work.
A colleague asks you to use unsafe practices when supporting an individual being hoisted.	Seeking support from your manager will ensure that you will be supported to not carry out these unsafe practices. This will also raise your colleague's awareness of unsafe practices and the consequences of these. This will ensure the safety and well-being of the individual you are supporting as well as you and your colleague's safety.

Evidence opportunity

4.5 How to ask for support

Discuss with your manager the agreed ways of working to follow when seeking support in two safeguarding situations where you have no experience or that are beyond your area of expertise. Obtain a witness testimony to ensure you can evidence this.

LO4 Knowledge, skills, behaviours
Knowledge: what legislation, policies and systems are in place for safeguarding and protecting individuals from abuse?
Do you know two Acts, national policies and local systems that relate to safeguarding adults from abuse?
Do you know what the safeguarding roles and responsibilities of the other agencies you work with are?
Do you know what sources of information, advice and support are available when safeguarding individuals?
Do you know what your agreed ways of working that relate to safeguarding adults say about your roles and responsibilities?
Do you know about different factors that have featured in reports into serious cases of abuse?
Do you know when to seek support in situations beyond your experience and expertise?
Did you know that you have just answered six questions about the legislative, national and local context of safeguarding adults?
Skills: how can you show that you can comply with safeguarding policies and procedures?
Do you know how to show in your working practices the main lessons learned from serious case reviews about safeguarding and protecting individuals from abuse?
Do you understand your employer's whistle-blowing procedures?
Do you know how to access information, advice and support about safeguarding individuals?
Do you know when to seek support in situations beyond your experience and expertise?
Did you know that you have just answered four questions about some of the skills you have in relation to effectively safeguarding and protecting individuals from abuse?
Behaviours: how can you show the personal qualities you have when safeguarding and protecting individuals from abuse?
Do you know how to work in partnership with others when safeguarding individuals?
Do you know how to respond assertively to situations beyond your experience and expertise?
Did you know that you have just answered two questions about a few of the essential behaviours that are expected from adult care workers when safeguarding and protecting individuals from abuse?

LO5 Understand ways to reduce the likelihood of abuse

Getting started

Think about someone you know that has care or support needs. This may be because of an illness or disability. Why do you think that they are more likely to experience some form of abuse? What do you think makes them vulnerable to abuse?

Now think about what you could do to reduce their likelihood of being abused? For example, how does the way you treat them impact on how they feel about themselves? Does it make them feel confident in themselves and valued? What else could you do to promote their safety and well-being?

AC 5.1 Explain how the likelihood of abuse may be reduced

You can explain how the likelihood of abuse may be reduced by:

- working with person-centred values
- encouraging active participation

- promoting choice and rights
- supporting individuals with awareness of personal safety.

The relevant safeguarding legislation, national policies and local systems you have learned about are what underpin your working practices in the care setting where you work. These together with the way you carry out your day-to-day role and responsibilities can reduce the likelihood of individuals being abused or neglected.

Working with person-centred values

Working with individuals with care or support needs involves working in ways that embed person-centred values. This concept is covered in more detail in Unit 211, Implement person-centred approaches in care settings. Working with person-centred values can reduce the likelihood of abuse. Some examples are listed below.

- **Treating individuals with respect** and showing that you value their individuality will reduce the likelihood of an individual being discriminated against and abused. Respect for individuals and their differences promotes confidence in those that you care for; they are more likely to challenge and speak up about abuse if they are more confident in themselves.

- **Promoting an individual's dignity** means taking precautions to ensure that they do not feel humiliated or intimidated. For example, you can promote an individual's dignity when they have had a bath by closing the door and placing a towel over them. Working in this way will reduce the likelihood of an individual being abused and make the individual feel comfortable about being supported with intimate care by workers. They will also become more aware of how care workers should support them and they will notice in future (and report) when the support they receive does not promote their dignity and rights.

- **Showing compassion** when working with individuals and their families means that you are showing genuine concern in their well-being. For example, you can make time to understand why an individual may be finding it difficult to settle in to their new care setting after living previously in their family home all their life. Working in this way will reduce the likelihood of an individual being abused because they will learn to trust and respect you and therefore be more likely to share any experiences of abuse or

neglect from others. The individual's family will also feel able to approach you with any concerns they might have.

Encouraging active participation

Active participation is a way of working that encourages individuals to be active participants in their care or support rather than passive recipients. It is a way of working that recognises that individuals with care or support needs have the right to participate in day-to-day activities as independently as possible. Encouraging active participation can reduce the likelihood of abuse happening in different ways. Some examples of this are included below.

- Supporting an individual's independence means that you are encouraging individuals to be actively involved in day-to-day activities at home and in their local communities. You can do this by supporting them to develop their skills in managing their money, learning how to cook, going shopping and socialising. Working in this way will reduce the likelihood of an individual being abused because they will not be seen as someone who can be exploited by others. It will also make the individual feel confident in their own abilities and believe in themselves.

- Encouraging individuals to be active in their care or support means working alongside them and letting them guide you as to what is important to them and how they want to be cared for. For example, you can develop an individual's care plan with them; this may mean providing them with all the information they need to decide what activities they would like to participate in – and those that they would not. Working in this way will reduce the likelihood of an individual being abused because using their care plan will ensure that the individual's history, preferences, needs and beliefs are taken into account. Both the setting and the individual will recognise when those needs are not met. Their care or support will be led by the individual rather than the care workers and will therefore make them feel in control of their own care or support. It makes the individual feel empowered rather than like someone who is always dependent on others.

Research it

5.1 Active participation

Carry out some research in the care setting where you work about how active participation is encouraged. You will find it useful to speak to your colleagues and your manager.

Discuss the techniques used, the reasons why these are effective and how they meet individuals' needs.

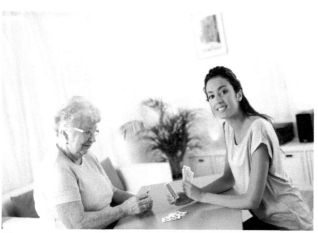

Figure 5.6 How do you encourage active participation?

Promoting choice and rights

Promoting individuals' choices and rights underpins all person-centred ways of working and is effective in reducing the likelihood of abuse happening because it encourages workers to put individuals' needs first and to focus on individuals' best interests rather than on what the workers think may be best. Some examples of how promoting individuals' choices and rights can reduce the likelihood of abuse are included below.

● Promoting an individual's choices means that you are encouraging individuals to think about the options available so that they can make their own choice. For example, by providing them with relevant information about the different ways they can travel to visit a friend, such as by rail, bus or taxi, in order that they can then consider all the information available to them and then make a decision based on what they prefer to do. Working in this way will reduce the likelihood of abuse because

it encourages individuals to be more bold and assertive not just in their behaviour but confident in themselves.

● Promoting an individual's rights means treating individuals as you would like to be treated, that is on equal terms, with all the same rights that you have. Working in this way will reduce the likelihood of abuse because you will be informing and raising individual's awareness about what is fair and equal treatment (in terms of their care or support), empowering the individual to feel in control and know when their treatment is not fair and equal.

Actively supporting individuals to fulfil their rights in your day-to-day working, for example by supporting their safety at home when mobilising and supporting their well-being at all times, will reduce the likelihood of abuse because you will be supporting their rights to be safe. In this way, they will develop their own understanding of their rights, how to stay safe and how they can be supported by those who work around them.

Supporting individuals with awareness of personal safety

Awareness of personal safety can be a very effective way of supporting individuals to be in control of their own safety and therefore reduce the likelihood of them being abused. Some examples of supporting individuals with awareness of personal safety are set out below.

● Promoting personal safety when working alongside individuals can be a very effective way to increase an individual's knowledge about how to stay safe. You can do this by providing information leaflets about the dangers that exist in the home, such as not opening the door to people they do not know, checking that the gas is turned off after using the cooker in the evening, not blocking fire escape routes with furniture and not leaving the windows open when leaving home. You can warn them of the dangers that exist in the community, for example remind them not to walk back on their own late at night. Working in this way will reduce the likelihood of abuse because you

5.1 Ways to reduce likelihood of abuse

Produce a leaflet that explains how the following can reduce the likelihood of individuals in the care setting where you work from being abused:

- working with person-centred values
- promoting choice and rights
- supporting individuals with awareness of personal safety
- encouraging active participation.

will be informing individuals about hazards so that they can take precautions to reduce the potential risks these may cause. There is more information about risk assessment in Unit 210, Health, safety and well-being in care settings.

- Supporting an individual's personal safety by involving them in working in safe ways will increase their awareness of personal safety by ensuring they always consider the dangers associated with different activities and the potential risks these pose. They can then use this information to make decisions that do not compromise their safety. Working in this way will reduce the likelihood of abuse because you will be actively supporting individuals to think about and make decisions that put their own safety first.

AC 5.2 Explain the importance of an accessible complaints procedure for reducing the likelihood of abuse

All organisations that provide care or support services are required to have a procedure in place to respond to complaints. A complaints procedure that is accessible means one that can be:

- available in different formats, for example Braille for individuals with vision loss; with signs and symbols for individuals with learning disabilities; in audio for individuals unable to read; in different languages to meet individuals' preferences
- available to all and located in places that can be accessed easily and without having to ask for permission to do so, for example in the entrance hall to a care setting

6Cs

(C)

Communication

Communication is essential for developing good complaints procedures. Effectively communicating your setting's complaints procedures involves ensuring that they can be used effectively by those who need them. You can ensure that this is communicated effectively by reporting when you have any concerns that an individual or someone else may not have understood your care setting's procedures. In this way these procedures can be adapted to meet the individual or someone else's needs and they can access the additional support they require to understand them. This will also increase the likelihood of them using it and decrease the likelihood of them not doing so, which may result in them continuing to be abused or neglected.

- explained and reinforced by the care staff on an ongoing basis in relation to its purpose, what it can be used for and how confidentiality will be maintained when it is used
- reviewed alongside the individuals and others it is aimed at, to ensure its effectiveness.

An accessible complaints procedure can reduce the likelihood of abuse because:

- it empowers individuals to respond to concerns they have about themselves and others
- it brings complaints out into the open so that they can be acted on through effective and clear **communication**
- it increases the confidence of individuals and others in the quality and safety of the care or support being provided – everyone knows that there is a way to report abuse if they need to do so
- it raises individuals' awareness of their rights to good-quality care or support.

Being able to raise concerns over safety or any risk of being abused is an effective and important way of ensuring that health and social care services or other agencies involved in safeguarding individuals are alerted to the potential of abuse happening so that they can act to prevent it.

Evidence opportunity

5.2 Consequences of not having an accessible complaints procedure

Reflect on the consequences of not having an accessible complaints procedure. What impact may this have on the likelihood of abuse happening? Why? Make notes to evidence your reflection. Remember to think about the impact that accessible formats, such as Easy Read, can have.

Then develop a flow diagram that explains how each stage of an accessible complaints procedure can reduce the likelihood of abuse taking place.

AC 5.3 Outline how the likelihood of abuse can be reduced by managing risk and focusing on prevention

Risk enablement is a way of working that reduces the likelihood of abuse happening by using techniques that encourage risk to be managed and focuses on the prevention of abuse.

How can you reduce the likelihood of individuals being abused by managing risk and focusing on prevention?

In AC 5.1, we discussed the different ways in which you can work to reduce the likelihood of abuse happening.

Risk enablement can reduce the likelihood of abuse because it involves using the following techniques and approaches, which you should implement.

Reflect on it

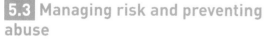

5.3 Managing risk and preventing abuse

Reflect on the consequences of not being able to manage risk effectively. How could this lead to abuse? Reflect on the importance of early prevention of abuse. What are the consequences of not doing so?

- **Encourage individuals to do what they can to protect themselves from being abused and harmed.** Empower them to be active participants and in control of their own care or support. For example, if an individual wants to move freely around their house on their own but has mobility difficulties, risk enablement would support the individual to mobilise safely around their home. You can do this by ensuring the individual has a walking aid and access to a personal alarm (that they can wear and use when on their own) in case of an emergency. Risk enablement enables individuals to do what they want safely; this makes individuals feel listened to and valued while maintaining their safety, thus reducing the likelihood of abuse taking place.

- **Empower individuals to complain when care or support goes wrong.** For example, if an individual knows that care workers must treat him or her with respect at all times then they will be more likely to complain when a care worker does not treat them with respect. As a result of risk enablement, the risk of them not having their rights respected or them being abused is less likely to happen.

- **Support individuals to understand and take managed risks.** For example, risk enablement can mean that an individual is supported to identify any risks that may be associated with an activity that they want to do and then decide whether, having assessed the benefits and consequences of the activity, they still want to do it or whether they need to consider other safety precautions. They can also understand how to manage risks.

- **Enable care settings to focus on the managing of risks and the prevention of abuse.** Risk enablement means that you promote the protection of individuals in your setting. For example, undertake safeguarding training (on the potential signs and symptoms that an individual is being abused) which can help identify abuse early on. You will become more aware of the factors that increase the likelihood of an individual being at risk of abuse and be able to help the setting focus on how the individuals' rights, safety and well-being can be promoted.

Caring for carers

Remember, you can reduce the risk of abuse happening by trying to prevent abuse before it starts and by spotting potential signs of abuse. If you see that carers are under immense pressure to support individuals, then you should offer support and advice to them. Stress and pressures do not mean that abuse will always happen, but spotting it means you are able to address it early on and be there for carers as well as individuals. Be empathetic and if your own work pressures mean that you cannot offer them support daily, then make sure that you tell them about support and services they can access. Not only could this reduce and prevent the likelihood of abuse, but it also means that you are able to build a good empathetic relationship with the carer, one where they feel supported.

Research it

5.3 Support carers in a practical way

Research the support that is available for carers. You could ask your manager about the sorts of practical support you could offer carers. For example, how can carers be supported with any practical equipment they may need? Do they need a stair lift in their home? Do they need help with daily tasks such as their shopping? Do they need any training for any tasks they do not have the skills to do?

How can you support them with this? How will this support the carer and the individual? How can this help to prevent abuse?

Evidence opportunity

5.3 Managing risk and preventing abuse

Read the Risk Enablement Policy in place in the care setting where you work.

Produce a one-page information handout or a poster that outlines how the likelihood of abuse can be reduced by managing risk and focusing on prevention.

LO5 Knowledge, skills, behaviours
Knowledge: why is reducing the likelihood of abuse important?
Do you know what person-centred values are and how they reduce the likelihood of abuse?
Do you know what rights an individual with care or support needs has and why supporting these can reduce the likelihood of abuse?
Do you know why an accessible complaints procedure is important and why this can reduce the likelihood of abuse?
Do you know how to follow your employer's risk enablement procedures for managing risk and preventing abuse?
Did you know that you have just answered four questions about the importance of reducing the likelihood of abuse?
Skills: how can you show ways of working that reduce the likelihood of abuse?
Do you know how to instil person-centred values in work practices and encourage individuals to be active participants in their care or support?
Do you know how to promote individuals' choices and rights, including to keep safe?
Do you know how to follow your employer's risk enablement procedures for managing risk and preventing abuse?
Did you know that you have just answered three questions about some of the skills you have in relation to working in ways that reduce the likelihood of abuse?
Behaviours: how can you show the personal qualities you have when working in ways that reduce the likelihood of abuse?
Do you know how to be respectful of individuals' choices and rights?
Do you know how to provide individuals with clear information about how they can promote their own personal safety by managing risks?
Do you know how to support individuals to be experts in their own care or support so that they can prevent abuse from happening?
Did you know that you have just answered three questions about some of the essential behaviours that are expected of workers to reduce the likelihood of abuse happening?

LO6 Know how to recognise and report unsafe practices

Think about an occasion when you witnessed something that was unsafe and made you feel uncomfortable. This may have happened at work or outside of your work setting. For example, you may have witnessed one of your colleagues not putting on gloves when supporting an individual to get washed and dressed or witnessed an individual out shopping with their relative and being spoken to in a patronising way.

How did this make you feel? Why? Did you do anything about it? Why?

Think about the benefits of reporting unsafe practices immediately? Now think about the consequences of not doing so. What will you do next time if this situation arises again and why?

AC 6.1 Describe unsafe practices that may affect the well-being of individuals

Being able to recognise unsafe practices when they occur and understand the procedures your care setting has in place for reporting these will help you to ensure that your ways of working focus on the prevention of abuse.

Unsafe practices are those that may lead to an individual, you, a colleague or visitor being placed in danger or at risk of being injured or harmed. Table 5.5 includes examples of three different types of unsafe practice that may occur in a care setting due to poor working practices, resource difficulties and operational difficulties.

All three types of unsafe practice can lead to an individual being subjected to abuse and neglect and therefore have the potential to affect their safety. Table 5.5 includes how unsafe practices may affect the different aspects of an individual's well-being.

Table 5.5 Unsafe practices and how they affect an individual's well-being

Unsafe practices	Examples of how the well-being of an individual is affected
Poor working practices	Poor health and safety practices may lead to accidents in the care setting and have the potential to cause both physical and mental harm to those involved.
	Not taking suspicions of abuse seriously may mean that individuals continue to be abused which can in turn affect their physical, emotional and mental well-being. If the abuse is financial then it will impact on their economic well-being and their trust in others. They may withdraw and become isolated thus having an effect on their social well-being.
	Unsafe practices when moving and handling may lead to individuals, you and your colleagues being injured or harmed physically. In turn, this will impact on the confidence of individuals and others and will have a negative effect on their emotional and mental well-being too.
Resource difficulties	Insufficient or a lack of equipment will mean that individuals' needs will remain unmet. For example, they may be injured, or their independence may be restricted which may in turn mean that their emotional and social well-being is affected because they may have to be more dependent on others.
	Insufficient workers to care for individuals will mean that individuality will not be recognised as there will be insufficient time to attend to every individuals' personal needs. This may mean that the support provided does not take into account their intellectual abilities, cultural and spiritual needs.
	A lack of regular training will mean that a carer's way of working may not reflect current best practice or legislation. They may fail in their duty of care to safeguard individuals, which will have a direct impact on their social, emotional and physical well-being.

➔

Table 5.5 Unsafe practices and how they affect an individual's well-being *continued*

Unsafe practices	Examples of how the well-being of an individual is affected
Operational difficulties	A lack of effective management means that no one is monitoring the care and support provided by workers. This means that the individuals may be subjected to abuse more easily which will impact negatively on their well-being physically, emotionally and socially.
	A lack of support for workers may mean that they cannot respond effectively to situations where they have insufficient expertise. As a result, abuse of an individual may go unnoticed. This can change how an individual feels about themselves, their confidence and their identity, e.g. in terms of their spirituality.
	Poor communication systems with other agencies may mean that the signs that an individual is being abused are not recognised or reported thus enabling the abuse to continue, causing a detrimental effect to the individual's well-being; this could be physically, culturally, emotionally or socially.

Reflect on it

6.1 Unsafe practices

Reflect on how unsafe practices can affect an individual's well-being. How do you think an individual may feel? Why? How do you think you would feel if that were you? Why?

Evidence opportunity

6.1 Unsafe practices and well-being

Develop two case studies for two different individuals who have different care or support needs. For each one write a description about how unsafe practices may affect their well-being.

Being able to recognise unsafe practices is essential for maintaining the safety and well-being of the individuals, your colleagues and others you work with. Not doing so can lead to individuals being abused, the likelihood of accidents occurring and the safety and well-being of individuals being affected which can in turn increase the likelihood of abuse happening.

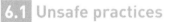

AC 6.2 Explain the actions to take if unsafe practices have been identified

The care setting where you work will have procedures in place for reporting unsafe practices that have been identified. It is your responsibility to ensure that you are familiar with these and to

Research it

6.2 Your job description

Research your job description, your job role and responsibilities. What do these say about your responsibilities towards the individuals you provide care or support to? Others who you work with?

Discuss how you can ensure that your ways of working are safe and fulfil your responsibilities to individuals and others. Make notes about your discussion.

report any unsafe practices that you observe or are told about.

Below is a list of some tips for the actions to take.

1 Follow your employer's procedures and agreed ways of working when unsafe practices have been identified so that the necessary action can be taken to prevent the unsafe practices from continuing to take place or injury or harm to individuals or others.

2 Constructively challenge (in a way that will be useful and beneficial) all unsafe practices so that the person that is carrying these out can understand the reasons why their ways of working are unsafe and how these could lead to the abuse and neglect of individuals or others. It is possible that they are not aware that their way of working is unsafe. Challenge the person constructively, in a calm way because you do not want them to react aggressively, or for them to feel embarrassed because they did not know their practice was unsafe.

3 Do not continue or carry out an activity that you think may be unsafe as this will place individuals at risk of abuse or put you and others in danger. Changing your practice will mean that your safety and that of others will be protected; individuals' well-being will also be protected.

4 Discuss your concerns with your manager so that your manager is made aware and so that the necessary actions can be taken. Your manager will be experienced in this area and so will be able to provide you with some useful advice and guidance as well as reassurance that you have followed the agreed ways of working of your care setting.

5 Record the concerns you have so that there is a permanent account on file of your concerns. This record will be particularly useful if, at a later stage, there is an investigation into a case of abuse of an individual or a review of the care setting's procedures for safeguarding individuals. Your record shows the actions you have taken when unsafe practices have been identified.

AC 6.3 Describe the actions to take if suspected abuse or unsafe practices have been reported but nothing has been done in response

You should ensure that your concerns about unsafe practices or suspected abuse that you have reported are followed through and addressed. This is very important and an essential part of your duty of care. Your care setting will have whistle-blowing procedures in place that will set out what you can do.

It is important that you show your **commitment** when following these through.

You could, in the first instance, discuss your concerns again with your manager and ask them to tell you what has been done in response. If your manager is unable to explain what has been done in response or you find out that your manager is also involved in the suspected abuse or unsafe practices identified, then you could report these to the next level of management in the organisation.

If you have reported your concerns to the next level of management and still nothing has been done, then you must persist and contact an outside agency such as the regulator of health and social care services, the Care Quality Commission (CQC) or the safeguarding team in adult social care services. If you are member of a trade union then you could also seek advice from your representative.

Following through your concerns about suspected abuse or unsafe practices when nothing has been done in response is essential for ensuring the safety and well-being of individuals. Case study 6.1, 6.2, 6.3 provides you with an opportunity to think about the impact of doing so and complying with your care setting's whistle-blowing procedures.

Case study

6.1, 6.2, 6.3 Unsafe work practices

Dave is a residential care worker who supports individuals with learning disabilities to live independently. Dave's work shift partner is Emma who is a senior residential care worker. During the morning shift, Dave observed Emma restrict an individual from leaving his room while explaining to him that this was in his best interests (because he had injured his leg and he had been told by his GP to rest). Dave noticed that the individual looked frustrated.

Dave felt uncomfortable about Emma's actions and so discussed his concerns with Emma. Dave constructively explained to Emma that he didn't feel that it was necessary to physically restrict the individual as it was his right to leave his room and not be confined in it. Dave also explained that he thought that this individual was able to make his own decisions.

Emma thanks Dave for his concerns and reassures him that there is nothing to worry about. She tells him that he should trust her, as she is the senior colleague, and work with her as he has done so for many years.

Discussion points

1 Dave's approach to challenging Emma.
2 Emma's response to Dave.
3 The actions Dave should take next and why.

Evidence opportunity

6.3 Actions to take

Consider what further action you would take if you had reported suspected abuse or unsafe practices in your care setting but nothing has been done in response.

Produce a flow diagram detailing the key actions to take when you have to follow up your report of suspected abuse and unsafe practices in your setting for a second time.

LO6 Knowledge, skills, behaviours
Knowledge: why is recognising and reporting unsafe practices important?
Do you know what unsafe practices are and how they can affect individuals' well-being?
Do you know why it is important to take action when unsafe practices have been recognised?
Do you know why it is important to take action when nothing has been done in response to reported unsafe practices?
Did you know that you have just answered three questions about the importance of recognising and reporting unsafe practices?
Skills: how can you report unsafe practices?
Do you know the actions you must follow if you have identified unsafe practices?
Do you know the actions you must follow if you have reported unsafe practices and nothing has been done in response?
Do you know how to record your concerns in line with your employer's agreed ways of working?
Did you know that you have just answered three questions about some of the skills you have in relation to effective reporting of unsafe practices?

→

LO7 Understand principles for online safety

Getting started

Think about all the online activities you and your friends participate in. For example, this may involve using a mobile phone to text your family and friends and/or surf the internet, using a tablet or PC to buy items online or to access social networking sites such as Facebook or Twitter. Have you ever experienced any problems with your safety online? If so, what happened? If not, what could happen?

Now think about an individual you know who has care or support needs. How can you make sure that you keep them safe while they participate in online activities?

AC 7.1 Describe the potential risks presented by individuals with care or support needs going online

Potential risks for individuals with care and support going online include:

- the use of electronic communication devices
- the use of the internet
- the use of social networking sites
- carrying out financial transactions online.

Whether you are an online expert or not, it is important that you are aware of the potential risks presented by individuals with care or support needs going online so that you can fulfil your duty of care to maintain their safety and promote their well-being.

The use of electronic communication devices

Individuals may increasingly use their mobile phones and tablets when they are out and about. It is important that individuals are made aware of the risks of others obtaining their security passwords to commit fraud or even being subjected to theft of their electronic devices.

Individuals are able to access websites and download apps such as Facebook, Instagram and Snapchat that enable them to comment on and share images with others. While these are ways for them to connect with others, they may also be subjected to unwanted comments, offensive images or be subjected to bullying online. Apps such as these also send information out about the individual's location, so others can see where the individual is; again, this may make them the target for abuse.

The use of the internet

The internet can be a great place to connect with others and share our lives whether it is through our updates, blogs or photos. However, because we may be sharing so much information, there is a danger that some of this may be abused or used dishonestly. Some of the potential risks that the internet poses are listed below.

- Individuals may use the internet and search engines such as Google to search for information about what is happening in their local communities and so that they can find out more about places to shop or eat out in. However, this sometimes requires sharing

Research it

7.1 Online safety in your setting

Carry out some research in the setting where you work. Find out how individuals use the internet. What sites do they use? How often? Produce a table with your findings.

Have the results surprised you? Say why you are surprised – or not.

For more information about data protection, see Unit 206.

Reflect on it

7.1 Social media

Reflect on the benefits to individuals with care or support needs of using social networking sites. Do you use social networking sites? If so, why?

your location to find good spots to eat – and the location is made public to others.

- Individuals need to be made aware of the risks of searching for information on unofficial sites that may contain offensive language. They also must be made aware about the risk of finding or being exposed to information that may be of a sexually explicit nature.
- Sharing financial details about their bank account – even if this is on a well-known or trusted website – can leave people open to fraud and theft (having their banking details stolen) if someone else is able to gain access to these details. See the section on 'Carrying out financial transactions online', below, for more information on this.
- Individuals can also play games online and may interact with their friends in this way. It is important that individuals understand that these games could become addictive and can lead to them spending many hours on these sites (becoming increasingly socially isolated from family and friends). They should also be informed about the risks that gambling websites pose as this too can become an addiction.

The use of social networking sites

Social networking sites such as Facebook and Twitter can be a source of positivity and enable individuals to keep in touch with family and friends. However, social networking sites also pose risks that individuals must be made aware of. As you will know, these sites can be a forum for people to share all the different things that

are happening in their lives, such as marriages, births and parties. The list is endless. It is human nature to compare our lives with those of others, but this can be harmful to people's health if they compare their lives too seriously. Individuals may also be excluded from certain online activities, such as 'live streaming' videos sent by some friends, which could make them feel devalued and upset. Of course, individuals may make new friends on these sites but it is important that they are aware that not all information friends share is true. They should also be made aware of the security measures and privacy settings that they can put in place to ensure that they are not exploited by people who do not know them.

Social networking sites such as those mentioned above also allow individuals to keep up to date with people in the public eye who they may admire such as their favourite group or actor. It is important that individuals remember that what is reported on these sites is not always true and therefore they must not let this influence who they are and how they live their lives.

Moreover, you should be aware that not all information available online, including news stories, will be objective; it may be incorrect, biased and not based on facts. In some cases, the stories may be completely made up. This can influence a person's view of the world and the people they interact with, so it is important that individuals are made aware of this as it is also a potential risk presented by the internet and social media.

Carrying out financial transactions online

Online shopping and banking have made our lives a little easier as we no longer need to visit the shops to buy clothes, or visit the bank to make a transfer, However, this too can pose risks for you and those you care for.

Individuals may pay bills, buy items and pay for their transactions online. The risks associated with this include unauthorised organisations (people and websites pretending to be lawful and asking for money) trying to commit fraud and steal from the individual. This can also happen via email. How many times have you read about email or internet scams where people have thought they were sending money to a trusted source or person, but later found out that this was a lie and had their money stolen as a result?

Often a password is required to carry out a financial transaction and people are usually required to confirm this if they are carrying out financial transactions online. If this is shared with others or obtained fraudulently by others, it can then be used to access individuals' money.

AC 7.2 Explain ways of reducing the risks presented by each of these types of activity

Working in ways that promote online safety is underpinned by the following key principles.

Reflect on it

7.2 Promoting online safety

Reflect on how you can work in ways that are open, constructive and show that you are genuinely interested when promoting online safety when working with individuals. Write up notes about your reflection.

- Educate individuals about online safety and be open – speak to individuals and tell them about the risks presented by using devices and internet sites.
- Be constructive – encourage individuals to assess the risks presented by using devices and internet sites and suggest ways that these can be overcome and how they can stay safe.
- Be interested – show individuals that you have a genuine interest in promoting their safety and well-being while they participate in online activities.

Table 5.6 includes some suggestions for how you can reduce the risks presented by electronic devices and internet sites. Can you think of any others?

Table 5.6 Promoting online safety

Online activities	Promoting online safety
The use of electronic communication devices	Inform individuals about the privacy settings that their electronic devices have and that can be switched on to protect their privacy to restrict the information that can be accessed by others.
	Inform individuals about the privacy settings that their electronic devices have and that they can switch on so that others are unable to access their device or contact them.
	Ensure individuals use passwords when using their electronic devices so that if they leave them unattended or forget them in a public place, it will be more difficult for others to access the device and the personal information it contains.
The use of the internet	Inform individuals that when using the internet they may meet people who are not who they claim to be, for example when playing games online.
	Remind individuals that they can block these people and report them.
	Remind individuals that they can also tell you.
	Also, inform individuals that if they receive emails from people that they do not know – perhaps asking for money or asking to meet them – then they should always tell someone about this. The people emailing may sound convincing or intimidating; so it is always best to check with someone else.

➔

Table 5.6 Promoting online safety *continued*

Online activities	Promoting online safety
The use of social networking sites	Ensure individuals remain on official social networking sites only and do not have private 'chats' with others away from these sites.
	Remind individuals not to give out any personal information about themselves including photographs that they do not want to be shared publicly.
	Remind individuals that they do not have to accept 'friend requests' and invitations from people that they know – or do not know – if they do not want to.
	Remind individuals that they can tell you about any concerns they have if they are being made to feel uncomfortable by any person on these sites.
Carrying out financial transactions online	Inform individuals that all financial transactions online should only be completed on official sites. Often official sites will start with 'https' and there will sometimes be a security certificate that appears on screen.
	Inform individuals that all financial transactions should be completed in privacy and not in public places so that others cannot see their personal information.
	Inform individuals of how to check whether organisations are who they say they are, i.e. by checking they are registered with professional bodies.

Identity theft

Remind individuals to keep their personal information, including their names and addresses, safe, both online and otherwise. Identity fraud is also an issue where personal information is used by others to pose as the person. This can result in theft under the individual's name and identity.

Staying up to date

If you do not have knowledge around online safety then this is something that you will need to research so that you can stay up to date with the latest developments. This is also something that you should discuss with your manager so that you can arrange training. You cannot be expected to advise others about online safety if you do not have knowledge in this yourself. You could ask someone who has expertise in this area to speak to individuals in the setting about this.

New developments

As technology continues to develop, increased online safety has become an issue – we can all become victims of online abuse and need to be aware of the risks.

It is clear that crimes around technology and digital information are increasing, but often

it will not even be criminals who will commit abuse online. Cyber bullying is an issue that you may have read about or seen reported in the media; it is where social media is used to abuse others. People have posted written comments, photos and videos to bully, hurt and embarrass others. More recently, the issue of revenge porn has been reported in the media, with people posting photos and videos of partners performing sexual acts, as revenge, perhaps at the end of a relationship.

Cameras on laptops can also be hacked so that others are able to view the person using the laptop on the other side. In 2017, there were reports of Bluetooth and WiFi enabled dolls that could enable strangers to spy on or talk to children who played with them.

You will need to be aware of stories such as these so that you can understand how to keep the people you care for safe online. Some of the people you provide support for may use the internet but may not understand the dangers around this. They may even be taking IT lessons to improve their knowledge. Obviously you cannot protect them from everything, however keeping them informed of the risks and supporting them with any concerns they have and telling them about the measures they can put in place to stay safe will reduce the risks of online abuse and help to keep them safe.

It is only by staying up to date with developments in this area that you can ensure that individuals are aware of the most recent developments and know about the various issues so that they can stay safe. This is an issue widely reported in the media so it is often hard to miss it. You should ensure that you educate yourself in this area so that you can then educate them. At the same time, do not assume that all individuals will not have any knowledge in this.

Online safety for the setting

Remember that it is not just the individuals in the setting that need to stay safe online, but also settings themselves. The NHS became a victim of hacking in 2016/2017 where hackers were able to gain access to patient records. Your setting will need to ensure that it has its own security measures in order to protect itself and to keep confidential information and data safe.

Research it

7.2 Agreed ways of working for online safety

Research your employer's agreed ways of working for online safety. Find out whether there are any training and development opportunities available so that you can provide support to the individuals you care for in the care setting where you work.

Evidence opportunity

7.1, 7.2 Risks

Produce an information leaflet showing the potential risks presented by the use of electronic communication devices, the internet, social networking sites and carrying out a financial transaction online. Make sure you also include information about the different ways you can reduce these risks.

AC 7.3 Explain the importance of balancing measures for online safety against the benefits to individuals of using electronic systems and devices

Promoting online safety does not mean that individuals are prevented or deterred from using electronic systems and devices but rather that they are informed of the risks, and are involved in assessing them and in making their own decisions about how to use these systems and devices safely. **Competently** working in this way is part of risk enablement (a way of working you learned about in AC 4.3) and also embeds person-centred values.

6Cs C

Competence

Competence in relation to promoting online safety refers to applying your knowledge and skills to ensure that you are able to communicate to individuals the risks and benefits that they face when using electronic systems and devices. You should tell them about how they can take control when doing so and keep themselves safe. You can also give them information leaflets, take the time to discuss the different risks with them and encourage them to ask you questions or share any concerns they have with you.

Reflect on it

7.3 Person-centred values when promoting online safety

Reflect on the person-centred values you have learned about. How can you instil these in your working practices when promoting online safety? Why is it important to do so? What are the consequences of not doing so?

The benefits to individuals of using electronic systems and devices are numerous and can include some of the following:

- **making new friends** – there can be more opportunities for meeting new people and being part of a group of friends. This can make individuals feel like they belong to a social group and can share their common interests with others.
- **learning new skills** – there are opportunities for developing new skills such as being able to communicate with others verbally and in writing. They can also be creative and express themselves through writing blogs, and posting pictures and online videos.
- **developing your knowledge** – there are opportunities for developing your knowledge about a range of different topics, and interests and study skills can be developed in this way.

Striking a balance between the risks associated with online safety and the above benefits means that the rights of the individual are promoted and their well-being enhanced. The reflective exemplar below provides you with some additional information about the importance of balancing the risks with the benefits of using electronic systems.

Reflective exemplar	
Introduction	I work as a personal assistant to John who has learning difficulties. I visit him once a week to support him to visit one of his best friends who lives locally.
What happened?	Last week, while supporting John to visit his friend he 'FaceTimed' another friend on his mobile phone. His friend began to tell him how unwell he was and also shared with him the personal difficulties he was having at the time with his family.
	I was aware that everyone on the bus was looking at us and could hear what John's friend was saying to him. I quietly pointed this out to John and told him to not 'FaceTime' his friend. John got very upset and when the bus stopped he got off the bus suddenly and accused me of treating him like a child, and not an adult.
What worked well?	I raised my concerns with John discreetly. I identified the risks of 'FaceTiming' another person in public.
What did not go as well?	Telling John about my concerns while we were still on the bus. I should have suggested to John that we get off at the next stop because I wanted to talk to him about something important. This way I could have talked through with him my concerns and supported him to understand the risks.
What could I do to improve?	I think I will need to put John's needs first rather than my own; it was my embarrassment on the bus that prevented me from handling this situation sensitively.
	I think I will need to reflect on the benefits that 'FaceTiming' has for John. I will suggest some suitable locations where he can 'FaceTime'. I will explain to him the reasons why I have identified these locations so that he can make his own decisions by choosing which one he prefers.
Links to unit assessment criteria	ACs 7.1, 7.2, 7.3

Evidence opportunity

7.3 Balancing measures

Discuss with your assessor the importance of balancing measures for online safety against the benefits to individuals of using electronic systems and devices.

Remember to think about how personalisation is relevant here.

LO7 Knowledge, skills, behaviours

Knowledge: what are the principles for online safety?

Do you know why it is important to discuss the risks of using electronic communication devices with individuals?

Do you understand the potential risks of carrying out financial transactions online?

Do you know how to weigh up online safety against the benefits to individuals of using electronic systems and devices?

Did you know that you have just answered three questions about the principles for online safety?

Skills: how can you reduce the risks of online activities to individuals?

Do you know how to prevent unauthorised people from accessing individuals' electronic communication devices?

Do you know how to support good practices for individuals using the internet and social networking sites?

Do you know how to inform individuals how they can carry out financial transactions safely online?

Did you know that you have just answered three questions about some of the skills you have in relation to promoting online safety when supporting individuals?

Behaviours: how can you show the personal qualities you have when promoting online safety?

Do you know how to provide information about online safety in a non-patronising way?

Do you know how to communicate clearly the risks of online activities to individuals?

Do you know how to encourage individuals' independence during online activities?

Did you know that you have just answered three questions about some of the essential behaviours that are expected of workers when promoting online safety?

Suggestions for using the activities

This table summarises all the activities in the unit that are relevant to each assessment criterion.

Here, we also suggest other, different methods that you may want to use to present your knowledge and skills by using the activities.

These are just suggestions, and you should refer to the Introduction section at the start of the book, and more importantly the City & Guilds specification, and your assessor, who will be able to provide more guidance on how you can evidence your knowledge and skills.

When you need to be observed during your assessment, this can be done by your assessor, or your manager can provide a witness testimony.

Assessment criteria and accompanying activities	Suggested methods to show your knowledge/skills
LO1 Understand principles of safeguarding adults	
1.1 Research it (page 151)	Produce a poster detailing your findings.
1.1 Evidence opportunity (page 151)	Write an account that explains what the term 'safeguarding adults' means, and addresses the points in the activity.
	You may find it useful to discuss the meaning of the term 'safeguarding' with a colleague in the care setting where you work.
1.2 Evidence opportunity (page 152)	Following on from your research, discuss your job role and responsibilities with your manager, who will be able to provide a witness statement. Follow the instructions in the activity and make detailed notes.
	You could also write a personal statement that describes your role and responsibilities in safeguarding adults in the care setting where you work. Explain, with examples, how your role and responsibilities relate to safeguarding individuals.
	You will find your employer's safeguarding policy, procedures, and agreed ways of working useful sources of information.

➔

Suggestions for using the activities	
1.3 Research it (page 155)	Produce an information handout as instructed in the activity.
	You could also present your findings in a written account.
1.3 Evidence opportunity (page 156) 1.3 Case study (page 155)	Produce a leaflet that describes the following terms: physical abuse, domestic abuse, sexual abuse, emotional/psychological abuse, financial/material abuse, modern slavery, discriminatory abuse, institutional/organisational abuse, self-neglect, and neglect by others.
	You could also produce a presentation, as well as a spider diagram that includes the definitions of all the different types of abuse and neglect named above.
	A case study has been included to help you think about the different types of abuse that can occur.
1.4 Evidence opportunity (page 156)	Produce the information handout as instructed in the activity.
	Or you could write a personal statement that describes the term 'harm'. Remember to include in your description how this term relates to safeguarding adults.
	You could also discuss the term 'harm' with your assessor, or your manager, who will be able to provide a witness testimony. Agree on a definition and on the key aspects it involves in relation to safeguarding.
1.5 Research it (page 156)	You could discuss your findings with a colleague and write an account to detail your findings and discussion.
1.5 Reflect on it (page 157)	Write a reflective account addressing the points in the activity.
1.5 Evidence opportunity (page 157)	Produce a list of two examples of appropriate restrictive practice and two examples of inappropriate restrictive practice. You should explain how the appropriate practices can be used to safeguard adults, and why the inappropriate practices are not appropriate.
	You could also prepare a presentation that describes restrictive practices when safeguarding individuals. Include examples of what these are, and how they can be used both legally and inappropriately.
	Or you could write an account that describes three examples of restrictive practices, how they are used with individuals with care or support needs, and the reasons why. Remember to include clear links in your account to safeguarding individuals.
LO2 Know how to recognise signs of abuse	
2.1 Evidence opportunity (page 162) 2.1, 2.2 Case study (page 164)	Produce a written account that identifies the signs and symptoms associated with each of the following types of abuse: emotional/psychological abuse, financial/material abuse, modern slavery, discriminatory abuse, institutional/organisational abuse, self-neglect, and neglect by others.
	You could also prepare a presentation or develop a spider diagram of the signs and symptoms associated with each type of abuse.
	The case study will help you to think about the range of signs and symptoms that may indicate that an individual has been abused.
2.2 Research it (page 163)	Produce a written account detailing your findings and address the points in the activity.

➜

Suggestions for using the activities	
2.2 Evidence opportunity (page 164) 2.1, 2.2 Case study (page 164) 2.2 Case study (page 163)	Discuss your findings with a colleague and produce a written account that describes the factors that can make older people and other individuals more vulnerable to financial abuse. Ensure you include a description of a range of factors that may contribute to an individual's vulnerability to abuse. When you discuss your findings with a colleague, you may also like to discuss the factors that can contribute to an individual being more vulnerable to abuse; you should try and cover both individual and environmental factors. The case studies will help you think about the different factors that can make an individual more vulnerable to abuse.
LO3 Know how to respond to suspected or alleged abuse	
3.1 Reflect on it (page 168)	Provide a short reflective account answering the questions in the activity.
3.1 Evidence opportunity (page 168)	Following on from your research, discuss the key actions to take if you suspect an individual is being abused. Your manager will be able to provide a witness statement. Discuss the importance of responding to suspicions of abuse, as well as the process to follow. Produce a factsheet that explains the key actions to take if there are suspicions that an individual is being abused. You will find your agreed ways of working a useful source of information about the steps that must be taken when responding to suspicions of abuse.
3.2 Research it (page 173)	You could discuss your findings with your manager. You could also provide a written account detailing your findings.
3.2 Evidence opportunity (page 173)	Discuss with your assessor the actions to take if an individual in your care setting alleges that they are being abused. Remember to explain the reasons for your actions. You could also produce a presentation or personal statement that explains the process to follow if an individual alleges that they are being abused. You will find your agreed ways of working a useful source of information about the steps that must be taken when responding to allegations of abuse.
3.3 Evidence opportunity (page 173)	Discuss with your assessor your role and responsibilities when preserving evidence of suspicions and allegations of abuse, and address the questions in the activity. You could also complete a spider diagram of the different ways to ensure that evidence of abuse is preserved. You will find your agreed ways of working a useful source of information about the ways that you can preserve evidence of abuse in the care setting where you work.
LO4 Understand the national and local context of safeguarding and protection from abuse	
4.1 Research it (page 176)	You could produce a poster with your findings or provide a written account.
4.1 Evidence opportunity (page 178)	Make some notes on your thoughts and then produce a one-page information handout. You could also complete a spider diagram or personal statement of examples of relevant legislation, national policies and local systems that relate to safeguarding and protection of individuals from abuse.

→

Suggestions for using the activities	
4.2 Evidence opportunity (page 179)	Discuss the roles of different agencies with your manager and obtain a witness statement. Then produce a leaflet that explains the roles of different agencies in safeguarding and protecting individuals from abuse.
4.3 Reflect on it (page 180)	Provide a reflective account.
4.3 Evidence opportunity (page 181)	Following on from your research, produce an information leaflet on the different factors that feature in the abuse and neglect. You could also complete a spider diagram or write a personal statement about the different factors that have featured in reports into serious cases of abuse and neglect. Or write a personal statement of the different factors that have featured in reports into serious cases of abuse and neglect.
4.4 Research it (page 182)	Discuss the key points with a colleague and make notes.
4.4 Evidence opportunity (page 182)	Develop a poster as instructed in the activity. Discuss sources of information and advice about your own role in safeguarding and protecting individuals from abuse, including whistle-blowing, with a colleague. Write a personal statement of the different sources of information and advice about your own role in safeguarding and protecting individuals from abuse, including whistle-blowing.
4.5 Evidence opportunity (page 183)	Discuss with your manager the agreed ways of working to follow when seeking support in two safeguarding situations where you have no experience or that are beyond your area of expertise. Obtain a witness statement to ensure you can evidence this. You could also complete a spider diagram of the different situations in which to seek support beyond your own experience and expertise. Or write a personal statement of the different situations in which to seek support beyond your own experience and expertise.
LO5 Understand ways to reduce the likelihood of abuse	
5.1 Research it (page 186)	Speak to your colleagues or your manager. Make notes about your discussion.
5.1 Evidence opportunity (page 187)	Produce a leaflet that explains how the likelihood of abuse can be reduced by working with person-centred values, encouraging active participation, promoting choice and rights, supporting individuals with awareness of personal safety, and encouraging active participation. You could also prepare a presentation or write a reflective account.
5.2 Evidence opportunity (page 188)	Develop a flow diagram as instructed in the activity. You could also write a personal statement that explains the importance of an accessible complaints procedure for reducing the likelihood of abuse. Discuss how an accessible complaints procedure can reduce the likelihood of abuse. You will find your complaints procedures and your manager useful sources of information.
5.3 Reflect on it (page 188)	Write a reflective account.
5.3 Research it (page 189)	Research the support that is available for carers and write down your responses to the questions in the activity.

→

Suggestions for using the activities	
5.3 Evidence opportunity (page 189)	Produce a one-page information handout or a poster that outlines how the likelihood of abuse can be reduced by managing risk and focusing on prevention.
	Or you could write a reflection of how the likelihood of abuse occurring in your care setting can be reduced by managing risk and focusing on prevention.
	You will find your risk enablement procedures and your manager useful sources of information.
LO6 Know how to recognise and report unsafe practices	
6.1 Reflect on it (page 191)	Provide a reflective account.
6.1 Evidence opportunity (page 191) 6.1, 6.2, 6.3 Case study (page 193)	Develop two case studies, as instructed in the activity.
	Or you could write a personal statement that describes unsafe practices that could affect the well-being of individuals.
	The case study will help you think about how unsafe practices can affect the well-being of individuals.
6.2 Research it (page 191)	Make notes about your discussion.
6.2 Evidence opportunity (page 192) 6.1, 6.2, 6.3 Case study (page 193)	Produce a table to illustrate different examples of unsafe practices that may arise in care settings, as instructed in the activity.
	You could also produce a presentation or spider diagram that explains the actions to take if unsafe practices have been identified. For each action, explain why it should be taken; include the consequences of not doing so.
	The case study will help you think about the actions that can be taken when unsafe practices have been identified.
6.3 Reflect on it (page 192)	Write a reflective account.
6.3 Evidence opportunity (page 193) 6.1, 6.2, 6.3 Case study (page 193)	Produce a flow diagram as instructed in the activity.
	Or you could write a personal statement of the actions to take if suspected abuse or unsafe practices have been reported but nothing has been done in response.
	The case study will help you think about the actions that can be taken when unsafe practices have been identified and nothing has been done in response.
LO7 Understand principles for online safety	
7.1 Research it (page 195)	Produce a table with your findings.
7.1 Reflect on it (page 195)	Write a short reflective account.
	An evidence opportunity for 7.1 is covered as part of the 7.2 Evidence opportunity, below.
7.2 Reflect on it (page 196)	Write up notes about your reflection.
7.2 Research it (page 198)	Write up notes to detail your findings.
7.1, 7.2 Evidence opportunity (page 198) 7.1, 7.2, 7.3 Reflective exemplar (page 199)	Produce an information leaflet showing the potential risks presented by: the use of electronic communication devices; the use of the internet; the use of social networking sites; and carrying out financial transactions online. Make sure you also include information about the different ways to reduce these risks.
	The reflective exemplar will help you think about the risks presented by online activity and the importance of balancing online safety against the benefits to individuals of using electronic systems and devices.
7.3 Reflect on it (page 198)	Write a reflective account.

→

Suggestions for using the activities	
7.3 Evidence opportunity (page 199)	Discuss the points in the activity with your assessor.
7.1, 7.2, 7.3 Reflective exemplar (page 199)	Or you could produce a presentation that explains the importance of balancing measures for online safety against the benefits to individuals of using electronic systems and devices.
	Discuss the importance of balancing measures for online safety against the benefits to individuals of using electronic systems and devices with your manager, who will be able to provide a witness testimony.
	The reflective exemplar will help you think about the importance of balancing online safety against the benefits to individuals of using electronic systems and devices.

Legislation	
Relevant Act	**It states that:**
Care Act 2014	there are ten different types of abuse that individuals may experience. It also defines safeguarding as individuals living safely, free from harm and abuse.
Health and Social Care Act 2012	health and social care services must work in partnership together to safeguard individuals effectively.
Equality Act 2010	a person must not be treated unfairly or discriminated against in relation to their protected characteristics. These are defined by the Equality Act as age, disability, gender reassignment, marriage and civil partnership, pregnancy and maternity, race, religion and belief, sex or sexual orientation.
Safeguarding Vulnerable Groups Act 2006	it established the vetting and barring scheme that prevents people who are not suitable to work with individuals with care or support needs from doing so; DBS checks are required of all those who work with individuals with care or support needs.
Mental Capacity Act 2005	it safeguards individuals who are unable to make choices and decisions for themselves because they lack the capacity to do so.
Modern Day Slavery Act	it is aimed at tackling slavery, servitude and forced or compulsory labour in the UK. It addresses issues such as human trafficking and the exploitation of people.
Human Rights Act 1998	everyone in the UK is entitled to the same basic human rights and freedoms. This includes individuals who have care and support needs. The Act supports individuals' rights to make their own choices and decisions, dignity, respect, to be treated fairly when accessing care or support services and to live safely and free from harm or abuse.
Data Protection Act 1998	it promotes individuals' rights to security over the use of their personal information by others and safeguards them from others infringing their rights to privacy over their personal information.
General Data Protection Regulation (GDPR) 2018	applies from May 2018 and introduces some new and different requirements for data protection. See Unit 203 for more information.
Public Interest Disclosure Act 1998	it established whistle-blowing procedures so that concerns over individuals' safety and well-being can be reported by workers free from fear or repercussions from their employers. You may make a disclosure about unsafe work practices or a crime.

See AC 4.1 for more information on legislation.

Resources for further reading and research

Books and booklets

Department of Health (2014) 'Positive and Proactive Care: reducing the need for restrictive interventions', Social Care, Local Government and Care Partnership Directorate

Ferreiro Peteiro, M. (2014) *Level 2 Health and Social Care Diploma Evidence Guide*, Hodder Education

Weblinks

www.cqc.org.uk Care Quality Commission (CQC) – information from the regulator of all health and social care services about the standards expected from care settings and workers providing care and support to individuals, information and guidance on the duty of candour and about whistle-blowing

www.elderabuse.org.uk Action on Elder Abuse – provides information, guidance and support regarding abuse that happens to older people

www.gov.uk The UK Government's website for information about current and relevant legislation for safeguarding individuals such as the Care Act 2014, Equality Act 2010

www.skillsforcare.org.uk Skills for Care – information about the Code of Conduct for Adult Social Care Workers, the Care Certificate and the Care Act 2014

Responsibilities of a care worker (202)

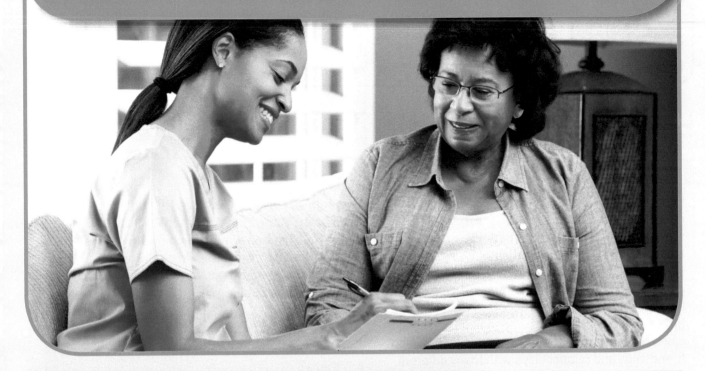

Credit value: 2
Guided learning hours: 16

About this unit

The best teamwork happens in **care settings** when there are good working relationships between individuals, their families, friends, advocates, team members, colleagues and other professionals, when everyone **works in ways agreed** with the employer and together in partnership as one big team.

In this unit, you will learn about what makes an effective working relationship, including the key differences between a working relationship and a personal relationship. You will also learn about what your employer expects of you, including

the reasons why it is important to work in ways agreed with your employer. In addition, you will be able to explore the opportunities to contribute and make sure the experience for the individuals you care for is a positive one.

Finally, you will learn about the benefits of working in partnership with others, the different skills and approaches needed for resolving conflicts and the range of sources of support available to you about partnership working and resolving conflicts that may arise.

Learning outcomes

LO1: Understand working relationships in care settings

LO2: Be able to work in ways that are agreed with the employer

LO3: Be able to work in partnership with others

LO1 Understand working relationships in care settings

Getting started

We have all experienced forming relationships with others throughout our lives. From a young age we begin to get to know and trust those closest to us such as our parents, grandparents, brothers, sisters, aunties, uncles and guardians. As we grow, our relationships with others develop and we begin to think about which people in our lives we have most in common with and make us feel good when we are around them. In this way, we develop friendships and relationships with many different people.

How many relationships have you had since you were born? Can you list them? Who is at the top of your list and why? Which relationships were the most successful? Were there any relationships that did not work out so well? Why didn't they work out?

Think about the relationships in your life today. Are these the same ones as you had when you were a child? What similarities and differences are there?

AC 1.1 Explain how a working relationship is different from a personal relationship

Relationships feature in all our lives and develop throughout childhood and into adulthood. According to the psychologist Abraham Maslow, the basic human needs we must all fulfil are love and belonging. Maslow defines these as including:

- friendship, for example a best friend who has known you since school
- intimacy, for example a partner who knows you in a loving and/or sexual way
- trust, for example a colleague at work who you can confide in and rely on
- acceptance, for example your sibling who accepts you for who you are
- receiving and giving affection and love, such as the relationship you have with your parents
- affiliating, in other words being part of a group, for example friends, family, at work.

These are the key ingredients of relationships and the reasons why relationships exist. They are the basis of our communications and interactions with others, they help us to get to know one another and form close bonds and they are the source of support through which the sharing of ideas takes place.

Relationships also play a crucial role in our overall well-being and how we see ourselves. For example, in times when we are not at our best, the relationships that we have can be a source of great emotional support, they can lift us up when we are not feeling at our most confident and can improve our self-esteem. Have you ever felt down and upset and had a reassuring conversation with a friend who has cheered you up? Does the feeling of being around people make you happier? As people, we like to feel included and a part of a bigger group and meaningful relationships are a key part of that, both in and outside of work.

Relationships can also vary according to the people involved and the context in which they are created in terms of whether they are personal relationships or work relationships.

Research it

1.1 Maslow's hierarchy of needs

Research Abraham Maslow's hierarchy of needs and produce a poster that outlines his five-tier model of human needs (often depicted as a pyramid). Think about how this relates to relationships in terms of what we give and receive from different relationships.

You will find the following link useful:

https://simplypsychology.org/maslow.html

Key features of personal relationships

Personal relationships can be formed with family, friends and partners. Figure 6.1 identifies some examples of who these types of relationships can involve.

Family

Personal relationships with family can mean different things to different people and can depend on who you trusted and relied on as you grew up. Family may be the people that you feel most comfortable with and with whom you feel you belong. You may grow closer over time, or you may find that you are less close as time goes by. A family may be related to you:

- by birth, for example you may have parents, brothers and sisters, aunts, uncles, grandparents
- by marriage, for example your partner
- or by adoption, for example your parents or guardian.

The meaning of family can also differ as there are various other structures. Family does not just refer to 'the nuclear family' consisting of a mother, father and children. Some families may be 'lone parent' families (just one parent), or there may be stepfamilies where one person may play the role of step-parent for example. There are also extended families that include grandparents, uncles and aunts who may also live alongside parents and children. You will find that you will work with a variety of family structures, so it is important that you understand the different relationships that exist.

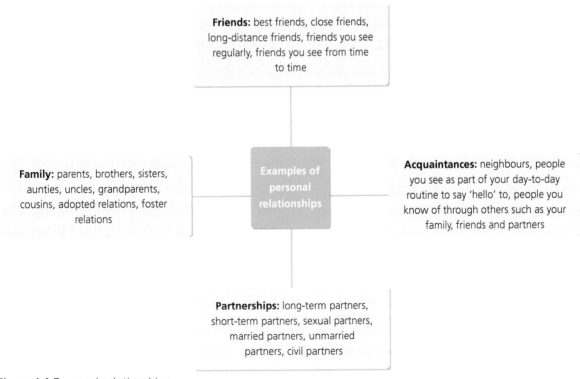

Figure 6.1 Personal relationships

6Cs

C

Care

Care involves putting others' interests before your own. This is because caring for someone involves being kind, thoughtful and approachable. A good carer does not just provide high-quality care as a one-off – but consistently, over and over again. You can show that you care by doing something kind for someone else, that shows you have thought about their needs and want to make a difference to their situation. It is an important quality required in both personal and professional relationships and especially important if you want to build positive relationships.

Reflect on it

1.1 Your relationships with family members

Think about what family means to you. Who do you consider to be your family? Why? Think about what all your relationships with family have in common.

Friend

This refers to a personal relationship with someone with whom you have a close connection or bond. If you think about who your friends are, they are usually people who you like, have things in common with and perhaps have shared similar experiences. For example, you may have a best friend who has known you since primary school and who you shared the same lessons at school with, went to each other's birthdays and other family celebrations, spent time with during the holidays and socialised together after work. Some friendships can last a long time, others come and go but it is usually our close friends that have most impact on our general well-being. Making a connection with others can be a skill (which will come naturally to some people but not to others) and it is often a skill that we have learned through

making the friends we have already. It is a skill you will need to draw upon in the care setting where you work.

Partnership

This refers to a personal relationship with a partner who you know intimately in a loving and/or sexual way. Partnerships are therefore different to relationships with family and friends because they usually develop out of affection and physical closeness. Partnerships also vary depending on our preferences and beliefs. For example, a civil partnership is a relationship only formed between two people of the same sex; civil partnerships and same-sex marriages are formally recognised in UK law and give people the same rights and responsibilities as heterosexual married couples.

Acquaintances

These are personal relationships, which may be frequent but not develop into anything more than an acknowledgement. Your next-door neighbour may be someone who you see every morning and say hello to but apart from that (and perhaps seeing them out in the area where you live) you have no other contact with them. Some relationships with acquaintances, however, can develop over time into friendships and even partnerships. For example, you may previously have only seen someone in the local shop every now and again but you may get to know them a lot better over time and find that you share the same interests. Similarly, you may only ever 'see' someone you went to school with on Facebook, but a message may lead you to getting back in touch and develop into a friendship beyond social media.

Key features of work relationships

Work relationships, as the term suggests, are formed with the people you interact with as part of your day-to-day work tasks. In care settings, work relationships are formed between those who work there and others, as Figure 6.2 shows; how many of the work relationships identified in the diagram have you formed in the care setting where you work? Are there any others not featured in the diagram?

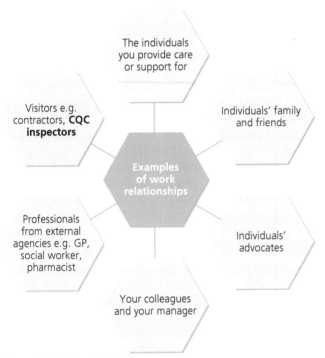

Figure 6.2 Work relationships

Key terms

CQC inspectors monitor and check the quality of **care settings**. They check whether care settings are safe, providing effective care, treating individuals with dignity and respect and meeting individuals' needs.

Care settings refer to adult, children's and young people's health settings and adult care settings. This qualification is concerned with adult care settings only.

Professional refers to carrying out your job in a skilful and knowledgeable way, showing behaviour that is moral and acceptable for the role that you are in.

Boundaries are the limits that you must work within when carrying out your job role.

Why are good working relationships important?

Having good working relationships is essential for:

- **providing good-quality care** and support because it means everyone works together to ensure individuals' needs are met
- **enjoying your work** and job satisfaction (there is nothing better than waking up in the morning and looking forward to going to work) – in addition, others who you work with will feel your positivity and commitment to the job and you will therefore be contributing towards a nice atmosphere
- **encouraging mutual trust and respect** – working together as one team will encourage you and your team members over time to build trusting working relationships with one another and learn to respect one another's ideas and contributions. You will also learn how to support one another.

Companies tend to focus on improving relations between team members, and may even organise team-building days in order to encourage positive relationships between staff. This is because they recognise the importance of effective working and how it can lead to a happier, productive workforce and (in a care setting) how it can improve the quality of service and support that we provide to individuals.

How do work relationships differ from personal relationships?

There are some important differences between relationships at work and personal relationships. You need to be aware of these so that you can carry out your role in a **professional** way. Table 6.1 outlines the main differences between personal and professional working relationships.

Table 6.1 The differences between a work and a personal relationship

A working relationship	A personal relationship
Working relationships are planned. In your care setting, you work with individuals and within a team in order to provide individuals with care or support; you do not choose the people you work with. You will work with those that you need to in order to fulfil the requirements of your job and provide the best care possible.	Personal relationships by contrast, such as those with friends, develop naturally and you choose who you want to be friends with.

Table 6.1 The differences between a work and a personal relationship *continued*

A working relationship	A personal relationship
Working relationships are structured. In your care setting, you and the team will have rotas and plans for how work activities are to be carried out including specific objectives and associated timescales for their completion. These are agreed before carrying out any work activities such as the support you provide to individuals in the mornings for their personal hygiene routines or during the day for eating and drinking, for example.	Personal relationships by contrast are not necessarily structured. The time you spend with family and friends will depend on your and their availability, it does not necessarily have to be planned. For example, you can be spontaneous and decide that you are going to give your friend a visit or decide during an evening visit to your family that you are going to stay overnight. You do not have to decide on a schedule or agenda for your meeting or how long the meeting will last.
Working relationships have clear boundaries in place. Your care setting will have guidelines (often written guidelines) that explain what is and what is not acceptable as part of your job role. This includes what is and what is not acceptable behaviour in the care setting where you work. You will be expected to demonstrate professionalism, work to a high standard to provide the best-quality support and fulfil your duty of care (see Unit 205, Duty of care). You will also have to ensure that you adhere to the codes of conduct in your setting. (Read about agreed ways of working on pages 218–23.) You will be expected to turn up on time for work, it will not be acceptable for you to always be late; you will be expected to be polite to individuals' families when they visit, it will not be acceptable for you to be rude to them.	Personal relationships, by contrast, (although there are unwritten rules of what is acceptable behaviour) do not have the same boundaries, i.e. ones that are written down that you must comply with. For example, you should not tell others anything that a friend has told you in confidence – but there is no contract to say that this is not allowed.
Working relationships are bound by agreed ways of working. In your care setting, you will have requirements set out by your employer including policies and procedures as well as codes of conduct which you must follow in relation to how you must behave when at work. • The care setting where you work may have a gifts policy in place that prevents you from accepting gifts of any kind from the individuals that you provide care or support to and their families. This is because others may think the reason you are being given a gift is because you somehow favoured these individuals and their families over others when providing them with care or support and as a result they have given you a gift. • The data protection policy and procedures in your care setting may prevent you from sharing personal information about the individuals that you work with outside of the care setting.	By contrast, in personal relationships you are not bound by any rules and can give a gift to anyone. This can be of any type or monetary value of your choice, in other words it can be as expensive or as inexpensive as you like. You can also share personal information about your family and friends with other family and friends, if you choose to do so –you are not bound by any confidentiality rules, only by your own conscience.
Working relationships include unequal balances of power. In your care setting, you will know personal information about the individuals you provide care or support to, such as their date of birth, their likes and dislikes and their family background, however they will not necessarily know any personal information about you. Individuals depend on you to have their care or support needs met, but you do not depend on them to have your needs met.	Personal relationships, by contrast, are more equal. Because everyone involved in the relationship shares personal information about themselves, this is one of the ways that close bonds are built.

	Dos and don'ts for maintaining professional relationships with the people you provide care and support for
Do	Try to keep things as professional as possible. Of course, it is good practice to be friendly, but you may be caring for a wide range of individuals, not just one, so making sure that you remain professional means that you will be able to provide equal care and support for all, and not be seen as favouring some over others. This can be a tricky task because it may be that while working together you feel rather close to the individual. However, remember that you are also a professional.
Do	Share information so that you are friendly and personable but do not overshare. It is important to share things with the individual that you care for, but being professional means that you do not go into too much detail. This oversteps the boundaries and means that you may be seen to favour some over others. Also, oversharing means that the relationship can become personal and there is a risk that it could be misinterpreted.
Don't	Accept gifts, money or anything in case it looks like you have favoured particular individuals. An individual may want to give you a gift as a thank you but it is important that you try not to accept these. An appropriate response may be 'Thank you very much, that is a lovely thought, but I really cannot accept. I'm sorry.' You could even say that you are not allowed to accept gifts and that you would be breaking the rules by doing so. Remember that providing the best possible care to some of the most vulnerable people is your top priority. You are there to provide care for them. Do not expect gifts or support in return for your work.
Don't	Tell the individual about your worries and problems. It is your responsibility to listen to them and help them with any issues they may have. Just because they tell you about their worries, do not use it as an opportunity to share your concerns. This is all part of maintaining a professional relationship.

Case study

1.1, 2.1, 2.3 Relationships at work

Aamna has worked as a support worker with five older individuals with learning disabilities in a residential care setting for ten years. Aamna has got to know every individual so well over the years that they always turn to her when they need support or advice; this even includes on her days off. This makes Aamna feel good about herself and gives her tremendous job satisfaction. Over the last few years Aamna has taken it upon herself to come in on one of her days off every two weeks to arrange outings with individuals to different places of interest including to the garden centre, cinema and bowling club. Aamna's manager is very impressed with Aamna's commitment to her job and sees her as a valued member of the team.

This week Aamna requested a meeting with her manager to inform her that, due to her husband being diagnosed with a serious illness, she will be resigning from her support worker role to care for her husband at home. Aamna's manager is shocked by her news and wonders how she is going to manage without her expertise. The individuals for whom Aamna provides support are very upset that she is leaving and do not want her to go – particularly because they liked her arranging their outings. One of the individuals is so upset that he has asked to meet with his social worker as he wishes to leave the care setting if he is no longer going to receive support from Aamna.

Discussion points

1 Have the boundaries between Aamna's working relationships become confused? If so, why have they become confused?
2 The individuals and colleagues in the setting have not taken the news of Aamna's departure well. Could this have been avoided? Suggest some different ways that the news could have been announced.

1.1 Personal and working relationships

Identify two people that you have a personal relationship with and two people you have a working relationship with.

For each person you identify write down:

- how well you know them
- when you see them, how often and the reasons why
- what you do together when you see them, how often and the reasons why
- what you know about them
- what they know about you.

Read through your comments to the above points. Explain the differences between the working relationships and personal relationships you have with these people.

AC 1.2 Describe different working relationships in care settings

Working together with others is part of your day-to-day role as a care worker. You will work with a variety of people, from colleagues and individuals that you care for, to their families, their advocates, GPs and other people and organisations outside the setting. For example, in a typical day, you may work with a colleague to provide support to an individual with an activity or communicate with an individual's advocate about arranging to meet with them, or you may work alongside an individual's social worker and GP to protect the individual from harm. Every one of the working relationships you have in the care setting where you work will be different. See Table 6.2.

Table 6.2 Examples of working relationships and aspects of what will be involved

Working relationships – people you will work with	Aspects of what is involved
An individual who you support in your care setting	Providing support with daily tasks such as with personal hygiene, eating and drinking, moving and handling, cooking and shopping.
	Supporting the individual to understand information in relation to their home, daily activities, finances.
	Enabling the individual to be part of their community, for example by supporting them to visit family and friends, encouraging them to socialise with others, supporting them to access local facilities such as the gym, leisure centre or shops.
An individual's mother who visits their relative on a weekly basis	Supporting the individual's mother to ask their relative about their week and activities.
	Providing the individual's mother with information about the care setting in relation to the services it provides, how many individuals live at the setting, how many staff are on each shift.
	Enabling the individual's mother to participate in some of the activities being organised at the care setting such as a summer fete open to all or a coffee morning open to individuals' relatives.
An individual's advocate	Discussing with the individual's advocate how an individual's communication needs have changed.
	Asking the individual's advocate for their advice on how to support an individual at a meeting about their care needs.
	Receiving information from the individual's advocate about the communication aids that the advocate uses to support the individual to communicate.

→

Table 6.2 Examples of working relationships and aspects of what will be involved *continued*

Working relationships – people you will work with	Aspects of what is involved
A colleague who works the same shifts as you in your care setting	Sharing with your colleague how you developed a successful group craft activity.
	Supporting your colleague who is having difficulties making themselves understood when communicating with an individual who has hearing loss.
	Agreeing with your colleague how to work together as a team to move an individual from a sitting to standing position.
Your manager	Discussing with your manager whether you can book some additional annual leave.
	Discussing with your manager your achievements at work and the areas you would like to improve on.
	Seeking guidance from your manager when you have witnessed a visitor speaking to an individual inappropriately.
An individual's GP	Telephoning the individual's GP to make an appointment.
	Providing the individual's GP with information about the individual's symptoms when they are feeling unwell.
	Finding out what support is available from the GP surgery for an individual who wants to stop smoking.
A contractor who has come to repair the sink in the staff room	Checking with the contractor before allowing him access to the premises – such as the purpose of his visit and his identity.
	Accompanying the contractor to the staff room to repair the sink in the staff room.
	Providing the contractor with all the necessary information in relation to the repair needed to the sink, i.e. where it is leaking, the length of time it has been leaking.

Team building and good working relationships

You cannot expect to understand how your colleagues work and how you can all work well together on day one. There will be times when you are able to all work successfully to meet an objective but there will also be times when you disagree with one another. This is all part of being in a team. In order to ensure that you try to work well with others, you should try to remember that good working relationships have key features, some of which we explore here.

Good communication

This includes both verbal and non-verbal communication and means communicating clearly with colleagues, clarifying your understanding of what has been communicated. When working in a team, you will need to ensure that everybody understands their role, and the part they will play in order to offer the best care possible to individuals in the setting. This will include effectively communicating in any discussions, making sure that you value what everyone else has to say, their views and opinions, and working together to reach a decision which is in the best interest of the individual (see Unit 205, Duty of care). In writing, this involves using respectful language and ensuring what you have written is true. For more information about good communication refer to Unit 203, Communication in care settings.

Good values

In working relationships, this involves treating others how you would like to be treated. In other words, treating the people you work with respectfully, being honest, polite, responsible and trustworthy. For example, you can show respect by being considerate of the opinions of colleagues, showing that you value their views and advice. You can show that you are trustworthy and honest by communicating correct, accurate information even if it means communicating something that you have done wrong. All of this helps to create strong trustworthy relationships, ones where people are open and supportive of one another.

Good understanding

This involves getting to know one another including one another's strengths and limitations and being willing to understand and learn more about one another's different roles and responsibilities.

Good support

This means supporting one another to work together as a team. This may involve putting a colleague's needs before your own or being prepared to give your time to a colleague who is finding it difficult to learn a new skill. Support involves giving and receiving skills, knowledge and experiences and also showing or displaying support for one another. For example, you not only work together to resolve issues, but also demonstrate your support for colleagues by speaking up. For example, if you feel a colleague has made a good point, then you can say 'Yes,

I agree with X, I think X has made a good point and we should consider alternating our team meetings between lunchtimes and evenings so that staff who work part-time can attend these too'. Of course, there will be times when there will be disagreements in the team but the best way to approach this is to listen carefully to all viewpoints and work together to reach a solution.

A good tip is to think about how you like to be supported at work, whether it is by your manager or by other colleagues. Do you sometimes want help and support when you are struggling with a task? Do you sometimes struggle with your workload and wish a colleague would help you? Do you wish someone would say 'well done' when you have done a good job? Remember that your colleagues feel the same way too. They sometimes feel that they have too much work to do – they too want some encouragement on days when they are not at their best.

Empathising can help to create strong professional relationships and in turn lead to a more productive and happier workplace if people feel supported and therefore motivated to do their job.

	Dos and don'ts for supporting colleagues
Do	Support one another if a colleague is struggling with a task. Maybe they are struggling with a moving and handling procedure. If so, help them. If you don't know how, then find someone who can help them.
Do	Share best practice. If something has worked well in practice, then share this with colleagues so that they can also learn from you. Likewise, if you have undertaken some training and found this helpful, share what you learned and encourage them to go on the course. Support one another to be better care workers.
Don't	Undermine or belittle a colleague. If you feel that they have done something incorrectly, it is useful to give helpful constructive advice. It is important that colleagues feel that they are part of a team and you cannot be part of a team if you constantly seek faults in others. Remember, however, that you must always tell your manager if you observe a colleague carrying out unsafe working practices.
Don't	Underestimate the importance of your colleagues just because you are busy. Value them! If someone is not well, or feels overwhelmed about something at work (or outside work), then be there for them. You could ask if they want to talk about the problem. Everyone is busy at work, but if you make time for one another, it will lead to more positive and supportive working relationships and a better working environment.

6Cs

C

Communication

Communication in a working relationship is essential for ensuring that you all work together as a team towards ensuring positive outcomes for individuals. Without good communication, misunderstandings may arise that may lead to an individual's care or support needs being unmet.

You can show good communication in your working relationships by:

- only writing down accurate information in your daily reports about the care you have provided to individuals
- remembering that if you have agreed with a colleague to do a task, then communicate this to your colleague when you have completed it.
- effectively communicating to support colleagues by being friendly and polite in your communications and by using encouraging and supportive language such as 'I thought you handled the situation with Mr Jones really well. I know it must have been hard for you especially because you have been really busy with other individuals, but you did really well.'

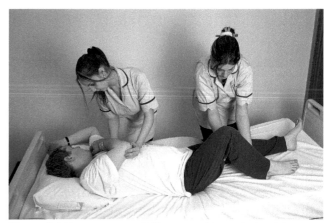

Figure 6.3 How can you tell if your working relationships are effective?

Evidence opportunity

1.2 Different working relationships

Building on your work from Evidence opportunity 1.1, develop an information handout about three different working relationships you have in the care setting. For each working relationship, provide some details about why it is important and what makes it effective.

L01 Knowledge, skills, behaviours
Knowledge: what is the difference between a working relationship and a personal relationship?
Do you know three key features of a working relationship? Can you provide some examples and describe what they involve?
Do you know three key features of a personal relationship? Can you provide some examples and describe what they involve?
Did you know that you have just answered two questions about how working relationships are different to personal relationships?
Skills: how can you show that you are developing effective working relationships?
Do you know how to communicate clearly with a colleague?
Do you know how to maintain a professional relationship with the individuals you care for?
Did you know that you have just answered two questions about good working relationships?
Behaviours: how can you show the personal qualities you have in developing effective working relationships?
Do you know how to show that you are reliable and professional when working alongside your colleagues and the individuals you care for?
Do you know how to be honest with your manager about how the team is working?
Did you know that you have just answered two questions about a few of the essential behaviours that are expected of all adult care workers when working with others in a care setting?

LO2 Be able to work in ways that are agreed with the employer

AC 2.1 Describe why it is important to adhere to the agreed scope of the job role

Your job role

Developing effective working relationships with others can only be achieved if you carry out all the tasks that form part of your job role; this is commonly referred to as 'the agreed scope' of the job role. In the care setting where you work, you will have a **job description** that sets out all the responsibilities you have agreed to with your employer.

These will include the following:

- **the responsibilities, tasks or work activities** that you must carry out as part of your job role. These might include:
  - providing support to individuals with daily living activities to meet their needs
  - maintaining accurate records of the support provided to individuals
  - attending all training provided.
- **how you must carry out your work activities**. This might include:
  - promoting individuals' rights such as privacy, dignity, independence
  - maintaining detailed and accurate records while protecting individuals' confidentiality at all times
  - putting into practice all training attended by using person-centred ways of working.

Key term

A **job description** is a document that outlines the purpose and responsibilities of your job role. You will find an example in Unit 207, Personal development in care settings.

- **who you report to**, such as your manager or team leader
- **who your supervisor is**
- **what your hours of work are**, for example flexible shifts, including evenings and weekends
- **how much you will be paid per hour**
- **where you must work**, for example in a variety of settings including in individuals' own homes, in residential care settings.

Job descriptions will vary depending on the job. They will also vary in detail: some may be brief with an outline of the job role and key responsibilities but good descriptions will detail the purpose of your role, responsibilities, different tasks you will be required to complete, and also the reasons for doing so. In this way you have a clear understanding of why you are doing what you are asked, and understand how it impacts on the individual and setting. For example, instead of saying 'assist at meal times', it would be more helpful to say 'assist at meal times and ensure that the meal meets the dietary requirements and needs of the individual.' Or instead of saying 'provide good care for individuals' it would be more helpful to say 'provide care that involves treating

	Dos and don'ts for adhering to the scope of your job role
Do	Comply with the agreed lines of reporting. For example, if you have a concern about an individual's well-being, then you should report your concerns to your manager in the first instance rather than going straight to the individual. Your job description will outline whom you will report to and you must work within these boundaries and the scope of your job.
Do	Only carry out work activities within your agreed hours of work. Do not assist an individual who wishes to go to the shops after your shift has ended without first seeking permission to do so.
Do	Work in locations agreed with your employer. Again this will be outlined in your job description and the scope of your job so do not, for example, provide support to an individual in your house or in the home of one of the individual's relatives rather than in the individual's own home.
Don't	Take part in work activities that have not been agreed as part of your job role and that you are not trained to do. For example, if your job description does not mention assisting individuals with medication, reviewing care plans or supervision of new members of staff, then you should not be expected to do this. You may of course receive training and as a result your job role and the scope of your role may change but this is something you should discuss with your manager before you undertake tasks that are not outlined in your job description.
Don't	Work in ways that are not person-centred. For example, by imposing your views and denying individuals their rights, or by documenting your opinions when recording the support provided to individuals.

Research it

2.1 Your job description

Find your job description for the care setting where you work. Identify the responsibilities you have agreed to with your employer, including what you must not do as part of your job role.

Discuss the scope of your job role with a colleague. How do your responsibilities compare to theirs?

individuals with compassion, dignity and respect and ensuring that they are involved in their care'.

Adhering to the agreed scope of your job role also involves working within the boundaries or limits of the job role. The 'dos and don'ts' table provides tips to make sure you work within the boundaries. Basically, if it is not part of your job description, then you should not be expected to carry out the task.

The importance of adhering to the agreed scope of your job role

Working within the agreed scope of your job role is essential for ensuring that you carry out your job responsibilities to the best of your ability. It is also very important for a number of other reasons set out below.

- **It ensures you are working at the correct level** – ensuring you adhere to the scope of your job ensures that you are working to your ability and doing the tasks that you are qualified to do. Doing tasks that you do not have any expertise or qualifications in risks the health and safety of those around you and yourself. You can of course gain knowledge and skills in those areas but it is best to stick to what you know before you start taking on responsibilities that are not outlined in your job description and those you have not discussed with your manager first.

- **It ensures you are only responsible and accountable for what you do** – all organisations need structures and a clear outline of what everyone does in the setting. That way, you are only accountable for those things that you are responsible for and not for others. It is also clear to management who is responsible for what tasks and so there are no misunderstandings (if you are all doing what you are responsible for). That is not to say you cannot assist colleagues; it just means you should not take on tasks that are not in the scope of your job.

- **It is how your employer will assess your competence** – during supervision meetings with your manager and as part of your appraisal at the end of the year your employer will discuss with you how you have performed in your job role. You will discuss whether you have carried out your work activities to the best of your ability, in line with your job role's requirements and your employer's expectations of you. By adhering to the agreed scope of your job role you will be more likely to show that you are doing what is expected of you and that you are doing this competently, i.e. to a high standard. You can find out more about supervision and appraisals in Unit 207, Personal development in care settings.

- **It is part of your duty of care** – you have a duty of care to ensure you provide the best possible care, and the support you offer is in the best interests of the individual. This concept is covered in Unit 205, Duty of care. For example, assisting an individual to move from their bed to their chair on your own when the moving and handling guidelines specify that two staff are present can have serious consequences for both you and the individual. You may lose your job for carrying out a task on your own that you do not have the agreement from your employer

to do. You may also injure your back during the move. Your actions may cause the individual to fall and fracture one of their limbs. Adhering to the agreed scope of your job role is therefore essential for your safety as well as the safety and well-being of individuals.

- **It ensures the health and safety of everyone** – you have a responsibility to ensure the safety of everyone you work with. Your responsibilities with regard to health and safety are covered in Unit 210, Health, safety and well-being in care settings. Not adhering to responsibilities around health and safety, such as reporting concerns, can have serious consequences. For example, if you do not report concerns about a colleague's unsafe working practices when preparing food, it could result in illness such as food poisoning for those in the setting (as well as visitors). It could even prove fatal if they already suffer from other illnesses. If you do not report your concerns your colleague will not be able to access the support and training they need. Both you and your colleague may also run the risk of losing your jobs. That is not to say you should spend your days worrying about what *might* happen, but it is a good idea to be mindful of the reasons why you should work within the scope of your job role and responsibilities.

- **It protects you from untrue allegations** – meeting with an individual on a one-to-one basis when it has been agreed that all meetings with this individual will take place in the presence of two members of staff can have

---

6Cs

C

Competence

Competence refers to your ability to apply the knowledge and skills you have learned to your day-to-day work activities. This is important because it means that you will only be carrying out work activities and working in ways that are set out in the agreed scope of your job role – activities that you have the knowledge and skills to carry out. You can show you are doing this by keeping a record of your professional development and discussing this with your manager during your supervision and appraisal meetings. You can also show your competence by obtaining feedback from the individuals and others you work with about how you carry out your work activities.

Evidence opportunity

2.1 Adhering to the scope of your job role

Think about three work activities that you are required to carry out as part of your job role. For each work activity, describe to your assessor why it is important you carry it out competently and within the agreed scope of your job role. What happens if you do not follow the scope of the job role?

serious consequences for everyone. You may be accused of something that you did not do, for example shouting at the individual. This will in turn mean that your employer will be required to conduct an investigation into what happened. The incident will also need to be reported to the individual's family and to the CQC, the external agency that regulates the services provided at the care setting. This may result in the individual requesting a move to another care setting, you losing your job and could even mean an end to your career in the adult social care sector. Again, this example is not designed to scare you, but you should remember that your job description has important reasons for everything that it outlines including the working methods you should follow. You shouldn't need to be too concerned about the consequences if you are following the rules and guidelines in your job description.

If the individual is your employer/if you are a private carer

If your employer is the individual to whom you provide care or support, or you work on your own as a private carer to an individual, then it is important that you understand and read through the guidance provided to you by the person who is employing you; this may be written formally and included in your contract of employment, or may be in the form of a personal plan of work that the individual has prepared. Some individuals and their families may also brief you verbally, and may ask you to approach them if you have any questions or concerns. You could also seek support from other carers you know or other lone workers who you meet when you attend training or conferences.

AC 2.2 Access full and up-to-date details of agreed ways of working

As you have learned, agreed ways of working refer to working practices that are used in the care setting where you work that have been agreed with your employer and set out how you will carry out your job role and its associated responsibilities.

Adult care settings are all different and therefore agreed ways of working vary between the different settings. However, all adult social care employers will have the following policies, procedures and guidelines in place.

- **Policies** are the general guidelines for the way you should work. Your setting will have many policies in place such as one for health and safety, one for handling information and one for dealing with visitors. The policies in your setting will comply with legislation and they will reflect the aims of the care setting. For example, in order to comply with the Data Protection Act 1998 or the new GDPR 2018 (see Unit 206, Handle information in care settings, AC 1.1 for more details) your care setting must have in place a policy that describes how it will ensure that individuals' personal information will be kept secure at all times when being used, recorded, stored and shared.

- **Procedures** set out in detail how you should work and the ways of working that your employer expects you to follow on a day-to-day basis to ensure the policies are being put into practice. Basically, the procedures detail the processes to follow! For example, data protection procedures describe your responsibilities for handling individuals' and others' personal information. Procedures explain how to follow the data protection principles, what to do when an individual requests access to their personal information and the process to follow when you have issues or concerns. This includes the people you must report these to, such as your manager or the data protection officer who has overall responsibility for managing data when there are issues or concerns. In your setting, there will be procedures for nearly everything you do, from moving and handling, to giving medication to individuals, to how to deal with an emergency such as a fire.

- **Guidelines** set out *precise* ways of working that your employer will expect you to follow for the care of specific individuals and work activities. For example, data protection guidelines may be in place for one individual who has given strict instructions that you are not to tell his family every time he has a fall because he does not want to worry them. It is important that you respect his right to have this personal data about him not shared with his family. Another example may include an individual who uses photographs to communicate with others. There may be specific guidelines in place to advise you on how to ensure that these photographs are kept secure and handled in a way that others do not have access to them. It may be that you need to ensure that communications only take place in a private area where others cannot have access to the photographs or you may need to ensure that when the photographs are being used they are placed in a holder that can only be viewed by you and the individual.

Agreed ways of working relate to many aspects of work in care settings, as Figure 6.4 shows.

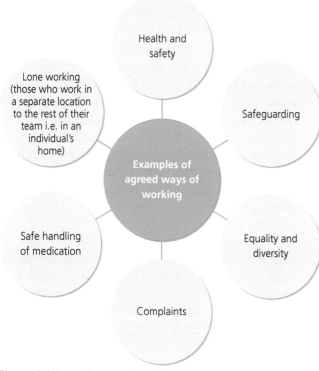

Figure 6.4 Agreed ways of working

Accessing agreed ways of working

Policies, procedures, guidelines and agreed ways of working are stored in adult care settings so that they can be accessed by workers. In this way workers can follow these when carrying out their work activities. You should remember that you will be observed while doing this as part of your assessment. In some care settings, they may be stored in the team leader's office, in others they may be stored in the staff room. In addition, there is usually a process that you must follow to gain access to them and although this varies across different care settings there are some general steps that you will be required to follow.

You should:

- request permission to access the documents from either your manager or team leader
- read them in a private area so that others who do not need to have access to them cannot pry
- confirm that you have read and understood them by signing and dating them when you have finished.

If there are any aspects of your employer's agreed ways of working that you do not understand or are unsure about then you must seek advice from your manager. Do not sign them indicating that you have understood them if you haven't, as doing so will mean that you may not be following them as you are legally required to do. This may mean not only the loss of your job but also that you will be placing everyone's health, safety and well-being at risk.

Full and up-to-date details of agreed ways of working

Having access to full and up-to-date information with respect to agreed ways of working is essential for ensuring that your work practices are safe, legal and up to date. Agreed ways of working need to be updated when there are:

- **changes to legislation** – so that you can ensure that your work practices comply with legal requirements. For example, when the new General Data Protection Regulation (GDPR) came into force from May 2018, care settings' agreed ways of working needed to be updated to reflect this. It is important you are aware of these changes and what they will mean for your working practices so that your practices remain legal.

- **changes to best practice** – so that you can ensure that your work practices are up to date, safe and reflect current best practice. For example, first aid procedures and the actions to follow for different health emergencies are always being reviewed and updated on a regular basis depending on current research. It is important you are aware of these changes so that any actions you take are safe and do not put yourself or others in danger or at risk of harm.

- **changes to individuals' needs** – so that you can ensure that your work practices are safe and promote individuals' health, safety and well-being. For example, an individual's guidelines with respect to the support they require for eating and drinking may change if the individual has developed swallowing difficulties. They may require support with ensuring that they are in a comfortable position when eating and they may only be able to eat soft foods and to take small sips when drinking (they may need to use a straw). It is important you are aware of the changes so that the support you provide is safe, meets the individual's needs and prevents the individual from choking.

The information in your employer's agreed ways of working must be complete and up to date so that it provides a true and accurate picture of the requirements expected of you in your job role. You can check agreed ways of working contain full and up-to-date details by:

- checking the legislation that supports these, for example legislation that supports the agreed ways of working may be included

- asking your manager; you could check with them whether you are reading and signing the most up-to-date version

- using your own knowledge of the individuals you provide care or support to. For example, if there is a change to an individual's condition and you notice that this has not been updated on the individual's guidelines. In this situation, you would report your concerns to your manager immediately.

Evidence opportunity

2.2 Accessing full and up-to-date details of agreed ways of working

Your work practices will be observed for this AC.

Find out who has the responsibility in the care setting where you work for maintaining and keeping the agreed ways of working complete and up to date.

1 Carry out some research in the care setting where you work. Find out where your setting's agreed ways of working are stored. Are they stored in one location? Find out the process you must follow to gain access to them. Why is this process in place?

2 Produce a poster with your findings.

Your working practices will be observed to ensure that you know how to check that the agreed ways of working you access contain full details and are up to date.

AC 2.3 Work in line with agreed ways of working

Working in line with your employer's agreed ways of working, as you have learned, is an essential part of your job role and ensures that you are carrying out your work responsibilities lawfully, safely and in line with current best practice; your work practices for working in line with your employer's agreed ways of working will be observed.

Below are some tips to help you work in line with your employer's agreed ways of working.

1 Ensure you find out where your work setting's agreed ways of working are, including how to gain access to them. Read them, and if there is something you do not understand, seek advice from your manager.

2 Ensure you only carry out work activities that have been included in the scope of your job role.

6Cs

C

6Cs

C

Courage

Courage involves being clear with others when mistakes have been made or unsafe practices have been witnessed. Taking no action is not an option. Doing so may mean that unsafe practices continue and potentially can place individuals, others and yourself in danger and at risk of harm. You can show courage by ensuring that you always follow agreed ways of working; in this way you will be setting a good example to others in your work setting and ensuring that you always report any unsafe practices you notice.

3 Attend all training and read all information updates provided to you by your employer. If you do not feel confident to carry out a work activity that you have been trained to do be honest with yourself and talk this through with your manager.

4 If you observe an unsafe working practice or if an individual, their family or a visitor brings something of this nature to your attention, ensure that you report it to your manager immediately. You will also need to make a record of these observations. Showing your **courage** in these situations will ensure that you promote your own and others' health, safety and well-being.

5 Be prepared to explain why you are carrying out your work activities in the way that you do, for example to the individuals who you are supporting with a daily activity or to a colleague you are working with, such as when you are both working together to assist an individual to mobilise.

6 Find out who you must report to when carrying out your work activities; ensure you do this and comply with any information or guidance that this person provides, for example this may be your manager or another senior member of the team.

7 Observe individuals, listen to their feedback (and the feedback of others) on how you carry out the work activities you are responsible for. Reflect on their feedback and use this to continue to improve your work practices.

Research it

2.3 Agreed ways of working and feedback

Carry out some research in the care setting where you work. Work with two colleagues, your manager and one other person; this could be an individual, another colleague, or a professional who visits the care setting.

Ask each person you have identified for their feedback in relation to the following:

- what they like about the way you carry out your work activities
- what work activities you carry out the best and why
- what work activities you carry out that could be improved and why.

Collate the feedback you have obtained and reflect on whether you always work in line with agreed ways of working. What could you do to improve?

Evidence opportunity

2.3 Work in line with agreed ways of working

You will be observed for this AC.

Identify two work activities you feel you are competent to carry out. Arrange for your assessor to observe you while carrying them out. Ensure that you can show that you are working within the scope of your job role and in line with your employer's agreed ways of working.

AC 2.4 Contribute to quality assurance processes to promote positive experiences for individuals receiving care

What is quality in care?

Good-quality care means that:

- an individual's experience will be positive, caring and enabling

- an individual's experience will meet their expectations as well as those of their family, friends or advocates
- care services will be safe
- care services will be effective.

What is quality assurance in care and how can you contribute to it?

Quality assurance means to ensure a high quality of care in the setting. It is about offering the best care and service possible and meeting the needs and requirements of those who use the services.

Below, we cover some of the different aspects involved in quality assurance.

Fact finding

This involves finding out about the care individuals receive, and will include the aspects of care that are working well for an individual and the aspects that require further development. Finding out this information means you can further improve the areas that are not working so well to ensure that individuals receive the highest quality of care. For example, an individual may express that they are pleased that they can request their care worker to arrive a little earlier or later in the mornings depending on what their plans are for the day. This works well during the week but they may find that this does not work as well at the weekends because sometimes the care workers may arrive quite late in the mornings.

You have a very important role to play in contributing to the quality assurance process and your practices will be observed. It is through quality assurance that you too can be part of an individual's positive experience of care. Below are some tips for how you can do this.

- **Focus** – start by deciding what you want to find out – and the reason why. Think about whether there are a few specific aspects of individuals' care needing improvement or whether there is just one aspect. For example:
  - care provided with eating (one aspect)
  - care provided overnight or over weekends (multiple aspects).

  Think about whether these aspects of care are specific to one individual or whether they apply to more than one individual. For example:

- providing support when communicating with a communication aid (one individual)
- risk assessment processes that are followed when supporting individuals on activities out in their local communities (more than one individual).

- **Work with others** – next, you need to decide who to involve in quality assurance processes and the reasons why. For example, if you are trying to find out why the new activities room in the care setting where you work is not being used as much as you thought it would be, you may want to involve the individuals who use the activities room because the activities room has been provided as a result of their request. You may also want to involve the care workers and activities co-ordinator who support the individuals to participate in the activities because they may also be able to share with you their observations about what individuals like or don't like about the activities room as well as what difficulties there may be, such as not enough lighting, too much noise, or not enough space for individuals who use wheelchairs. You may be aware that from time to time some of the individuals' relatives will also provide support during activities; you may identify who these are and ask them too for their views.

- **Take action** – you need to consider the methods available and which ones you think will be most suitable to use to find out the information you want to know. For example, you will need to consider whether you want to have a discussion with individuals in pairs, in small groups or on a one-to-one basis. You may opt to use questionnaires that can be completed over email or sent out in the post to relatives and others. Again, you will need to think about what kind of information you want to collate; for example if you would like to hear the opinions and suggestions of the individuals then a discussion may be better, whereas if it is factual information you need, questionnaires that contain specific questions may work better.

Contributing to quality assurance processes to promote positive experiences for individuals receiving care means having open discussions where there is an honest exchange of information

Commitment

Commitment to quality assurance is necessary to ensure that you and others promote a positive experience for the individuals who receive your care. This means not being afraid to find out how effective the care or support you provide is and then making the improvements that are necessary to meet individuals' and others' expectations. You can do this by showing that you are genuinely interested in finding out about the experiences, the views and opinions of everybody involved and by taking on board all the feedback you receive. You can regularly review and monitor the care or support you provide to all individuals.

and ideas, obtaining feedback from all those involved and reflecting on this. It also involves a high level of **commitment** from you to ensure that quality assurance processes continue to be maintained and are effective.

Taking action

This involves listening to what is being said or observing what is happening, using this information as the basis for making improvements to the care provided, discussing it with colleagues and putting this into action. For example, an individual's family may tell you that they have noticed that when their relative has their afternoon coffee in their room it often arrives lukewarm but that this never happens if the resident has their afternoon coffee in the lounge. You decide to take action by informing your manager as well as the chef in the kitchen. As a result, new coffee pots are bought so that when the coffee is served to residents in their rooms it retains its heat. It is also agreed for a team member to check 15 minutes or so after the coffee has been taken to the resident's room that it is to the individual's liking.

Monitoring

This involves assessing how well a service is running including how well the care being provided to individuals is working. For example, in the situation described above about the individual having a hot drink in their room, it will be important to check that the measures that

have been put in place to resolve the situation are *still working*. For example, you may want to check with the individual and their family by asking them at regular monthly intervals directly about their experiences. You could speak with the chef and the care workers to find out their views about how the new coffee pots are working. You could also take on board any other suggestions shared with you for further improving the situation.

Monitoring whether the CQC's fundamental standards are being met is a responsibility of all services that provide individuals with care. It is important that services are regularly checking on the quality of the care or support being provided, i.e. is it tailored to individuals' needs and preferences? Are individuals' rights to dignity and privacy being upheld? The safety of the care or support being provided also needs to be checked regularly. Does it promote individuals' health and well-being, and safeguard them from abuse – for example, by ensuring that risk assessments are completed and that staff are trained, qualified and competent to provide care and support?

Quality assurance is not:

- **one size**: all individuals receiving care are different, with their own values, beliefs, views and experiences.
  - For example, when finding out about individuals' experiences of care you may ask one individual directly by discussing this with them but you may have to make arrangements for another individual who has communication needs to have their advocate present so that they can ensure that the individual's views and preferences are expressed.
- **a one-off**: promoting positive experiences for individuals receiving care does not just happen once a year or on one occasion; instead it is an ongoing process.
  - For example, ensuring that the activities provided in the care setting where you work are safe is an ongoing process as it involves daily, weekly and monthly checks. You can't stop checking that they are safe or only assess activities for any risks they present once, it has to be done every time the activity is provided to ensure it does not place yourself,

individuals and others in danger or at risk of harm. This is part of your duty of care.

- **an exercise**: promoting positive experiences for individuals receiving care is not about filling in questionnaires and about ticking boxes on forms; quality assurance is a process.

Following your employer's agreed ways of working is an integral aspect to your job role. For example, you don't assess how well you do this by answering a short questionnaire about your own working practices; you do this by discussing this with your manager in supervision meetings and by seeking feedback from your colleagues, the individuals you provide care to and their families, friends and advocates.

Case study 2.4 will help you consider the different factors you need to take into account when contributing to the quality assurance processes in the care setting where you work.

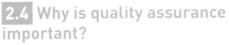

Reflect on it

2.4 Why is quality assurance important?

Think about the reasons why quality assurance is important for the care setting where you work. What are your expectations for providing quality care in your job role and care setting? Why do you think this is important?

Research it

2.4 Quality assurance processes in your setting

Carry out some research in the care setting where you work about the quality assurance processes that are in place for promoting positive experiences for individuals receiving care. Produce an information handout with your findings.

You will find it useful to speak with your manager and access the quality assurance policy and procedures that are in place in your work setting.

Case study

2.4 Contributing to quality assurance processes

Michael is a day care centre worker. As part of his role, he works in a team of four to support the activities provided for young adults with learning disabilities by encouraging and enabling the individuals to participate. The team met last week to discuss the activities being provided because they do not seem to be as well attended as before and the team are unsure as to the reasons why.

The team has agreed to involve all the members who attend the activities as well as those who used to attend but have stopped doing so. This also includes involving individuals' relatives who from time to time support the activities and also the activities worker who leads on the outdoor activities at the weekend.

Michael and his colleague will be interviewing the individuals who attend and have decided that due to their range of needs, they will interview

them one by one. Michael has developed a set of questions that he plans to use with individuals, he has also adapted these to include photographs and signs as some individuals are unable to read and others prefer to communicate through signs. Michael's colleague has also arranged for an individual's advocate to be present during the interview as the individual feels less anxious in a one-to-one situation when someone he knows well and trusts is present.

Questions

1 Why is it important for the team to find out the reasons why individuals are not attending the activities?
2 Why did Michael and his colleague take into account individuals' needs when making arrangements for interviews?
3 What other methods could be used by the team to obtain feedback from all those involved?
4 How could Michael and the team continue to monitor how the activities are working?

LO2 Knowledge, skills, behaviours
Knowledge: why is it important to adhere to the agreed scope of your job role?
Do you know the consequences of not carrying out the work activities you are responsible for?
Do you know why it is important to seek guidance if you do not feel able to carry out any aspect of your job role?
Did you know that you have just answered two questions about the importance of only working within the agreed scope of your job role?
Skills: how can you show that you are working in ways that are agreed with your employer?
Do you know how you can find out if you are accessing the most up-to-date details of your employer's agreed ways of working?
Do you know how to ensure your work practices follow your employer's agreed ways of working?
Do you know how to contribute to quality assurance processes so that the individuals you work with have a positive experience of care?
Did you know that you have just answered three questions about some of the skills you have in relation to working in line with your employer's agreed ways of working?
Behaviours: how can you show the personal qualities you have when working in ways agreed with your employer?
Do you know how to be confident and speak up if individuals are not having a positive experience of care?
Do you know how to show your commitment to consistently making sure that you are working in line with your employer's agreed ways of working and that you can promote a positive experience for individuals in care?
Did you know that you have just answered two questions about a few of the essential behaviours that are expected of all adult care workers?

LO3 Be able to work in partnership with others

AC 3.1 Explain why it is important to work in partnership with others

Your job role in adult social care will involve working alongside a wide range of different people and organisations that have different roles and responsibilities. This may include the individuals you provide care or support to, their families, friends, advocates or others who important to them, your colleagues, other team members such as your manager and other professionals from other organisations such as social workers, mental health nurses, dieticians, dementia care nurses, GPs.

Working in partnership with others is more than just working alongside them. It involves becoming 'a team'. This can only happen when you are all committed to:

- sharing a common set of values – to support individuals' independence, to safeguard individuals from harm, to respect individuals' unique differences
- agreeing goals – to enable positive outcomes for individuals (which may be agreed over both short and long periods of time)
- communicating effectively – communications must be open and honest, timely and regular both with individuals and others, which includes both verbal and written communications. (You may find it useful to refer to Unit 203, Communication in care settings and Unit 206, Handle information in care settings.)

Working in partnership brings many benefits for you, the individuals who require care, as well as others both inside and outside the organisation. Most importantly in a setting, working effectively as a team and in partnership means that you all have the shared goal of providing the best support possible for individuals.

Working in partnership and working effectively together can have the following benefits.

- You all improve and develop your understanding of different ways of working, share knowledge and best practice. For example, a colleague may show you a more effective way of communicating with an individual who has hearing loss.

- A stronger team creates a better working environment where you all feel supported. For example (similar to what we mentioned above), working in partnership with others involves sharing skills, knowledge and getting to know one another. This enables team members to learn from one another and share good ideas.
- Understanding one another's roles and responsibilities will avoid duplicating one another's work so that staff make better use of their time. You may also share resources, such as meeting venues, which can reduce costs and encourages everyone to meet together.
- You all work together to provide person-centred care. Individuals receive care that is co-ordinated and meets all of their individual needs (they will receive better services).

AC 3.2 Demonstrate ways of working that can help improve partnership working

As you will have learned there are many benefits to partnership working with others and so it is important that you are able to recognise this and show you are able to demonstrate different approaches and methods that can help improve partnership working. For this assessment criterion you will be observed as part of your assessment.

Below are some useful tips to help you do this.

1 **Be clear about your own roles and responsibilities** and show your understanding of the role and responsibilities of all those who you work in partnership with. This encourages mutual trust and respect because it involves recognising and encouraging your own and others' contributions.

2 **Communicate well** and consistently by being honest, listening actively, showing a genuine interest. This also means making sure that the different 'partners' are kept informed of any information that they should know. This is essential for learning from one another, sharing ideas and working practices and ensuring your relationships are open and honest. You may find it useful to refer to Unit 203, Communication in care settings.

3 **Work to shared goals and objectives** so that everyone is working together to support individuals to achieve their goals. Working to shared goals and objectives also means that everyone will be working as one team consistently to provide good-quality care.

4 **Involve others in planning, discussions and decision making** so that partners feel included and everyone can come to an agreement about the best course of action together. This also means that you can draw on everyone's expertise and that the different areas of expertise inform the decision. For example, you may need to make decisions about an individual's medication with the help of your manager, the individual's GP and their family.

5 **Be a role model** to others by being professional and trustworthy, by using positive language and showing positive behaviours, such as open communication, being punctual and polite. This is essential for others respecting you and looking to you to lead by example.

6 **Be supportive** by showing you have a genuine interest in individuals' well-being and showing that you recognise and value others' contributions, values and beliefs, which may be different to your own. Value the people you work with, what they bring to the team, draw on their knowledge and expertise, show that

you value them in team meetings, or even during one-to-one meetings.

7 **Show your passion, commitment and enjoyment of working together** with other people to achieve positive outcomes for individuals. This is essential for enabling everyone involved to feel comfortable and motivated to work with you.

8 **Agree to work together as one team.** This is essential for achieving agreed goals and involves you obtaining and providing information about the progress of the goals, whether there have been any difficulties in achieving them, what needs to be done to resolve these difficulties. This involves sharing good practices as well as learning together from mistakes made.

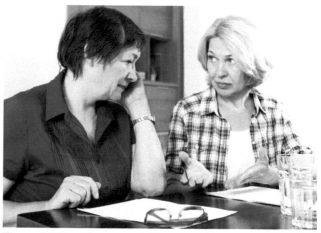

Figure 6.5 How do you work in partnership with others?

Evidence opportunity

3.2 Demonstrate ways of working that can help improve partnership working

Demonstrate to your assessor a situation that involves you working in partnership with others in the care setting where you work. For example, this may be working with a colleague when moving and positioning an individual, or meeting with an individual and their family to discuss the care the individual is receiving from you. Alternatively it might be carrying out a group activity working alongside your colleagues and other professionals such as music therapists or drama teachers.

AC 3.3 Identify skills and approaches needed for resolving conflicts

Working in partnership in care settings with different people and organisations can at times be challenging. Although everyone is working towards agreed goals, disagreements may result over how to achieve these goals due to people's different ideas about how to deal with situations.

If conflicts are not managed effectively then this can be very damaging to how the team works together, communication can break down, causing resentment, and people may stop sharing information, which in turn may lead to the care and support not meeting individuals' needs.

Therefore, it is important that you are aware of the main skills and approaches needed for resolving conflicts that may arise in your care setting. The main skill that you need to resolve conflicts is good communication abilities. If someone disagrees with you, or if you disagree with them, the best way to resolve the issue is to have an open and honest discussion where you can both discuss your differences in a calm way.

You should openly state what the issue, conflict or disagreement is. Each of you should listen to what the other person (or people) have to say and put forward your thoughts and opinions. You may need to involve others who have more experience in the area that is the cause of the dispute.

You can then try to find a way to resolve the conflict. This should not be an argument or a debate. It should be a discussion where the best interests of the individual, the setting or best practice are at the heart of the matter.

Table 6.3 on page 232 includes some examples of the main skills and approaches that you can use when you discuss and try to resolve conflicts.

Research it

3.3 Conflicts

Carry out some research in the care setting where you work. Speak with your colleagues about some of the conflicts that have arisen in the team and how these have been resolved. Find out what happened for two of these conflicts. Why did they arise? Who was involved? How did they make everyone feel? Discuss your findings with your manager. Reflect on how you felt doing this activity. Did you feel uncomfortable or awkward about asking these questions? Why might you feel awkward?

Reflect on it

3.3 Consequences of not resolving conflicts

Reflect on the two conflicts you researched earlier that arose and were resolved in the care setting where you work. Reflect on the consequences should these not have been resolved. Why would these have impacted negatively on the team and the care and support provided to individuals?

Table 6.3 Skills and approaches needed for resolving conflicts

Skills required for resolving conflicts	Approaches required for resolving conflicts
Empathy: Show that you are able to put yourself in someone else's shoes. This can help you gain a better understanding of others' views and feelings and it also encourages mutual respect as the other person knows that you are taking their view into account.	**Use effective communication**: For example, it is important to show that you are genuinely interested in what others are saying; you can do this by using positive body language such as nodding, smiling and maintaining eye contact, by actively listening and trying to understand others' views. This also encourages a willingness to work together.
Assertiveness: Show that you are confident and able to make clear your views and the reasons why. This will inspire confidence, as it will show that you are capable of making reasoned judgements and know what you are talking about. This also encourages mutual trust.	**Be positive**: It is important to show that you are being constructive and taking into account others' views and beliefs. You can do this by acknowledging what others are saying by repeating their views back (to show that you have understood) and by using respectful language. This encourages mutual respect.
Honesty: Be honest when sharing information and communicating with others. This will show that you have a genuine interest in individuals' well-being and promoting positive outcomes. This also encourages others to approach you and encourages open communications.	**Make the conflict the difficulty** rather than the individual or a member of the team. Focus on the conflict rather than on a person. This avoids making it personal and stops anyone feeling like they are to blame. (You can do this by not using negative language or making negative comments about specific individuals or members of the team.) This encourages positive teamwork as everyone knows that while you may disagree, you are still a team working together to resolve an issue.
Enthusiasm: Show your willingness to work in partnership with others. This can help with team building and will show that you genuinely care about working with them and not simply because it is part of your job.	
Negotiation: Show your ability to communicate with others to reach a mutual agreement or compromise. This can help with putting ideas for improvement into practice. This also encourages mutual trust, respect and open communications.	

Key terms

Empathy is the ability to understand how someone else may be feeling, or understand another person's way of thinking.

Negotiation means reaching an agreement through discussion.

Evidence opportunity

3.3 Skills and approaches needed for resolving conflicts

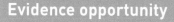

Think of a time when conflict arose in the care setting where you work. Write down the skills

that would need to be shown, and the working approaches that could be taken, in order to resolve this conflict.

AC 3.4 Access support and advice about partnership working and resolving conflicts

Your practices will be observed for this assessment criterion.

As partnership working and resolving conflicts involves working with many different people and

organisations there may be times when you may need to seek support or advice. This may be when:

- an individual's family wants you to disclose personal information about their relative that they do not have a need to know – this means that the individual's family may be frustrated with you that you are not disclosing this information as they may feel they have a right to know as they are related to the individual and you are not

- you have been asked to complete a work activity that you do not feel competent to carry out – this means that you may feel anxious that if you don't carry it out this may result in your employer thinking that you are not skilled enough for the job role you have been employed to carry out – but on the other hand you know that you also have a duty of care
- you have been asked to support an individual with an aspect of their care that is not agreed as part of the individual's care plan – this may cause tensions between you and the individual – at the same time you know that you have to work within the agreed scope of your job role.

Being able to recognise the types of different situation and when you must ask for support and advice is just as important as knowing how to do so. There will be procedures in the care setting where you work for how to do this and you must ensure that you comply with these agreed ways of working when seeking support and advice about partnership working and resolving conflicts. If you have tried to resolve the issues with the people concerned or feel unable to approach those involved directly then there are other options available to you.

Sources of support and advice available within your work setting can include an experienced colleague who you trust, your manager or someone else in a senior position. These colleagues, due to their experience, may have come across a similar difficulty or conflict before and will also have the skills and expertise to be able to assess the best ways to resolve the situation quickly and satisfactorily.

It is important not to delay seeking support and advice because not doing so may lead to these difficulties becoming worse, tensions increasing and the quality of care and support provided to individuals being affected negatively.

If you are unable to access the support you need or are dissatisfied with the advice offered by your manager then you must contact the next level of management within the care setting where you work. For example, this may be a more senior manager or the owner.

If you are still dissatisfied with the response you receive from senior management, then you may need to seek advice from independent external sources. Sources of support fall into two categories: those relevant to the care being given to an individual, and those that relate to employment issues. CQC is the regulatory body for care and would be able to assist with care-related issues; the Advisory, Conciliation and Arbitration Service (**ACAS**) would be able to assist with employment-related issues.

The reflective exemplar that follows will help to draw your attention to the importance of always taking action when there are difficulties with partnership working or resolving conflicts.

Key term

ACAS is an independent organisation that provides impartial and confidential advice to employees for resolving difficulties and conflicts at work.

Research it

3.4 Policies and procedures in your setting

Research the procedures that are in place in the care setting where you work for seeking support and advice about partnership working and resolving conflicts. Develop a poster with your main findings.

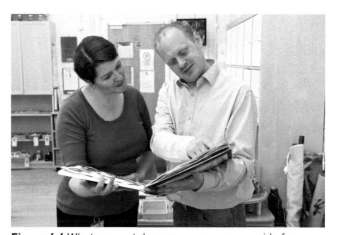

Figure 6.6 What support does your manager provide for resolving conflicts?

Reflective exemplar	
Introduction	I work as a personal assistant to Gemma, a young lady who has cerebral palsy and episodes of depression. My duties involve supporting Gemma with personal care tasks such as showering, dressing, eating and drinking.
What happened?	Yesterday morning I arrived as usual to support Gemma with her personal hygiene and saw that she was smoking cannabis in bed. I asked Gemma what she thought she was doing smoking cannabis, an illegal drug, and she told me that she had been doing this for a while as it helped her physical body spasms and reduced the pain she was in.
	I explained to Gemma politely that I didn't think this was appropriate as it wasn't good for her health and well-being. Gemma told me that it was her home and she could do what she liked and that as she employed me as her personal assistant I would have to continue with assisting her with her personal hygiene routine.
	I explained to Gemma politely that I didn't agree and left immediately without telling anyone so as not to cause any more conflict.
	The next day I found out from the office that after I had left Gemma, she telephoned her advocate and her parents to tell them that she was very unhappy with me as her personal assistant because I did not treat her as an adult and did not respect her beliefs. I was also informed that Gemma had requested a different personal assistant.
What worked well?	I was polite and I communicated calmly with Gemma in this difficult situation.
What did not go as well?	I should not have left without telling anyone. I should have sought advice straight away and communicated that I was doing so to Gemma.
	Also, I should have explained clearly to Gemma my duty of care towards her and showed more compassion in understanding her situation, i.e. that she was in pain. Perhaps I could have suggested alternative remedies that are available to help Gemma.
What could I do to improve?	I think I will need to familiarise myself again with the procedures to follow if I experience this type of situation again.
	In addition, I plan to discuss this situation with my line manager and request some further training in how I can be more confident and assertive when dealing with conflicts at work.
Links to unit assessment criteria	ACs 3.2, 3.3, 3.4

Evidence opportunity

3.4 **Accessing support and advice about partnership working and resolving conflicts**

Write a reflective account of how you would seek support and advice in relation to a conflict or a difficulty with partnership working at work. Ensure that you are able to show how you identified the most appropriate source of support and advice, what you reported and recorded, the reasons why, as well as a positive outcome.

LO3 Knowledge, skills, behaviours
Knowledge: why is it important to work in partnership with others?
Do you know why partnership working is essential for teamwork?
Do you know why effective care to individuals cannot be achieved without partnership working?
Do you know the skills and approaches needed for resolving conflicts?
Did you know that you have just answered three questions about the importance of working in partnership with others?
Skills: how can you show that you have the necessary skills for improving partnership working, resolving conflicts and accessing support and advice?
Do you know how to demonstrate shared values and agreed goals that can help improve partnership working?
Do you know how to show effective skills and approaches for resolving conflicts?
Do you know who to go to for support and advice in the care setting where you work if asked to do a work task that you do not feel competent to carry out?
Did you know that you have just answered three questions about some of the skills you have in relation to working in partnership with others effectively?
Behaviours: how can you show the personal qualities you have when partnership working and resolving conflicts?
Do you know how to behave with sensitivity if an individual wants you to care for them in a way that has not been agreed as per their care plan?
Do you know how to approach a colleague assertively if you witness them using unsafe practices?
Did you know that you have just answered two questions about a few of the essential behaviours that are expected to be able to work in partnership with others and resolve conflicts at work?

Suggestions for using the activities

This table summarises all the activities in the unit that are relevant to each assessment criterion.

Here, we also suggest other, different methods that you may want to use to present your knowledge and skills by using the activities.

These are just suggestions, and you should refer to the Introduction section at the start of the book, and more importantly the City & Guilds specification, and your assessor, who will be able to provide more guidance on how you can evidence your knowledge and skills.

When you need to be observed during your assessment, this can be done by your assessor, or your manager can provide a witness testimony.

Assessment criteria and accompanying activities	Suggested methods to show your knowledge/skills
LO1 Understand working relationships in care settings	
1.1 Research it (page 209)	Write notes to detail your findings.
1.1 Reflect on it (page 210)	Write a short reflective account.
1.1 Evidence opportunity (page 214) 1.1, 2.1, 2.3 Case study (page 213)	Answer the questions in the activity and provide a written account. Or you could write a personal statement that explains the main differences between a working relationship and a personal relationship. Remember to include examples of both in your personal statement. Discuss with your manager the boundaries that are established in working relationships and how these differ to personal relationships. They can provide a witness testimony. You will find the case study useful when thinking about boundaries at work.

Suggestions for using the activities	
1.2 Evidence opportunity (page 217)	Develop an information handout as instructed in the activity.
	Or you could develop a presentation that describes different working relationships in care settings. For example, you could begin by thinking about your care setting and detail the different working relationships that exist and the reasons why.
	You could also discuss with your manager how the working relationships you have in the care setting where you work are different to those your manager has. Find out what each working relationship involves. Your manager will be able to provide a witness testimony.
LO2 Be able to work in ways that are agreed with the employer	
LO1 Understand working relationships in care settings	
2.1 Research it (page 219)	Provide a written account addressing the points in the activity.
2.1 Evidence opportunity (page 221) 1.1, 2.1, 2.3 Case study (page 213)	Describe the points mentioned in the activity to your assessor.
	You could also write a personal statement or prepare a presentation that details the reasons why it is important for you to adhere to the agreed scope of your job role. You could include in your statement the consequences of not doing so.
	The case study is a useful source of information.
2.2 Reflect on it (page 222)	Write a short reflective account.
2.2 Evidence opportunity (page 223)	Complete the activity and produce a poster.
	You must make arrangements for your work practices to be observed so that you can show how you access full and up-to-date details of agreed ways of working in the care setting where you work. You could also collect a witness testimony to support your observation.
2.3 Research it (page 224)	Provide a written account addressing the points in the activity.
2.3 Evidence opportunity (page 224) 1.1, 2.1, 2.3 Case study (page 213)	You must make arrangements for your work practices to be observed so that you can show how you work in line with agreed ways of working in your care setting. Arrange for your assessor to observe you while you carry out two activities, as instructed in the activity.
	You could also collect a witness testimony to support your observation.
	The case study is a useful source of information.
2.4 Reflect on it (page 227)	Provide a short reflective account.
2.4 Research it (page 227)	Produce an information handout as instructed in the activity, or provide a written account.
2.4 Evidence opportunity (page 228) 2.4 Case study (page 227)	You must make arrangements for your work practices to be observed so that you can show how you contribute to quality assurance processes to promote positive experiences for individuals receiving care. Demonstrate to your assessor how quality assurance ensures the care an individual receives is of the highest quality. Demonstrate how you have put this into practice as outlined in the activity.
	You could also collect a witness testimony to support your observation.
	The case study is a useful source of information.
LO3 Be able to work in partnership with others	
3.1 Evidence opportunity (page 229)	Develop a PowerPoint presentation as instructed in the activity.
	Or you could write a personal statement about the reasons why it is important to work in partnership with others in the care setting where you work.
	You could also discuss the importance of working in partnership with others and the consequences of not doing so with a colleague, which will inform your understanding.

➡

Suggestions for using the activities	
3.2 Evidence opportunity (page 230)	Demonstrate to your assessor a situation that involves you working with others as instructed in the activity.
3.2, 3.3, 3.4 Reflective exemplar (page 234)	You must make arrangements for your work practices to be observed so that you can demonstrate different ways of working that can help improve partnership working. The reflective exemplar will help you with how to show best practice. You could also collect a witness testimony to support the observation of your work practices.
3.3 Research it (page 231)	Provide a written account to answer the points in the activity.
3.3 Reflect on it (page 231)	Provide a reflective account addressing the points in the activity.
3.3 Evidence opportunity (page 232)	Provide a written account answering the points in the activity.
3.2, 3.3, 3.4 Reflective exemplar (page 234)	You must make arrangements for your work practices to be observed so that you can demonstrate different skills and approaches that you use to resolve conflicts. The reflective exemplar will help you to think about different skills and approaches you can use. You could also collect a witness testimony to support the observation of your work practices.
3.4 Research it (page 233)	Develop a poster with your findings.
3.4 Evidence opportunity (page 234)	You could provide a written account as suggested in the activity.
3.2, 3.3, 3.4 Reflective exemplar (page 234)	You must make arrangements for your work practices to be observed so that you can show how you access support and advice about partnership working and resolving conflicts.
	The reflective exemplar will help you to think about different skills and approaches that you can use.
	You could also collect a witness testimony to support the observation of your work practices.

Legislation	
Relevant Act	**It states that:**
Civil Partnership Act 2004	you can get married or form a civil partnership in the UK if you are: 16 or over, free to marry or form a civil partnership (i.e. single, divorced or widowed), not closely related. Only same-sex couples can form a civil partnership. You need permission from your parents or guardians if you are under 18 in England, Wales and Northern Ireland.
Data Protection Act 1998	employers must ensure the secure handling of all information and data. Adult care settings therefore have policies, procedures and agreed ways of working in place to ensure that individuals' personal information is kept secure and handled lawfully when recorded, used, stored and shared.
General Data Protection Regulation (GDPR) 2018	In May 2018, the General Data Protection Regulation (GDPR) came into force. It provides detailed guidance to organisations on how to govern and manage people's personal information and this will need to be included in the care setting's policies, procedures, guidelines and agreed ways of working.

Resources for reading and research

Books

Davies, C. Finlay, C. and Bullman, A. (2000) *Changing Practice in Health and Social Care*, Sage Publications

Ferreiro Peteiro, M. (2014) *Level 2 Health and Social Care Diploma Evidence Guide*, Hodder Education

Hawkins, R. and Ashurst, A. (2006) *How to be a Great Care Assistant*, Hawker Publications

Knapman, J. and Morrison, T. (1998) *Making the Most of Supervision in Health and Social Care*, Pavilion Publishers

Weblinks

www.acas.org.uk Advisory, Conciliation and Arbitration Service (ACAS) – providing workers with impartial and independent advice for work issues

www.cqc.org.uk Care Quality Commission (CQC) – information about the standards expected from care settings and workers providing care and support to individuals

www.skillsforcare.org.uk Skills for Care – information about the knowledge, skills and behaviours expected from adult care workers

Handle information in care settings (206)

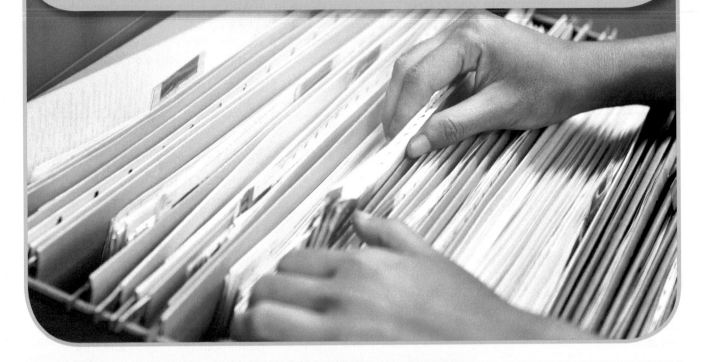

About this unit

Credit value: 1
Guided learning hours: 10

Handling information in **care settings** is a big responsibility. There is a lot of information to document about every individual in a care setting and this is held in different files and reports. The information we record about individuals is personal and private to that individual and so it is very important that these documents are handled with care. These are legal documents and need to be completed, stored and shared by following **agreed ways of working** and legal requirements.

In this unit, you will learn about the legislation that relates to the recording, storage and sharing of information in care settings. You will also develop your understanding of the reasons why it is important to have secure systems in place for recording and storing an individual's information and how you can access guidance and advice about handling that information in your care setting. You will also understand what to do and the actions to take if you have any concerns or are worried about recording, storing and sharing information.

Finally, you will be able to develop your skills around keeping records that are up to date, complete, accurate and legible, and how to follow policies and agreed ways of working for recording, storing and sharing information.

Learning outcomes

LO1: Understand the need for secure handling of information in care settings

LO2: Know how to access support for handling information

LO3: Be able to handle information in accordance with agreed ways of working

Key terms

Care settings can be residential homes, nursing homes, domiciliary care, day centres, an individual's own home or some clinical healthcare settings. Full definitions of each of these terms are included in the glossary.

Agreed ways of working are your employer's or setting's policies and procedures. In this unit, the agreed ways of working that we discuss are to do with handling information. The 'agreed ways of working' may be documented less formally if you are working for smaller employers, including the guidance on handling information.

LO1 Understand the need for secure handling of information in care settings

Getting started

Think about all the conversations that you and your friends or family have. Do they ever tell you something private or personal about themselves that they do not want others to know? Do you make sure that you keep that information safe and do not tell others?

How would they feel if you told someone or passed on that information without asking them? Think about how you would feel if you told your friends something private about yourself and did not want them to tell anyone else.

Now think about the information that you tell people about yourself, and more specifically the more official information such as private and **personal information** that you tell your doctor, or a nurse.

Then think about how they might record, store and share this information. You may not want them to pass this on to others without your permission. Why do you think it is important that they record, share and store this information in a safe way? Think about the reasons. Is this because the information is personal and private? Is it because you do not want others to have access to this information? Have you ever wanted to see the information that they have recorded about you? How would you feel if you asked to see the information that the people who care for you had recorded only to be told you are not allowed to see it?

Thinking about this will help you to understand why it is important to handle information securely in care settings.

AC 1.1 Identify the legislation that relates to the recording, storage and sharing of information in care settings

Handling information in a care setting involves:

- recording accurate information about individuals so that you and your colleagues can provide good-quality care or support that meets individuals' needs

- storing information about individuals securely if you are to ensure that you maintain their **confidentiality** (see page 241 for definition)

- sharing information about individuals safely and in a way that respects individuals' rights to privacy and in agreement with who it should be shared.

Information and legislation

Information in a care setting is needed for different reasons:

- for making decisions and planning the care and support for individuals
- to get to know individuals, for example their backgrounds, cultures, needs, wishes and preferences
- to find out about the individuals' support networks, such as their families, friends and advocates
- to provide information to other professionals, for example the GP, pharmacist, social worker
- to provide information about individuals to your colleagues to ensure consistent care and support
- to provide an audit trail for actions (this would be particularly important in any investigation about abuse or an incident).

The term 'legislation' in the UK means a set of laws that are put forward by the Government and made official by Parliament. Legislation in relation to recording, storing and sharing information is very important because it:

- sets out the **rights** and **responsibilities** of all those who live and work in care settings

- requires accurate information to be recorded about individuals
- requires information about individuals to be stored securely
- requires information about individuals to be shared securely.

In your role as a care worker you will need to know and understand the different pieces of legislation that exist in relation to the recording, storing and sharing of information in care settings so that you are able to carry out your duties to the best of your ability. Showing your **competence** involves putting into practice your knowledge and skills of how to record, store and share information effectively.

Table 7.1 includes information about relevant pieces of legislation.

Research it

1.1 Why are laws needed?

Research the reasons why laws are needed and how they are developed in the UK. See the UK Parliament's 'Making Laws':

www.parliament.uk/about/how/laws/

Key terms

Personal information refers to information that is personal to the individual such as their name, date of birth, weight, care needs.

Confidentiality refers to maintaining the privacy of sensitive or restricted information such as information about an individual's diagnosis of a health condition.

Rights are legal entitlements to something, for example, to have the information held about you by an organisation kept secure.

Responsibilities are the legal (ones that you are legally required to fulfil like working to the requirements of the Data Protection Act 1998 or the General Data Protection Regulation 2018) and moral duties and tasks that you are required to do as part of your job role. Examples include writing information in an individual's record book clearly, only noting factual information, completing records fully and accurately so that it can be read and understood.

Competence means to effectively apply the knowledge, skills and behaviours you have learned.

Competence

Applying your knowledge and skills in relation to handling information is essential for high-quality care and support. This is because you need accurate information to plan how to meet individuals' care or support needs.

You can do this by showing that you can write accurate reports about individuals, keep individuals' reports in a safe place in the care setting where you work, and share information about individuals only when you have permission to do so. See AC 1.2, page 246, for more information on competence.

Key term

Processing, in this unit, refers to handling information, i.e. recording, storing and sharing information.

Research it

1.1 Legislation for recording, storing and sharing information

For more information about these pieces of legislation, you will find it useful to access:

www.gov.uk

Also see the website of the Information Commissioner's Office (ICO), which is an independent body in the UK established to uphold information rights:

https://ico.org.uk

Table 7.1 Legislation for the handling of information in care settings

Legislation	What is it and how does it relate to handling information securely in care settings?
Data Protection Act 1998	This Act is the main piece of legislation that protects the rights of people who have personal information recorded, used, stored and shared by organisations. It also established how personal information can be used.
	Under this Act, all information you use in your care setting, must be:
	• collected and used or **processed** fairly and lawfully, for example you can do this by obtaining the individual's permission
	• used and held only for the reasons given when obtained, for example you can do this by making sure that if information is requested for an individual's care plan it should only be used for their care plan
	• adequate, relevant and not excessive, for example if information about an individual's communication needs is required then, you should make sure that it is specific and relevant to the individual's communication needs only
	• accurate and kept up to date, for example you can do this by making sure that information held is checked by the individuals concerned and by others who know them
	• removed when necessary, for example you can do this by making sure that when information is no longer needed, it is deleted
	• collected and used in line with the person's rights, for example you can do this by informing individuals what information is being collected, the reasons why and how it is being used

→

Table 7.1 Legislation for the handling of information in care settings *continued*

Legislation	What is it and how does it relate to handling information securely in care settings?
General Data Protection Regulation (GDPR) 2018	• kept safe and secure, for example you can do this by ensuring all paper-based and electronic information is accessed only by those who have permission to do so, ensuring it is stored securely by being locked away when not being used and is password-protected • verified before transfer to other countries without adequate protection, for example you can do this by ensuring information is not transferred to other countries without the individual's permission as these countries may not have legislation in place in relation to how personal information about individuals is used and stored. The Act also allows people the right to see the information about themselves, which means that individuals can ask to see the information should they wish to do so. The Act also protects people from having their information accessed by other people. In May 2018, the Data Protection Act was replaced by the General Data Protection Regulation (GDPR). The **GDPR** gives individuals greater rights over their personal information: • Organisations will have to demonstrate how they have obtained individuals' consent when handling information. • Individuals will have the right to give and to withdraw their consent for processing information. • Individuals' rights and interests must be safeguarded when information is being processed, i.e. to rectify inaccurate personal data. • All public authorities must have a named data protection officer who is responsible for ensuring the organisation is complying with the GDPR and is the main point of contact.
Human Rights Act 1998	This Act sets out the rights and freedoms that everyone in the UK is entitled to in a series of articles and every article relates to a different right. Under this Act people are entitled to the following rights in relation to the handling of information. • Article 8 – The right to respect for your private and family life, home and correspondence such as letters, telephone calls and emails • This article states that personal information about an individual must be kept securely and not shared without their permission; except in certain circumstances, such as in the case of a medical emergency where information about an individual's condition is required. • Personal information about a person includes, for example, official records, photographs, letters, diaries and medical records. • You should be aware of these rights, because in your role you will gather information about individuals as you discuss and plan with them the care or support they would like.
Freedom of Information Act 2000	This Act promotes the right of people to request information held about them by public authorities such as government departments, schools, colleges and universities, health trusts, hospitals and doctors' surgeries and the police. This right is referred to as the 'right to know'. Under this Act, as a care worker you must: • support individuals' rights to access and view information that has been recorded about them (unless there are reasons to keep it confidential), such as care files, medical reports, documents, letters, test results, minutes of a meeting held about their care needs. • You should remember this when you are recording information about individuals as they may access the files and will be able to read what you have said. You should remember that this Act does not allow people to access the personal data of other people, only their own.

➜

Table 7.1 Legislation for the handling of information in care settings *continued*

Legislation	What is it and how does it relate to handling information securely in care settings?
Care Act 2014	*'Information, information, information – without it, how can people be truly at the heart of decisions? Information should be available to all regardless of how their care is paid for. There are some things that should be universal – information is one.'* *Department of Health, 'Care Act Factsheet 1: General responsibilities of local authorities: prevention, information and advice, and shaping the market of care and support services', April 2016* The Care Act places duties and responsibilities on local authorities when providing care or support services. As a care worker, you should: • provide the information and advice individuals need to make good decisions about their care and support, for example you will need to provide information and advice on the types and range of care and support available to individuals, how to access the care and support available, how to access independent financial advice • provide information and advice to individuals in a way they can understand, for example by making it available in different formats such as in Braille, in a different language, using signs and pictures, by working closely with professionals and services to help individuals to understand the information provided.
Health and Social Care Act 2008 (Regulated Activities) Regulations 2014	The 2014 Regulations established the fundamental standards that identify the standards of care that care workers are expected to meet at all times. They also established the **duty of candour** that requires care workers to be **open** and **transparent** with individuals and their representatives such as their advocates or families, regarding their care and treatment. Under this Act, as a care worker, you must: • use personal information about individuals in care settings in line with your organisation's requirements so that the care provided to individuals is safe, effective and of a high quality • promote **openness** by supporting individuals and others to raise any concerns and complaints they may have • promote **transparency** by allowing information about the organisation's services and their outcomes to be shared, e.g. with individuals, their families.

The Caldicott Principles

The Caldicott Principles are a set of seven principles that were developed in the 1990s following a review into the use of patient information across the NHS. Organisations should adhere to these principles to ensure that patient-identifiable information is protected and only used when necessary. Although these guidelines are not the law as such, it is important that you are aware of them. For more information, take a look at: www.igt.hscic.gov.uk/Caldicott2Principles.aspx

Key terms

GDPR refers to the General Data Protection Regulation. This is a set of data protection laws that protects individuals' personal information. This superseded (or replaced) the Data Protection Act 1998 in May 2018.

Duty of candour refers to the standards that adult care workers must follow when mistakes are made. This means being open and honest.

Open or **openness** is being truthful and approachable.

Transparent or **transparency** is making the same information available to everyone.

1.1, 3.2 Legislation for recording, storing and sharing information

List three pieces of personal information that you know about for one individual in the care setting where you work.

Think about how these three pieces of information are recorded. Are they in writing? Or are they stored electronically? Where are they stored? Is this information shared with other people in the care setting where you work? If so, who?

Identify the legislation that is relevant to how these three pieces of information are recorded, stored and shared in the care setting where you work.

AC 1.2 Explain why it is important to have secure systems in place for recording and storing information in a care setting

As you will have learned it is important to have secure systems in place for recording and storing information in a care setting to comply with or follow legislation. Not doing so will mean that you are not carrying out your responsibilities competently.

If you are not recording and storing information properly, the information that others in the setting may need to access about individuals will be of poor quality. If the information is not accurate or correct, this can lead to mistakes happening and unsafe care and support being provided to individuals.

The individuals that you care for also need to be confident that the information that they give to you will be recorded and safely secured. This involves showing compassion when handling their personal information – in other words, thinking about how you would feel if it were your personal and private information and how safely and securely you would want it to be handled. If they do not trust that this will happen, it could stop

them from giving you information, or affect the things that they decide to tell you.

It is important that individuals in your care setting understand that you will only share the information they have given you if you have their permission to do so. Any information that you do share about them with your colleagues, or other professionals, will only be shared in private to ensure its confidentiality and that it is on a need-to-know basis (this is covered in Unit 203, AC 4.3). When making a decision about what information can be shared and not shared on a 'need-to-know' basis, the individual's personal situation must always be taken into account as well as their best interests. You can only do this if you know the individual. When making a decision to share or not share information on a 'need-to-know' basis, the pros and cons must be fully explored and a decision made in the individual's best interests only.

You will also need to keep in mind any capacity issues – does the individual have capacity to make the decision to share or not share details? The issue of capacity is covered in Unit 211, LO3.

It is also important that the individuals understand that sometimes you have to share information about them without their permission – a process referred to as 'breaching confidentiality'. For example, if an individual tells you that they are going to harm themselves or someone else. You would need to share this kind of information without their permission, probably with your manager, because not doing so may mean that they will put themselves and others in danger; something that you cannot allow to happen.

Compassion is central to keeping individuals' personal information secure as doing so involves showing your kindness towards individuals and upholding their rights to dignity, respect and being taken seriously.

Secure systems for recording and storing information

Recording and storing information must always be done in ways that ensure the security of

6Cs

Competence

Competence means carrying out your work tasks to the best of your ability and while applying the required knowledge and skills. Here it would mean that you are able to effectively handle, record, store and share information without compromising the confidentiality of these documents and the privacy of the individual. You could for example show this by making sure that if you need to share confidential information, and have been given permission to do so by the individual, then you only share this in private, perhaps in a private meeting room.

Compassion

Compassion here means being able to provide care and support, with kindness when working with individuals' personal information. In order to do this, you will need to be able to empathise, and understand what it is like to share your own personal information, and how you would like it to be treated. What would it be like to have your personal information shared without your permission, or what would it be like if your personal medical records accidentally went missing?

You should show individuals that you care about and understand that their personal information is important and must be treated sensitively at all times. You can do this by thinking about the words you use when sharing written and verbal information about individuals, i.e. they should be respectful, positive and appropriate. For example, you can show respect by asking them if it is okay for information to be shared with others.

---

the information being held. This is because individuals have rights to have their personal information kept private and safe and you have a duty to uphold these.

Secure systems for hard-copy or paper-based files

What is the meaning of 'secure systems'? What do they look like in a care setting? Below are some key features of secure systems for paper-based and electronic records and information. To make sure that the systems in your setting are secure, you should make sure that private information and files are:

- **kept locked.** You should make sure that any files are kept in a filing cabinet, or a drawer that is locked, and not left anywhere that others may be able to easily access or see them. Keys should be held with a named member of staff to ensure that only those who have permission can access the information. It is also important that you do not take personal information about individuals anywhere with you as you could accidentally misplace or lose this, which may mean other people have access to the information. For example, if you are supporting an individual to learn how to travel independently on public transport, it is important that you do not complete your daily records while travelling; you can do this safely when you return to the care setting. The consequences of losing information could be serious. 'Identity theft' is a crime and has become a bigger issue in recent years. This is when people steal other people's personal details to commit **fraud** (see page 248 for definition). They may pretend to be that person in order to perhaps buy goods, or get loans in that person's name. This has also increased with the sharing of information on the internet, which means that the protection of all personal data has become a very important issue.

- **safe from damage.** Files should be protected from water, fire damage and theft. This may mean that they are kept in waterproof document folders, or in locked filing cabinets as mentioned.

- **easy to retrieve when required.** This means that you should be able to find what you are looking for fairly easily. You can do this by using an index, for example which could be in alphabetical order, under individuals' surnames, in a named file if held on a computer.

- **backed up.** This means that if you have hard-copy or paper files, then you should make sure that this information is also stored electronically so that if you lose the paper files you have the information stored somewhere else as well.

- **understood by those who have access to it and those who will be using it.** Files and the information in them must be presented in a format that can be understood clearly. Handwriting, for example, must be neat and legible; it should be dated so that it is clear when the records were written. Even if you make notes quickly on a notepad, make sure you transfer them to a safe place; then destroy the notes so others cannot read them, by shredding them, for example.

- **monitored regularly for their effectiveness.** This means that you and your colleagues should review and feed back on how well the systems in place are working. What is working well when it comes to recording and storing information? What is *not* working well? This includes being open and honest about when things go wrong. This will mean that if some things are working particularly well or effectively in terms of keeping information safe and secure, they still need to be maintained or improved if necessary.

Your setting will have its own policies and you should make sure that you are aware of these.

Secure systems for electronic files

Where files are stored electronically (on a computer), you should make sure that private information and files are:

- **password protected.** If files are stored in a computer, then the computer and files should be password protected, and with different passwords for those with different levels of access to ensure that only information that is needed is accessed by those with permission to do so. Passwords should be changed regularly. This is another measure you can put in place to make sure that files are secured, and to make sure that no one without permission is able to access files. And remember, do not write passwords down.

- **firewall protected.** Computers that store personal details, data and information should be protected by a 'firewall'. This is a piece of software that protects the computer and the information stored from people outside who do not have permission to access the network or the information that is stored on the computer. It can also stop people 'hacking' into the computer and possibly stealing information. Hacking occurs when people access a computer without permission, and possibly misuse the information.

- **anti-virus software protected.** Firewalls can also stop other internet viruses from infecting the computer. They can be installed as part of anti-virus software which will stop any harmful virus from entering your computer. You may know from experience of having a virus on your laptop or computer that viruses can harm documents or files that you have stored. You may even have had your computer or laptop repaired or fixed and lost files. How serious might this be if a virus infected a computer in your care setting? While anti-virus software may not stop all viruses, it is definitely something that should be installed on computers in your setting as this can stop important information and files from being lost.

- **backed up.** You must make sure your computer is regularly 'backed up' and keep copies of paper documents as well, in case the electronic copies are lost. They should also be stored safely.

Research it

1.2 NHS hacking scandal 2017

Research the famous global cyber-attack that took place in January 2017, which affected more than 100 countries and had serious consequences for the NHS and its hospitals across the UK. Doctors were unable to access electronic information held on IT systems unless a ransom was paid. This meant many operations were cancelled as patients' personal information about allergies and health conditions, for example, could not be accessed. Results of patients' blood tests and x-rays could not be obtained and patients could not be admitted or discharged from hospital without access to their information that was held electronically.

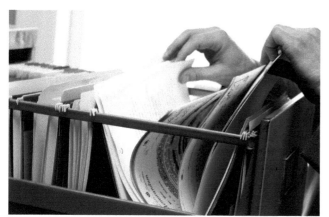

Figure 7.1 How do you store records in the care setting where you work?

Key terms

Fraud means deliberately misleading a person to commit an unlawful act, for example pretending to be an individual's relative on the telephone so that you can obtain personal information about the individual.

Comply or **complying** means to follow and ensure you are working in line with your employer's agreed ways of working.

Agreed ways of working you will find it useful to refer back to the definition of this term provided earlier on, on page 240.

Reflect on it

1.2, 3.2 Complying with agreed ways of working

Reflect on the impact that *not* complying with your employer's agreed ways of working for recording and storing information can have.

● How can this affect you? How could it affect your job as an adult care worker? Or your future career working with adults?
● How could this affect your colleagues and the way they carry out their roles and responsibilities? How could this affect the way the whole team works together?
● What would happen to the individuals who receive care and support from you? What about their working relationship with you and the team? What would happen to the quality of care they would receive?

Now that you understand the meaning of secure systems, let us think about other reasons, apart from **complying** with legislation, why it is important to have secure systems in place for recording and storing information in a care setting.

To **comply** with or follow **agreed ways of working**:

● One of your responsibilities as an adult care worker will be to read and understand what your employer's agreed ways of working are in relation to recording and storing information.
● Complying with or following your employer's agreed ways of working correctly will mean that you will be following best practice.
● Not following your employer's agreed ways of working can have serious consequences for you, your colleagues at work and the individuals for whom you provide care and support. For example, you may lose your job, you will prevent your colleagues from providing the care the individual needs, and the individual may not have their unique needs met.

Your responsibilities and the consequences of not having secure systems in place

Protect the privacy of individuals' personal information

- As an adult care worker, you are responsible for protecting the privacy of all personal information that you record and store about individuals.

- Protecting the privacy of individuals' personal information will mean that you will be supporting individuals' rights to have their personal information kept private at all times. This will help you to form a relationship with the individual based on trust.

- Not protecting the privacy of individuals' personal information can have serious consequences as individuals may lose their trust in you because you are not keeping their information safe. It may stop them from sharing further information with you. Individuals' personal information could also be accessed by those who do not have permission to do so which places individuals in danger and/or at risk of harm and abuse. See page 246 for information on identity theft.

Prevent unauthorised access to individuals' personal information

- It will also be your responsibility to stop or prevent those who are not authorised, or do not have permission to access individuals' recorded and stored personal information, from doing so.

- You can keep individuals' personal information safe and secure by ensuring that you provide access to only those people with whom it has been agreed 'need to know' the individual's personal information. This means that the only people that this information is shared with are those that the individual has agreed can have access to their information.

- If you do not take steps to stop unauthorised people gaining access to individuals' personal information, there can be serious consequences. These include individuals' rights to privacy and respect not being upheld and personal information falling into the 'wrong hands'. This can in turn lead to individuals being put at risk of **harm** and **abuse** (see page 250 for definitions). It will take **commitment** from you to make sure that these safe standards are maintained on an ongoing basis and as part of your responsibilities. It will also take **courage** to recognise and admit when you have made mistakes.

6Cs

Commitment

Commitment means to be dedicated or devoted to doing something. Here it would involve being dedicated to ensuring individuals' personal information is maintained securely. This is for all the reasons that we have discussed in this section. In this way, individuals will be able to experience care and support that improves their lives and is focused on their individual needs and preferences. You can show your commitment to ensuring that information is kept safe by keeping the information that individuals share with you safe and not disclosing it to anyone else (unless it has been agreed previously). You can also show your commitment by raising any concerns about handling information with colleagues and your manager.

Courage

Courage here would involve you making sure that you speak up for individuals if you are aware that they may be put at risk of danger, harm or abuse and provide them with the necessary support. It is your duty to ensure their safety and well-being. You can do this by being observant and listening to what you are told and ensuring you report and record all concerns that you have or that others tell you about. If, for example, you feel that another member of staff has breached an individual's confidentiality without a good reason, you would need to consider whether to speak to your manager about this, and speak up for the individual.

Key terms

Harm can mean distress, pain or injury. An adult at risk of harm may be an individual with care or support needs who is unable to protect themselves and is at risk of abuse or harm. This may include individuals with learning disabilities, mental health needs and older people.

Abuse means to treat someone in a cruel way, by causing physical or emotional suffering. Someone who has been abused has experienced mistreatment by another person or persons that violates their human and civil rights.

Research it

1.1, 1.2, 3.2 Security of personal information

The Information Commissioner's Office (ICO) is an independent organisation that was set up to support information rights in the UK. Its job is to look at how information is handled. It has produced a guide for those who have day-to-day responsibility for data protection.

Research the part of the guide that provides information about how to manage the security of the personal information you hold, 'Information security (Principle 7)':

https://ico.org.uk/for-organisations/guide-to-data-protection/principle-7-security/

Discuss with a colleague how this compares to how you manage the security of personal information you hold in your work setting.

Prevent individuals' personal information getting lost or misplaced

This is similar to what we have discussed above, about ensuring that personal information is not accessed by people who have not been authorised. However, it is also your duty to ensure that information does not get lost or misplaced.

- As an adult care worker, you are responsible for keeping individuals' personal information safe and preventing it from getting lost or misplaced. For example, you will need to ensure it does not get lost in the care setting, or outside of the care setting. This means not taking private documents outside of the setting.

- Keeping individuals' personal information safe will mean that you will be supporting individuals' rights to respect and security for their personal information by not letting it be accessed by those who do not have permission to do so.

- Not preventing an individual's personal information from getting lost or misplaced can have serious consequences, for example if a hospital consultant needs to know the medication an individual is taking in a medical emergency.

Ensure the provision of safe care and support to individuals

Overall, you will need to have secure systems in place in order to ensure individuals are provided with safe care and support. As an adult care worker, you will be expected to develop the knowledge, skills, values and behaviours to ensure the provision of safe care and support to individuals.

Recording and storing individuals' personal information securely will mean that you will be able to support individuals to be in control of their care and support needs to live the lives they want safely and independently. If individuals trust you and your abilities, they will be able to trust that all information held about them is recorded accurately and kept safe.

Not ensuring the provision of safe care and support to individuals will have serious consequences for the continuity of their care and support and will in turn impact negatively on their lives. For example, if information is not recorded accurately, the people you work with will not be able to provide care that continues to meet individuals' needs in a consistent way and so their needs may remain unmet.

Evidence opportunity

1.2 Secure systems for storing and recording information

Produce a leaflet that provides individuals with information about the secure systems that exist in the care setting where you work.

Your leaflet must identify two secure systems you use for recording information and two systems you use for storing information. Then explain the reasons why these systems are important. You could also think about the consequences of not having these secure systems in place.

Case study

1.2, 3.2 The importance of keeping personal information secure

David works as a personal assistant and provides support to Joe, a young adult who has **autism**, to help him live a full and active life. David carries out a wide range of tasks such as providing assistance with meal preparation, going shopping, meeting friends, attending appointments and going on holiday. As part of his role David is required to keep Joe's personal information secure and respect Joe's right to privacy.

After supporting Joe with his shopping, David begins recording the tasks he has completed with him this morning in the **daily report book** while having a cup of coffee in the garden. While doing so, Joe's sister arrives, walks through to the garden where David is and sits down next to him. A few moments later the front doorbell rings and Joe asks David to come to the front door. David leaves the daily report book on the garden table and asks Joe's sister to keep an eye on it for him as he will only be a few minutes.

Five minutes later, David returns to the garden and finds Joe's sister reading through the daily report book. Joe's sister tells David that she has read that Joe has chosen not to prepare healthy meals and wants to know the reasons why. David explains politely to Joe's sister that she does not have the right to read through the daily report book as the information it contains about Joe is personal to him. Joe's sister replies, 'What do you mean? I'm his sister, of course I have a right.'

Discussion points

In pairs or small groups, ask each other the following questions.

1 Do you agree with Joe's sister? Why?
2 How could David have improved his recording in the daily report book and the way he stored Joe's personal information?
3 Why is it important for David to have secure systems for recording and storing Joe's personal information?

Key terms

Autism is a condition that affects how people perceive the world around them and interact with others. This can cause difficulties when communicating, interacting and socialising with others.

A **daily report book** is a record that is completed by adult care workers and includes information on the tasks, care and support provided on a day-to-day basis to individuals.

LO1 Knowledge, skills, behaviours
Knowledge: why is handling information in care settings important?
Do you know why you must keep personal information about individuals in care settings secure?
Do you know why you must respect individuals' personal information?
Do you know about the legislation that relates to the recording, storage and sharing of information in care settings?
Did you know that you have just answered three questions about the Data Protection Act 1998 and the legal requirements that are in place for handling information in care settings?
Skills: how can you show that you are complying with legislation for handling information?
Do you know how to record information about individuals while maintaining their rights to privacy?
Do you know how to store information about individuals securely?
Did you know that you have just answered two questions about a few of the skills that you will need to have when recording and storing individuals' personal information?
Behaviours: how can you show the personal qualities you have when handling information?
Do you know how to support individuals' dignity when you are recording information?
Do you know how to respect individuals' personal information?
Did you know that you have just answered two questions about a few of the essential behaviours that are expected of all adult care workers?

LO2 Know how to access support for handling information

Getting started

Think about an occasion when you were worried or anxious about someone or something and were unsure what to do about it. Who did you go to for guidance and advice? Why? What do you think would have happened if you didn't seek their guidance or advice?

Now think about how an individual in a care setting may feel if they approached you with a concern they had about how their information was being handled and you did nothing. Why do you think they would feel this way? How might it affect your working relationship with them?

AC 2.1 Describe how to access guidance, information and advice about handling information

As you will have already learned, current legislation requires that you comply with your different responsibilities in relation to handling individuals' personal information in care settings including when recording, storing and sharing information about individuals.

You cannot of course be expected to know everything about handling information but it is your responsibility to find out about anything you are unsure about or any concerns you have over the recording, storing or sharing of individuals' personal information. Figure 7.2 shows some examples of questions that need answering.

There are many different sources of guidance, information and advice about handling information. Who you go to will depend on: the question you have, where you work and the care setting you work in. In the first instance, you must go to your manager or to a senior member of staff in the care setting where you work. The Information Commissioner's Office (ICO) can provide up-to-date information about legislation; this can be useful for checking whether you are following legislation and guidelines for handling information.

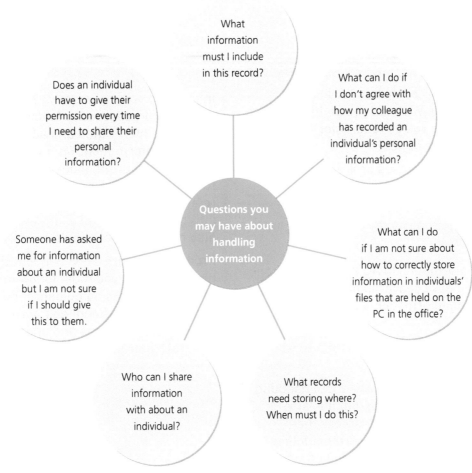

Figure 7.2 Questions about handling information

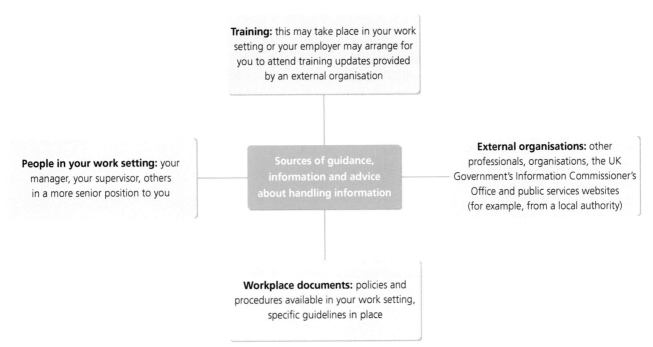

Figure 7.3 Sources of guidance for handling information in care settings

Reflect on it

2.1 Sources of guidance

Reflect on how the sources of guidance for handling information identified in Figure 7.3 compare to the sources that are available in your care setting. Who can you go to for guidance? Who can you go to for information? Who can you ask for advice?

Are these the same sources or are they different? Why do you think this is?

Figure 7.3 will help you identify the different sources of guidance.

There is more information in AC 2.2 on the actions to take when you have concerns over recording, storing or sharing information.

Examples of when to seek help and who to ask

It is important to know who to ask about handling information in your care setting, but it is also important that you know how to access the support you need. The process you must follow for accessing this support will depend on your job role and responsibilities as well as the agreed ways of working that are in place for the care setting where you work.

- If you are a care worker in a residential care home and want to know how you can access the communication page of an individual's care plan then a senior care worker could guide you with how to access it.
- If you are a personal assistant working in an individual's home and want to know more information about how the records you complete are stored securely then the individual could provide you with this information.
- If you are an activities worker in a nursing home and want to seek advice about the personal information that was disclosed by one individual about another during one of your activities sessions, then the manager of the nursing home could provide you with advice.

Evidence opportunity

2.1, 3.1, 3.2 Accessing guidance, information and advice about handling information

In the care setting where you work, find out about the procedures to follow for accessing guidance, information and advice about handling information. You may find it useful to speak with your manager and your colleagues. Reading your work setting's procedures in relation to how to record, store and share information as part of your day-to-day role will also help you with completing this activity.

Produce an information handout that details the procedures you must follow in your work setting for accessing guidance, information and advice about handling information. You can use diagrams and photographs to illustrate your information handout.

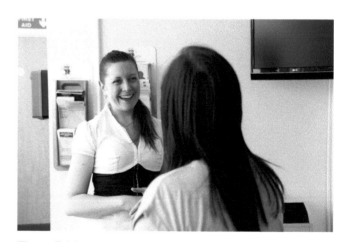

Figure 7.4 Are you a team player?

AC 2.2 Explain what actions to take when there are concerns over the recording, storing or sharing of information

You already know about the procedures you must follow in your care setting for accessing guidance, information and advice about handling information, but do you know what to do when you have concerns over the recording, storing or sharing of information? Do you know when to take action and the reasons why you may need to take action?

Every care setting will have a procedure in place that details the action to take when there are concerns over the recording, storing or sharing of information. You will need to look at the one at your setting so that you can find out what it says you must do when you need to know; who to go to, when and how the actions you take must be recorded.

Concerns and actions

In a care setting, where information is constantly being recorded, stored and shared, there may be times where not everyone will be following the correct procedures and you may be concerned about how information is recorded and stored. You must take action when there is an issue that is worrying you. Remembering these best practice points will help you with taking the correct actions over concerns that you and/or others may have.

Concerns

Recording of information: you may be unsure about the correct form to use or about how much information to include. You may have noticed that one of your colleagues has recorded inaccurate information about an individual. An individual's advocate may raise concerns over how information has been recorded, such as the privacy of the individual not being respected.

Storing of information: you may have concerns over the filing system used for individuals' personal information because you may be experiencing difficulties in retrieving information quickly. You may not know where to find individuals' personal information that is held electronically and whether you can access it. An individual may raise concerns over whether their information is being held securely.

Sharing of information: you may have concerns over whether you can share an individuals' personal information. You may have concerns regarding sharing information over the telephone, or discussing individuals' personal information

with professionals from other organisations. An individual may raise concerns over personal information being shared with their family.

Actions: step by step

Always record your concerns and the information that has been reported to you immediately so that you do not forget the important details of what happened. This will ensure your record is an accurate one and includes all the necessary information.

You must include only the facts as well as the date and time of the concerns so that the information is a true record of what happened. Remember to sign and date your record so that you can show that you are responsible for adding the information.

Report your concerns to your manager; ensure you explain your concerns fully and that you do so in a private area to ensure you maintain the confidentiality of this information.

If you do not think that your concerns have been addressed then report them to someone more senior in the organisation. You can do this verbally or in writing.

Figure 7.5 shows an example of the type of information you may be required to provide. Your work setting will have a 'concerns form' that you will be required to use; you should familiarise yourself with this.

If your concern has still not been addressed then you can seek advice from other organisations outside of your care setting including the Information Commissioner's Office (ICO) and the independent charity Public Concern at Work that provides free confidential advice to people who are not sure whether, or how, to raise concerns about practices that they have seen at work.

You could also report your concern to the Care Quality Commission (CQC), which regulates adult care settings.

Reporting your concerns to external organisations can feel scary and daunting but is necessary if you have exhausted your own care setting's procedures for doing so and your duty to do so is supported by legislation.

Concerns form

Section 1: About you

Name:

Address:

Tel: Email:

Section 2: Information about your concern

Do you work for the organisation? Yes/No

Have you complained to your manager? Yes/No

If yes, please provide date of complaint and details:

If no, please provide reason(s) why:

Have you had a response from your manager? Yes/No

Date of response and details:

Section 3: Details about your concern

Who are you complaining about?

What are you complaining about?

How has this affected you?

How has this affected others?

Figure 7.5 An example of a form that you may be required to fill in when you have a concern

Research it

2.1, 2.2 Concerns and actions

Research two adult care settings' procedures for the actions to take when there are concerns over recording, storing or sharing of information. You may want to start by researching the procedures in your setting, and then look at the procedures in another setting, for example. You could ask your line manager about the procedures in your setting. You will find it useful to use the internet to carry out your research as there may be examples of good practice available from different organisations that provide care or support services.

How did your research of both care settings compare? Were there many similarities or differences between these?

The 'dos and dont's' table that follows includes some best practice points to remember when taking action over concerns in relation to handling information.

It is also important that you think about and understand the process to follow when you have a concern so that you can ensure you are taking the correct actions and that you also know what to do when you have been given the wrong advice. Table 7.2 highlights a couple of examples of how concerns can be handled.

	Dos and don'ts when dealing with concerns
Do	Record all concerns you have or that are raised with you.
Do	Report all concerns you have or that are raised with you.
Do	Listen to and treat all concerns seriously.
Do	Take action immediately when you have concerns or when these are raised with you.
Don't	Ignore concerns you have or that are raised with you.
Don't	Forget or be afraid to report all concerns you have or that are raised with you.
Don't	Make judgements about the concerns you have or that are raised with you.
Don't	Delay or do nothing when you have concerns or when these are raised with you.

Table 7.2 Examples of how to address concerns

Concern:

An individual tells you they overheard a colleague talk about another individual's care needs in the corridor.

The action you take	Manager's response	Does the manager's response address the concern?	Is further action required?	The next step
You report it to your manager verbally and explain to the individual why you are doing so. You do not record your concern.	Your manager tells you that she will apologise to the individual and explain that your colleague's actions were not intentional.	Your manager's response has not addressed your concern because the manager: • is assuming that your colleague's actions were not intentional • has not asked you to record what the individual has said • has not said that she will be speaking to both the individual and your colleague about what happened. Your manager must record the complaint and report it to the ICO.	Yes	You must record what the individual disclosed to you. You must report this to a more senior person in your organisation. You could seek further advice and guidance from the ICO.

Concern:

You find an individual's daily report notes on the coffee table in the entrance hall.

The action you take	Manager's response	Does the manager's response address the concern?	Is further action required?	The next step
You immediately return the individual's daily report notes to their allocated secure location, i.e. the filing cabinet in the office, and ensure this is locked. You record your concerns and report this to your manager.	Your manager thanks you for your immediate action, your report and record, and explains that you have taken all the correct actions. The manager explains that she will now inform the individual and their advocate of the breach of confidentiality to their personal data.	Yes, because the manager confirms that the correct actions to take are to report and record your concern and to safeguard the individual's personal information by returning the report notes immediately to a secure area where it cannot be accessed by those who are not authorised to do so.	No	It is important to remember to follow the same procedure next time something like this happens but make your manager aware that this has happened before.

2.2 Best practice when handling information

Reflect on the reasons why it is important to follow best practice when handling information. What are the consequences of:

- not recording the concerns others have raised with you?
- not reporting immediately the concerns you have?
- not being able to judge whether or not a concern is serious?
- doing nothing when you have concerns?

Evidence opportunity

2.1, 2.2, 3.2 Concerns about handling information

Discuss with your assessor three different types of concerns that may arise in the care setting where you work, over the handling of individuals' personal information. Next, discuss the recording and reporting actions that you must follow for each of these concerns, the reasons why these actions must be taken as well as the consequences if they are not.

Did your discussion include the best practice points you learned about earlier on?

Understanding the correct actions to take when there are concerns is therefore very important so that you can make sure that you know what to do in the different situations that may arise in your care setting. Good **communication** underpins the recording, storing and sharing of all information. It involves, for example, writing details clearly and accurately and effectively communicating concerns.

6Cs

Communication

Communicating effectively both verbally and in writing and when following agreed ways of working is central to working well together as a team and developing good working relationships. This is because without doing so you will not be able to interact with one another positively and understand how to work together.

In a care setting, you will need to effectively communicate any concerns when you are worried about an issue around recording and storing. Even if you are worried about offending someone, it is still important that you speak up, so that the issue can be addressed. This will enable individuals to trust you with their personal information and feel able to approach you with their concerns. For example, if you have a concern about how a senior colleague is handling an individual's information, you could discuss this with your manager in confidence. In this way, you have shared your concerns and your manager can take the necessary action that will ensure this individual's information is safeguarded and that your senior colleague is applying only best practices when handling information.

Case study 2.1, 3.1, 3.2 will help you with applying the knowledge you have learned about handling concerns correctly in the care setting where you work.

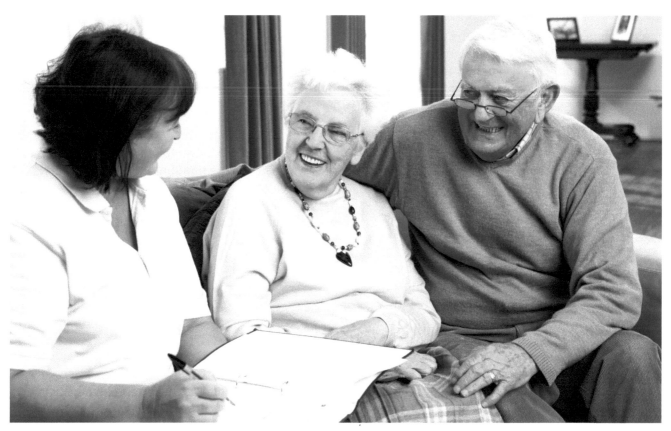

Figure 7.6 Are you a good communicator? What skills make you a good communicator?

Case study

2.1, 3.1, 3.2 Handling information, concerns and actions to take

Mia is new to working in an adult care setting. As part of the introduction to her job as a care assistant providing support to older adults in a day centre, her employer has arranged for her to observe and work with a more experienced colleague, Sylvie, who has worked with the organisation for seven years. Today, Mia is observing Sylvie assisting an individual with their meal at lunchtime.

Sylvie begins by explaining to Mia that she must first check with the individual, Ken, how he is and what he is having for lunch. Ken tells Sylvie that his throat is sore and that he is not very hungry but would like to have something small to eat such as a salad or sandwich. Sylvie listens to Ken and then explains that she is going to share his lunch request with the kitchen so that

this can be prepared for him, and asks Ken for his permission to do so.

Ken looks away and then speaking slowly tells Sylvie that he's not sure whether she should do this because last week when he mentioned that his throat was sore and wanted something to eat that wasn't on the menu the kitchen staff told him that he was being difficult and didn't understand how busy they were. Ken added that this was said in front of everyone in the main lounge and that he felt very embarrassed.

Sylvie listened carefully to Ken's concerns about her sharing this information with the kitchen staff but explained how it was his right to make his own choices and express his own preferences over what he would like to eat at lunchtime. Sylvie also explained that it was Ken's right to have had this conversation held with the kitchen staff in private and not in front of everyone in the

→

main lounge. Sylvie added that she would like him not to feel embarrassed or awkward about raising his concerns and agreed with him that it would be a good idea to complete a complaints form.

Mia observed Sylvie and Ken find a private room and Sylvie assisted Ken to think about what his concerns were over how his requests for lunch were shared by the kitchen staff. Sylvie then wrote down Ken's concerns on the complaints form and ensured she used his words to explain what these were. Ken signed and dated the form and Sylvie placed it in a sealed envelope. Sylvie went with Ken to the day centre manager's office and gave her the complaints form. Ken then thanked Sylvie and asked to speak with the day centre manager in private and so Sylvie left.

Sylvie then returned to the staff office and in private explained to Mia that all complaints in relation to the kitchen must be made in writing to the day centre manager using the complaints form.

Questions

1 What actions did Sylvie take in relation to Ken's concerns over the handling of his personal information?
2 Why did Sylvie take these actions?
3 Thinking about your work setting's procedure for taking actions when there are concerns over the handling of individuals' information, what actions would you have taken? Would you have done anything differently?

L02 Knowledge, skills, behaviours
Knowledge: why is it important to know how to access support for handling information?
Do you know who to seek guidance from in your care setting about handling information?
Do you know why it is important to seek information and advice about handling information in a timely manner when a concern is raised?
Did you know that you have just answered two questions about the agreed ways of working for handling information in the care setting where you work?
Skills: how can you show that you are complying with your care setting's agreed ways of working when you have concerns over handling information?
Do you know who to go to in the first instance when you have concerns over the recording or storing of individuals' personal information?
Do you know what to do if the method sharing of an individual's personal information does not meet your care setting's agreed ways of working?
Did you know that you have just answered two questions about a few of the skills you have in responding to concerns about the handling of information?
Behaviours: how can you show the personal qualities you have when reporting concerns about handling information?
Do you know how to support good communication when reporting your concerns?
Do you know how to speak up for individuals if you have concerns about the handling of their personal information and who you can go to for guidance?
Did you know that you have just answered two questions about a few of the essential behaviours that are expected of all adult care workers?

LO3 Be able to handle information in accordance with agreed ways of working

AC 3.1 Keep records that are up to date, complete, accurate and legible

Different records in your setting

As we have discussed, as part of your role as a care worker, you will also have responsibility for recording various information about the individuals that you care for. Your setting will hold information about individuals located in different records and reports and you must complete these correctly to comply with both legislation and your organisation's agreed ways of working.

You will need to be able to demonstrate you understand this assessment criteria in the care setting where you work.

There are many different records and reports that are kept in care settings. Examples of some of the main ones used are:

- care or support plans that detail individuals' needs, choices and support required
- daily reports that provide information on the daily tasks completed with individuals

- health profiles that provide information on individuals' health needs, conditions and allergies
- medication records that provide details on the medications individuals take, including the dose, how often they are taken and how to take them
- menus that provide information on individuals' nutritional requirements and preferences
- **fluid balance charts** that provide information on individuals' fluid intake and output
- **moving and handling charts** that provide information on the **equipment** the individuals use and the support required to move from one position to another
- activity records that provide information on the activities completed with individuals
- **risk assessments** that detail the potential and actual risks to individuals and others, and how to manage them safely
- accident reports that document accidents that have taken place in the work setting
- **health and safety checklists** (see page 262 for definitions) that provide information on the health and safety checks completed in the care setting
- a visitors book that provides information on those that have visited the care setting.

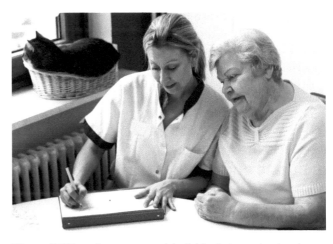

Figure 7.7 How do you support individuals to understand records about them?

Key terms

Fluid balance charts are used to record the amount of fluid being taken into and leaving (in the form of urine) a person's body, to monitor their hydration, which is necessary for their well-being.

Moving and handling charts are used to record the methods and equipment to be used with an individual for safely moving them from one position to another.

Moving and handling equipment includes hoists, bath lifts and slide sheets.

Risk assessments are used to record the **hazards** associated with tasks, the risks that have the potential to cause harm, ways of removing the hazards or controlling the risks when the hazards cannot be removed.

A **hazard** is a danger, or something that poses a danger.

Health and safety checklists are used to record safety checks that are made in the environment such as ensuring fire alarms are working, windows locked securely and the first aid box is complete.

Up to date refers to ensuring records contain information that reflects current information.

Complete refers to ensuring records contain full details and all the information that is necessary.

Accurate refers to ensuring records contain factually correct information.

Legible refers to ensuring records are written in a way that they can be easily read and understood.

Reflect on it

3.1, 1.2 Different types of records

Reflect on the records you have in the care setting where you work. Think about the different types of records that there are such as written (paper-based) and electronic records. Do you have access to all these records? If not, why not?

Can you make a list of the records that you use on a daily basis? Think about when you make entries, store these records and share the information they contain. Explain why it is important that you follow agreed ways of working with regard to keeping up-to-date, complete, accurate and legible records.

Why we record and why it is important records are up to date, complete, accurate and legible

All the records that you access and complete in the care setting where you work are legal documents. This is because they fully document the care and support provided to individuals, record all decisions taken and how those decisions were made.

Because records may be referred to in the future, it is important that they are **up to date**, **complete**, **accurate** and **legible**. This will also be helpful to the next person who accesses the records, such as a colleague or the individual's GP. Not only will your notes inform the care they give to the individual, but if they are up to date, accurate, complete and neatly recorded, it will also save them time from having to find out when the information was recorded or trying to make sense of what you have written. The information that these contain is very important for ensuring the provision of high-quality, safe and effective care to individuals.

All the information that is maintained and stored must also adhere to the Data Protection Act and its requirements you learned about earlier on in this unit because individuals' information contains personal details that they would want to be kept private and safe; not doing so may mean that others may try to unlawfully gain access to it. For example, the information documented may be about an older adult who is returning home after being in hospital, a young adult who has developed mental health needs or an individual with learning disabilities who would like support to find a job and there are concerns about their safety. Those issues/details would need to be recorded so that the appropriate actions can be taken to ensure that the individual's safety and well-being can be safeguarded.

It is therefore important that when completing your records, you do this correctly and in line with the agreed ways of working in the care setting where you work.

Keeping records up to date

This is important because individuals' needs and preferences can change. Not doing so can mean that individuals' information becomes out of date and does not provide a true picture of the support they require, the care needs they have, their preferences for how they want to live their life. This may then mean that the care and support that you provide does not meet an individual's needs and can result in it being unsafe. If documents are dated, then it will be clear for you or the next colleague who accesses the record to see when the information was recorded. They can then update the record by adding a new entry, signing and dating this.

Keeping records that are complete

This is important because not doing so can mean that important information about for example a change in an individual's health condition may not be recorded. This can mean that the individual is not provided with the correct care and their health condition may as a result worsen. Not writing down records completely can therefore have serious consequences for individuals but can also mean that you risk putting your own job and career at risk.

Writing accurate records

This is very important for ensuring that all information included provides a true picture of what really happened. Not doing so can mean that important decisions about individuals are made based on inaccurate information. For example, recording that you feel that an individual was looking 'a bit down' when you supported him to get dressed in the morning is your opinion and may not lead to any further action being taken. However, recording that the individual told you he was feeling 'a bit down' when you supported him to get dressed in the morning is fact and would therefore lead to further actions being taken. This might include asking the individual to find out the reasons why he was feeling 'a bit down', booking an appointment with his GP and close monitoring of how he was feeling

by the team. You should therefore ensure that the records are facts, not your own personal thoughts and opinions. This will help to ensure your records are accurate. The Data Protection Act allows people to view any information/records held about them and so it is important to ensure the information you include is accurate, as well as complete and legible.

Ensuring records are legible

This means that individuals, your colleagues and others accessing your records must be able to read your handwriting and understand what you have written. Not doing so may mean that important information about individuals is not understood, that misunderstandings arise and that the required care and support are not provided when individuals need this. It also means that colleagues may spend more time trying to work out what you have written. How would you feel if you accessed a record and could not read what was written? Would this make you worried that you may miss important information simply because the writing was not clear and legible?

Overall, making sure that records are up to date, complete, accurate and legible will help to ensure that you and your colleagues can carry out your job effectively, and efficiently. You will not have to spend time looking for certain information if the person who last completed the record did this clearly. This will be especially helpful if the matter is urgent. If the information that has been included is legible, accurate and useful it will also inform the care that you give to the individual. In turn, the individual will receive good-quality care, which is provided by the information that has been included in their records.

Remember that the GDPR replaced the Data Protection Act 1998 in May 2018 (see AC 1.1 on page 243).

How to keep up-to-date, complete, accurate and legible records

You can **keep records up to date** by recording all information:

- as soon as possible – making an entry into an activity record as soon as you have completed an activity such as cooking a meal with an individual
- regularly – making an entry into the daily report at the end of *every* shift

- consistently – documenting information about individuals in *all* records that you use.

You can **ensure records are complete** by recording all information:

- with all the necessary details, for example write out a **risk assessment** in full, identifying clearly the **hazards**, potential risks and the ways you have agreed with the individual to manage these before supporting them to go shopping

- with the date, time and your signature – including these at the end of your daily report entries will mean that you have made it clear that this is your record in full and prevents someone else adding to it. It also means the next person to access the record can see who added to it and when

- as soon as possible – completing records as soon as possible after you have finished a task or after an accident has occurred will ensure that you do not forget to include important information and will provide a true picture of what happened.

You can **ensure records are accurate** by recording all information:

- with the facts only – information recorded in an accident report must be based on what you have seen and heard (fact) not on what you think or feel (opinion). You should also make sure that you can justify what you have written, in other words you should have clear reasons for what you have recorded

- with the relevant details only – including the necessary details and the information that is required. Relevant information on an individual's support plan will mean that the key areas of support are clear and easily understood by your colleagues so that they can provide consistent care

- relating to the individual only – you should also ensure that you only write about the individual and not anyone else in their notes so it is clear that the information relates to that individual only

- as soon as possible – updating records as soon as possible after a task has been completed will mean that you will be more likely to include the most relevant and important information only.

You can **ensure records are legible** by recording all information:

- clearly – information recorded on an individual's care plan must be written using neat handwriting so that it can be read easily

- correctly – information recorded on electronic records for individuals should be written using the correct spelling and grammar so that it can be easily understood by those who access and read them

- in permanent ink – information recorded in the daily report for an individual must be written using permanent ink that cannot be erased or altered; if you make an error on a paper-based record then put a single line through it, so that the error is still legible and it is clear what you wrote

- concisely – try not to write too many paragraphs. Bullet points are often a good way to convey information and will save time for the next person who needs to read the records. You should cover all important and correct information and be clear but if you can be concise, even better!

Evidence opportunity

3.1 Keeping records

Identify three records you have completed in your work setting and show these to your manager. For this assessment, the criteria you will need to demonstrate is that you are able to keep records that are up to date, complete, accurate and legible. Your work practices will be observed.

Next, discuss with your manager whether the information you have recorded in them is:

- up to date
- complete
- accurate
- legible.

You will need to be able to explain to your manager the reasons why these have been completed correctly.

Are there any improvements that you can make to the way you keep records? Identify what these are and then discuss with your manager what action you are going to take. This activity will be best evidenced through a witness statement.

AC 3.2 Follow agreed ways of working for recording information, storing information and sharing information

All care settings will have agreed ways of working in place for the procedures adult care workers are expected to follow when recording, storing and sharing information. It is important that you find out what these are in the care setting where you work so that you can ensure that your work practices are correct and that you are following the requirements of current legislation and the agreed ways of working for the care setting you work in. You should ensure that you work collaboratively, i.e. with colleagues. Working consistently with your colleagues means that the quality of the **care** provided will be of the same quality for the individual irrespective of who provides it; it will be consistent care.

Your work practices will be observed for this assessment criterion.

Following agreed ways of working for **recording information** means that you must:

- know the different types of records you can access and complete them as part of your day-to-day responsibilities

- know when information has to be recorded and the reasons why
- show that you can record information using the correct process.

Following agreed ways of working for **storing information** means that you must:

- know the whereabouts of all paper-based and electronic information – how this is stored and the reasons why
- show how to access manual and electronic information using the correct process
- show how you maintain the security of all information stored using the correct process.

Procedures for **sharing information** mean that you must:

- know what information about individuals can or cannot be shared with others and understand the reasons why
- show when and how information can be shared with others
- show the checks you make before sharing information with others.

Your setting will advise you on its policies and procedures when it comes to sharing information, and the 'dos and don'ts' table on the next page gives you some suggestions for best practice.

6Cs

Care

Care involves showing that you genuinely have the best interests of the individual at heart and want to make a positive difference to their life. As a care worker, you are committing to providing good-quality care every time you work with each individual. You can do this by showing your respect towards every individual and by working hard every time you go to work to provide good-quality care. You must have the best interests of the individual in mind when you record, store and share information. You can do this by following agreed ways of working and best practice.

Reflect on it

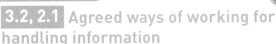

3.2, 2.1 Agreed ways of working for handling information

Think back over the sources of guidance, information and advice about handling information that you have learned about. Where can you find out about the agreed ways of working for recording, storing and sharing information in the care setting where you work? Reflect on both internal and external sources of information that you can access.

Why is it important that you know about these sources of information?

265

	Dos and don'ts for recording, storing and sharing information
Do	Share information on a need-to-know basis only, i.e. if someone has requested information about an individual's participation in an activity, you do not have to give them the individual's entire history.
Do	Check the identity of the person requesting the information before you share it, i.e. what their role is, why they have requested the information, and what information they will need to know in order to carry out their job and provide informed care.
Do	Check with your manager in the first instance if you are unsure about what information you can share – and who to share it with.
Do	Show compassion and empathy. If relatives really want to find out information, and want you to share this with them, you should explain that you understand their situation but that you really cannot share the information unless the individual says so. This will also help to create a more positive relationship with the individual's family and will show them that your priorities are the care and wishes of the individual first and foremost.
Do	Seek consent. (The new GDPR 2018 legislation puts a strong focus on consent.) You should only share information if you have permission from the individual to do so. When it comes to sharing information with workers directly involved in their care in the setting, you do not need to gain permission to share information. When information is going to be shared with those outside the setting, for example GPs and social workers, you do need to gain permission to share information with them. However, when family members have requested information, particularly if it is private and confidential then you will need to get permission from the individual. If you do not seek permission from the individual, the individual may not trust you with other important information that may be beneficial to their care if they feel that you cannot be relied on to keep the information confidential.
Don't	Inadvertently share information when speaking to others, i.e. to colleagues at lunchtime, or to an individual's friends and family you meet while shopping outside of the work setting.
Don't	Give out information to anybody that you do not know. If an outside organisation, or someone that you have never come across before, requests information, even if they seem trustworthy, you should always ask to see some ID or proof of who they are. If you are unsure who is requesting information, you should check with colleagues in case they know the person who has requested the information. You should never feel like you have to give out information straight away if you do not know the person, even on email or on the telephone. Take your time to confirm the identity of the person before sharing information. If you are not careful, then information could end up in the hands of individuals that should not have access to it.
Don't	Share information unless you have permission to do so, i.e. with outside organisations such as the media.
Don't	Automatically share information with those who have the individual's best interests at heart unless you have permission to do so, e.g. an individual may request that their family is not told about a minor fall they have had because they do not want to worry them.
Don't	Think that you cannot share information without the individual's consent. This is because sometimes it is in the individual's best interests to safeguard them from danger. For example, an unlawful act may need to be reported and the police and courts may request information about this. In this case, you would need to share information regardless of whether the individual agrees.

Remember, keeping up-to-date, complete, accurate and legible records involves showing that you can keep records that:

- read easily
- ensure a permanent record of information
- contain clearly written information
- organise information in a logical way
- record information in a way that it can be easily retrieved when needed
- detail information accurately and fully
- specify the facts only.

Security and privacy of records

Records that need to be left in individuals' rooms will usually be kept safe in a drawer or cupboard, out of sight. Other records will be held in the file for example. In residential settings, some records such as the care worker's daily report may be left in the individual's room but where they choose; this might be in their drawer or cabinet. The individual can read the report, and their family may also access it with their permission. If a record contains sensitive information, for example about an allegation towards a staff or family member, then a separate confidential report would be made about this.

Agreed ways of working and things to think about

Your setting and manager will make you aware of the types of things you will need to consider when you record, store and share information, but it is good practice to think about what the purpose of the information is: why are you recording this? Who do you need to share this with? Is this private information? If it is confidential, should you share it? If you share it, should you record that you have shared it? Is it an urgent matter? If it is urgent, is it better to pick up the phone rather than send an email? Your setting will be able to let you know about these things, but it is good practice to think about and ask yourself these questions.

Table 7.3 Methods of communicating in different situations

Situation and the information you need	Method of communication
Private and confidential matter You need to send the GP information about an individual's health and you also need to gain access to the individual's medical records.	It may be best to communicate verbally, i.e. speak to your manager in the first instance because you can discuss what information needs to be shared and why. You can then speak to the GP in order to receive feedback and advice from them. It can be an exchange, rather than you just sharing information with the GP. (The GP is also able to share their expertise with you.) Not only does this mean that the individual's private information is kept confidential, but it also means that receiving expert knowledge can inform the support you offer the individual and therefore the care you provide will be of a high quality. If the matter is not urgent, and you are not seeking the GP's expertise, but rather just records from them, then you could send a letter marked 'private and confidential'. Again, before doing so you should discuss this with your manager in the first instance who can guide you regarding what details to ask for, how to write the letter, i.e. using letter headed paper from the care setting, or email. Marking a letter private and confidential means that the information is only accessed by the person to whom the letter is addressed. This also means that the individual's privacy is maintained and remains secure.
Urgent matter An older individual needs admitting to hospital as a matter of urgency.	The best course of action would be to phone for an ambulance. The individual may not wish you to do so but your duty of care to them would override this. As this is an urgent situation, direct contact is required so that the individual's care needs are met and the individual is not at risk of being placed in any danger. For example, being left on their own at home, if they are unable to manage may lead to the individual not eating or drinking or having a fall.

➡

Table 7.3 Methods of communicating in different situations *continued*

Situation and the information you need	Method of communication
Non-urgent matter An individual asks you if they can have their meal this evening half an hour later as a good friend is visiting them at the same time the evening meal is served.	As this is a non-urgent matter but important to address it would be appropriate to ask the kitchen staff to change the time when this individual's meal is served in the evening. This can be communicated verbally and quickly. A note on the menu could also be made to remind the kitchen staff that a change of time for this individual's meal has been agreed.

Evidence opportunity

3.2 Agreed ways of working

You must make arrangements for your work practices to be observed. Show your assessor how you follow the agreed ways of working in your care setting for recording, storing and sharing information.

You will find it useful to refer back to ACs 1.1, 1.2, 2.2 and 3.1 for more information.

Methods of communication, information and situations you may encounter

The reflective exemplar provides you with an opportunity to explore in more detail how to follow best practice when handling information in a care setting and ensures it is in line with agreed ways of working.

Reflective exemplar	
Introduction	I work as a care worker with older people in a residential home. My duties involve supporting individuals with personal tasks such as showering, dressing, eating and drinking as well as assisting individuals to take part in social and recreational activities such as meeting with family and friends, shopping and gardening.
What happened?	Yesterday afternoon, my manager arranged for a team meeting to take place in the staff's training room for all the care workers who work in the residential home. My colleagues and I were all feeling a little anxious because we wondered why the meeting had been called at short notice and why all the care workers were asked to attend.
	The manager began by explaining that the reason for the meeting was to share best practice amongst the care workers for writing in records and reports. The manager added that she had noticed that the team had been working very hard and that as a result the quality of report writing at the home had significantly improved but how there was still room for more improvements to be made.
	We began by discussing the areas of best practice that were consistently being followed by all care workers. In relation to recording information, we were all ensuring that we were doing so in private and before our shifts had ended; the information being recorded was written clearly and included sufficient detail. In relation to storing information, we were all ensuring that we were following the alphabetical system that was in place for filing individuals' records which meant that information was being retrieved more quickly and easily now than before. The manager added that this was particularly useful for occasions when individuals' families and other professionals had requested information.
	In relation to sharing information, discussions took place around the different methods that are used in the home for sharing individuals' information including in meetings, on a one-to-one basis, in writing, over email, text and telephone. The manager reminded the team that when sharing information over the telephone, appropriate checks must be done to check the identity of the person requesting the information, and added that if anybody was unsure, care workers were not to give out any personal information and were to instead seek advice from her.

Reflective exemplar	
What worked well?	It was pleasing to hear that we are all working consistently well together as a team when handling information and that our working practices had improved, in particular in relation to keeping and storing records.
What did not go as well?	The practices being followed by the team for sharing information need further improvement particularly in relation to verifying or confirming who we are sharing information with and ensuring when we are unsure that we do not give information out but instead seek further guidance and advice from the home manager.
What could I do to improve?	I think I will need to re-read the home's procedure for sharing personal information about individuals and ensure that I understand when I can share information and when I cannot. If there are any areas I am unclear about I will talk these through with the home manager. I am also going to be more careful when giving out information to others over the telephone and will follow the agreed ways of working for checking the caller's identity.
Links to unit assessment criteria	ACs 1.2, 2.1, 3.1, 3.2

LO3 Knowledge, skills, behaviours
Knowledge: why is it important to be able to handle information in line with agreed ways of working?
Do you know why it is important to write information in records accurately and keep them up to date?
Do you know why it is important to write records clearly and in full?
Did you know that you have just answered two questions about best practices that adult care workers follow when completing records?
Skills: how can you show that you are complying with your care setting's agreed ways of working when recording, storing and sharing information?
Do you know how to record and store information in accordance with the agreed ways of working in the care setting where you work?
Do you know how to share information with your colleagues and others in the care setting where you work?
Did you know that you have just answered two questions about a few of the skills you have in relation to following agreed ways of working in the care setting where you work?
Behaviours: how can you show the personal qualities you have when following agreed ways of working about handling information?
Do you know how to share information about individuals in a positive way?
Do you know how to work with your team members when handling information about individuals?
Did you know that you have just answered two questions about a few of the essential behaviours that are expected of all adult care workers and that you are legally required to show under the Data Protection Act 1998?

Suggestions for using the activities	

This table summarises all the activities in the unit that are relevant to each assessment criterion.

Here, we also suggest other, different methods that you may want to use to present your knowledge and skills by using the activities.

These are just suggestions, and you should refer to the Introduction section at the start of the book, and more importantly the City & Guilds specification, and your assessor who will be able to provide more guidance on how you can evidence your knowledge and skills.

When you need to be observed during your assessment, this can be done by your assessor, or your manager can provide a witness testimony.

Assessment criteria and accompanying activities	Suggested methods to show your knowledge/skills
LO1 Understand the need for secure handling of information in care settings	
LO3 Be able to handle information in accordance with agreed ways of working	
1.1 Research it (page 241) 1.1 Research it (page 242)	Make notes detailing your findings.
1.1, 3.2 Evidence opportunity (page 245)	Provide a written account addressing the points in the activity.
	You could complete a spider diagram of different examples of current legislation related to the recording, storage and sharing of information in care settings. You could also prepare a presentation about the legislation.
	You could also discuss with your assessor the care setting where you work, and think about the legislation that is in place that underpins your work practices for recording, storing and sharing information.
1.2 Research it (page 248)	Write down your findings.
1.2, 3.2 Reflect on it (page 248)	Write a reflective account addressing the questions in the activity.
1.1, 1.2, 3.2 Research it (page 250)	Discuss your findings with a colleague and make notes detailing your research and discussion.
1.2 Evidence opportunity (page 251) 1.2, 3.2 Case study (page 251)	Produce a leaflet as instructed in the activity.
	You could write a personal statement that details the secure systems for recording and storing information in a care setting and include the reasons why these are important.
	You could also discuss with your assessor the care setting where you work and explain why it is important to have secure systems for recording and storing information. You could discuss examples of the consequences of not doing so and the impact of these on the individuals, you and your colleagues.
	The case study will help you.
LO2 Know how to access support for handling information	
LO3 Be able to handle information in accordance with agreed ways of working	
2.1 Reflect on it (page 254)	Write a reflective account.

➜

Suggestions for using the activities	
2.1, 3.1, 3.2 Evidence opportunity (page 254)	Produce an information handout as instructed in the activity. Remember that you can use diagrams and photographs to illustrate your handout.
	Write a personal statement about occasions that could arise in relation to handling information when you may require additional guidance, information and advice. Remember to include examples of the range of internal and external sources available to you and how you can access these.
	You could develop a presentation that details the steps to follow for accessing guidance, information and advice about handling information in the care setting where you work. You could also discuss with your assessor the agreed ways of working that must be followed in the care setting where you work. The written procedure from your care setting can be used as the basis of your discussion.
2.1, 2.2 Research it (page 256)	Write up your research findings.
2.2 Reflect on it (page 258)	Write a reflective account addressing the points in the activity.
2.1, 2.2, 3.2 Evidence opportunity (page 258) 2.1, 3.1, 3.2 Case study (page 259)	Discuss the points in the activity with your assessor.
	Discuss with your assessor the actions to take in the care setting where you work when there are concerns over the recording, storing or sharing of information. Remember to explain why these actions are necessary. The written procedure from your care setting can be used as the basis of your discussion.
	You could also write a reflective account about an occasion when you had concerns over the recording, storing or sharing of information. Explain the actions you took and the reasons why. The case study will help you. You could also collect a witness testimony to support your reflective account, and work product evidence such as the concerns report/form you completed.
LO3 Be able to handle information in accordance with agreed ways of working	
LO1 Understand the need for secure handling of information in care settings	
LO2 Know how to access support for handling information	
3.1, 1.2 Reflect on it (page 262)	Write a reflective account.
3.1 Evidence opportunity (page 264) 2.1, 3.1, 3.2 Case study (page 259)	Complete the activity and obtain a witness statement from your manager. Address the points in the activity.
	You must make arrangements for your work practices to be observed so that you can show your assessor how you keep up-to-date, complete, accurate and legible records in the care setting where you work.
	To support your observation work, you could also show your assessor evidence of different records you have completed in your care setting. Remember to show through your work practices how you are following the care setting's agreed ways of working for keeping records. The case study will help you.
3.2, 2.1 Reflect on it (page 265)	Write a reflective account.
3.2 Evidence opportunity (page 268)	You must make arrangements for your work practices to be observed so that you can show your assessor how you follow the agreed ways of working in your care setting for recording, storing and sharing information. The case studies in this unit will help you to identify best practice when recording, storing and sharing information. You could also collect a witness testimony from your manager to support the observation of your work practices when following agreed ways of working for handling information.

Legislation	
Relevant Act	**It states that:**
Data Protection Act 1998	information and data must be processed fairly, lawfully, used only for the purpose it was intended to be used for, be adequate, relevant, accurate and up to date, held for no longer than is necessary, used in line with the rights of individuals, kept secure and not transferred to other countries without the individual's permission. It established how personal information must be recorded, used, stored and shared.
General Data Protection Regulation (GDPR) 2018	Also see GDPR on page 243.
Human Rights Act 1998	everyone in the UK is entitled to the same rights and freedoms. In relation to the handling of information Article 8 established the right to respect for your private and family life, home and correspondence.
Freedom of Information Act 2000	individuals have the right to request information held about them by a wide range of public bodies, such as local authorities and hospitals.
Care Act 2014	local authorities must provide comprehensive information and advice about care and support services in their local area so that individuals can make informed decisions about their care and support. The information provided must be able to be understood by individuals.
Health and Social Care Act 2008 (Regulated Activities) Regulations 2014	personal information about individuals in care settings must be used in line with your organisations' agreed ways of working. It promotes transparency by supporting the sharing of information with individuals and their families.

Resources for further reading and research

Books

Clark, C. and McGhee, J. (2008) *Private and Confidential? Handling Personal Information in Social and Health Services*, Policy Press

Ferreiro Peteiro, M. (2014) *Level 2 Health and Social Care Diploma Evidence Guide*, Hodder Education

Weblinks

www.cqc.org.uk Care Quality Commission (CQC) – record-keeping requirements and standards

www.equalityhumanrights.com Equality and Human Rights Commission – information on the Human Rights Act 1998

www.gov.uk The UK Government's website for information about current legislation including factsheets about the Care Act 2014

www.ico.org.uk Information Commissioner's Office (ICO) – the UK's independent body set up to uphold information rights provides guidance on handling personal information

www.nice.org.uk National Institute for Health and Care Excellence (NICE) – guidance on record-keeping standards

www.rcnhca.org.uk Royal College of Nursing, First Steps for health care assistants – guidance on keeping records

www.scie.org.uk Social Care Institute for Excellence (SCIE) – e-learning resources on good and poor record keeping in care settings

www.skillsforcare.org.uk Skills for Care – e-learning resources on the Care Act 2014

Implement person-centred approaches in care settings (211)

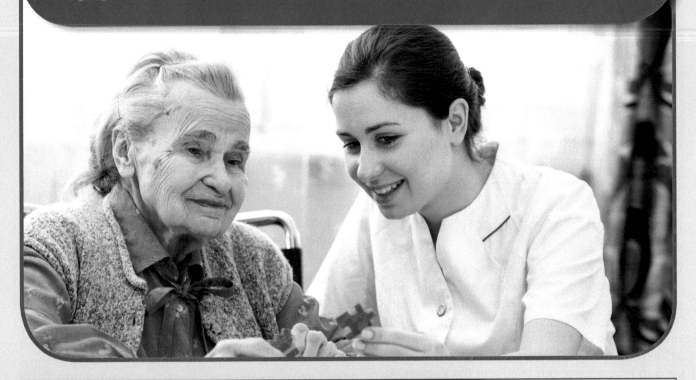

About this unit

Credit value: 5
Guided learning hours: 39

Person-centred care involves individuals with care or support needs being actively involved in the planning and provision of their care. Working in a way that embeds person-centred values is crucial for ensuring individuals are in control of their care or support.

In this unit, you will also learn about person-centred approaches for care and support, how you can work in a person-centred way and how you can establish consent when providing care or support to an individual. Encouraging active participation and reducing the barriers that may arise as well as supporting individuals' right to make choices and considering how this can be done in line with best practice and risk assessment processes are another two aspects of person-centred working that you will be able to use your skills to practise.

You will also understand the importance of supporting individuals' well-being and learn more about how you can do this effectively in your role.

Learning outcomes

LO1: Understand person-centred approaches for care and support

LO2: Be able to work in a person-centred way

LO3: Be able to establish consent when providing care or support

LO4: Be able to encourage active participation

LO5: Be able to support the individual's right to make choices

LO6: Be able to support the individual's well-being

LO1 Understand person-centred approaches for care and support

Getting started

Think about what makes you an individual and different to your family and friends and others you know. For example, it may be your personality or your beliefs. Imagine how you would feel if your beliefs were not taken into account by the people who know you? Why would you feel this way? Imagine how you would feel if you had the same beliefs as a member of your family and because of this you were both treated in exactly the same way rather than as different individuals? Why is it important to be treated like an individual?

AC 1.1 Define person-centred values

Your values are unique to you, they make you who you are and influence what you do and how you do it. If you have already read the unit that focused on your personal development (Unit 207) you will know that values represent what we believe to be important to us; they also guide us with how we live our lives and the decisions we make.

The care and support that you provide as an adult care worker is also underpinned by a set of values. These are commonly referred to as 'person-centred' values. Person-centred values mean placing the individual or person you care for at the centre or heart of everything you do. By making sure that these values underpin your work, the care you provide will be:

- focused on the individual and represent their unique needs, wishes and preferences
- focused on enabling the individual to be in control of their life including how they want to live it
- focused on enabling the individual to plan for the care and support they would like (including changes that may arise in the future).

The person-centred values that underpin high-quality care and support are set out in Table 8.1. You will need to show that you can apply these to the way that you practise in your **care setting**.

Key term

Care settings refer to adult care settings as well as adult, children and young people's health settings. This qualification, however, focuses on adult care settings.

Table 8.1 The person-centred values that underpin high-quality care and support

Person-centred values	What they mean in relation to providing care and support
Individuality *Treating people as individuals*	This means supporting and encouraging an individual to be their own person. This can include assisting an individual to dress in the way they want to. It means understanding that everyone is different and unique. The people you care for may have similar impairments or conditions but they will all have different needs and preferences. For example, not all individuals will want assistance with eating and drinking – some individuals with physical disabilities may be able to eat and drink independently while others may require support to eat and drink or use adapted cutlery to do so.

Table 8.1 The person-centred values that underpin high-quality care and support *continued*

Person-centred values	What they mean in relation to providing care and support
Rights *Helping individuals to understand and access their rights*	This means supporting and encouraging an individual to understand what they are entitled to. For example, ensuring individuals' rights are met and that there are no barriers to stop them from accessing their rights. Having a disability or being in a wheelchair should not be a barrier to joining in activities and fear of upsetting a care worker should not be a barrier to making a complaint. Not being able to read or read English should not be a barrier to signing a form. Instead, you should support individuals to access their rights and ensure activities allow everyone to participate. You must make sure that individuals are aware of the process for making complaints and are supported to make a complaint should they need to. You must make sure that you support anyone who cannot read to understand what they are signing before they do so.
Choice *Enabling individuals to make choices*	This means supporting, encouraging and empowering an individual to make their own choices and decisions. Everyone is entitled to make their own choices in a care setting. Individuals should choose how they would like to be supported and be given information about what options are available in order to make informed decisions. For example, you should tell individuals about the different care and support services that are available in their local area so that they can decide which one is best for them.
Privacy *Allowing individuals to have privacy*	This means showing respect for an individual's personal space and personal information. For example, this could include something as simple as knocking on the door of an individual's room before entering; or making sure that individuals can spend some time alone if they want to; that they are given privacy should they request it when family members visit. Or, that they are able to privately carry out personal care should they want to.
Independence *Supporting individuals to be independent*	This means supporting an individual to be in control of their life by doing as much for themselves as they are able to. This could, for example, include encouraging an individual to find out about the range of services that are available to them to enable them to remain living in their own home. Supporting individuals also means assessing the risks that they face but ensuring that they understand these and are able to live as independently as possible.
Dignity and respect *Treating individuals with dignity and respect*	This means treating people well and showing respect for their views, opinions and rights. Respect for individuals involves taking into account their differences and valuing them as individuals with their own needs and preferences. It also means promoting an individual's sense of self-respect by ensuring they do not feel humiliated or embarrassed in any way. Although you are there to support them, individuals should still feel that they are in control of their lives and treating them with dignity and respect is a big part of this.
Care *Providing care to individuals – this is also one of the 6Cs*	Providing care is of course perhaps the key person-centred value that underpins your role. But, more specifically, it means providing care in a way that is consistent, sufficient and meets the needs of the individual. For example, one of your responsibilities will be to support an individual with their meal times. However, in order to make sure that you provide good-quality care and fulfil this duty adequately, you will need to ensure that the meal is prepared in a way that meets their dietary and nutritional requirements, is enjoyable and you may also need to support them in eating and drinking should they need it.

→

Table 8.1 The person-centred values that underpin high-quality care and support *continued*

Person-centred values	What they mean in relation to providing care and support
Compassion *Showing compassion and kindness – this is also one of the 6Cs*	This means providing care to an individual in a way that shows kindness, consideration, empathy, dignity and respect. For example, this might mean taking time out from a busy shift to sit with an individual who has received some sad news.
Courage *Speaking up for individuals – this is also one of the 6Cs*	This means providing care in a way that is morally acceptable, to do the right thing for the individuals we care about, and to constantly improve and change ways of working if this means improved, more efficient ways or working. It also includes speaking up if you have concerns about practice at work or about an individual. This could include speaking up for an individual who is being abused and is too scared to report it.
Communication *Communicating effectively with individuals – this is also one of the 6Cs*	Good communication is key to providing high-quality care and support and to effective team working. It includes actively listening to what the individuals have to say and is necessary for building strong relationships with them and colleagues. Unit 203 covers communication and you may like to refer to it for more on communication in the care setting.
Competence *Working effectively and efficiently with individuals – this is also one of the 6Cs*	Being competent in your job role means having the knowledge, skills and expertise to provide high-quality care and support. It means understanding the needs of the individuals you care for and providing effective care to meet their needs. For example, this could include applying the knowledge and skills you have learned in relation to moving and handling to assist an individual to move safely from one position to another.
Partnership *Working together with individuals and others*	This means working together, alongside the individuals for whom you provide care and support. This will ensure that they are at the centre of the care you provide and are in control of the care they receive. It also includes working with others, their families, your colleagues and those outside the organisation. This is essential for the provision of high-quality person-centred care. You might want to look at Unit 202, Responsibilities of a care worker, AC 3.1 and 3.2, which cover partnership working.

6Cs

Courage

Courage is speaking up for an individual if they are at risk – this is an important responsibility that all adult care workers have.

Commitment

Although commitment is not covered in the table above, it is one of the 6Cs. Being committed to the people we care for is a key part of our role. This means being committed or dedicated to continuously improving the quality of care that we offer individuals so that their experience is a positive one.

It means dedication to providing care that has the person at the centre and is underpinned by person-centred values. It also means striving to improve your practice to ensure it is person-centred. How can you show you are committed to providing person-centred care and support in your current job role? How have you contributed to an individual's positive experience of accessing care and support? Look at Table 8.1 and think about how you apply person-centred values in your role.

Research it

1.1 Person-centred values in different care settings

Research two different adult care settings. For each one, find out what care and support services it provides. Then, see if you can find out what person-centred values underpin the care and support each provides to individuals.

You will find the internet useful for carrying out your research. You may also be able to visit two different care settings in your local area and speak with the care staff who work there.

Record your findings. Ensure that you include a) the type of adult care setting, b) the services it provides and c) the person-centred values that are applied.

Did you notice any difference between the care settings? Were all the person-centred values that you learned about in the table above included?

Evidence opportunity

1.1 Person-centred values

Write down two care and support tasks you carry out on a day-to-day basis in the care setting where you work (for example, assisting individuals with washing, dressing, eating, drinking, budgeting, shopping and attending appointments).

For each task, identify two person-centred values that you apply and describe how you do this.

Being **committed** (see 6Cs box on page 276) to improving the experience of individuals who access care and support by making sure it is underpinned by person-centred values will be expected from you as an adult care worker.

AC 1.2 Explain why it is important to work in a way that embeds person-centred values

Embedding person-centred values in your everyday work practice is central to providing person-centred care. As you know, person-centred care is about

providing support that keeps the individual as the focus. This involves supporting the individual to be in control of their life and the decisions they make both in relation to now and in the future. These person-centred values will underpin everything that you do. Everything from meal times to personal routine tasks and activities that they participate in will need to have the individual and their preferences at the centre.

Working in a way that embeds person-centred values is important and benefits individuals because:

- by involving individuals in the care they receive and supporting them to make their own choices and decisions, you will allow them to live as independently as possible, helping them to feel in control of their lives and to feel more confident. It is worth thinking about how you would feel if someone made decisions about your life for you. (What if someone else made the decisions about where you lived, what you ate and what medicine you did or did not want to take.) Everyone is allowed the right to make their own choices, including those in care settings and taking away this control denies people their right to make choices and live the way they want to.

- it can make a positive difference to individuals' lives as the care and support you provide will reflect individuals' needs, views and preferences. It will be in line with what the individual wants, again enabling individuals to live how they want to.

You will also be able to find out more about individuals' unique likes, dislikes, abilities and preferences and can tailor your care to meet their requirements. This will show individuals that you respect and value them. It will show you have a genuine interest in them and that you care.

Working in a way that embeds person-centred values also benefits you and other adult care workers because:

- it ensures you are meeting the expected standards – embedding person-centred values in your work practices means that the way you provide care and support to individuals will meet the standards that are expected of you as an adult care worker, i.e. showing you have the right values and behaviours

- it ensures you provide high-quality care and support – embedding person-centred values in your work practices means that you are following best practice which will in turn impact on the quality of the care and support you provide, i.e. showing you are able to support individuals to be in control of their lives, including their care and support will lead to the provision of safe and effective care and support.

- it ensures you promote partnership working – embedding person-centred values in your work practices means that you will be getting to know how to work alongside individuals and others who are involved in their lives, such as, their families, other professionals and services, i.e. showing you are able to work as part of a team for the best interests of individuals.

> **Research it**
>
> **1.2 Legislation and embedding person-centred values**
>
> Research how key pieces of legislation, such as the Human Rights Act 1998 and the Care Act 2014, can help with embedding person-centred values when providing care and support to individuals. Produce a written account of your findings.

Not working in a way that embeds person-centred values in adult care settings is unthinkable and must be avoided. Figure 8.1 provides you with some of the consequences of not embedding person-centred values in your working practices.

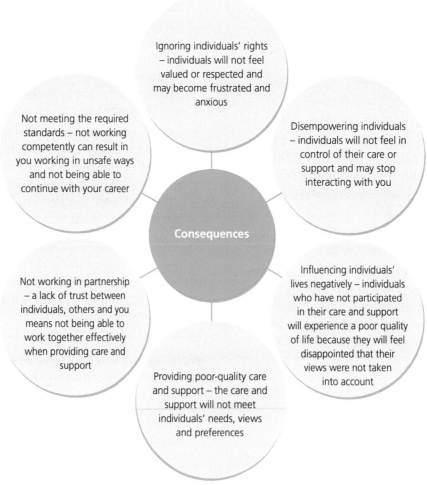

Figure 8.1 Consequences of not embedding person-centred values

Imagine you are an experienced adult care worker and have been asked by your manager to write some guidance for a new member of staff about why it is important to work in a way that embeds person-centred values.

Write down how you would explain what person-centred values are. Which ones do you think you would say are the most important? Why? Ensure you explain all of this in your written work.

What examples could you use to explain how to work in ways that embed person-centred values.

Or, you could reflect on an occasion when you were cared for or supported. For example, this may have been an occasion when you were unwell or when you received sad news. How did the care or support you received help you? Think about how you would have felt if the person providing the care or support did not embed person-centred values. Why do you think you would have felt this way?

AC 1.3 Explain why risk-taking can be part of a person-centred approach

Risk-taking as part of a person-centred approach

Taking risks is part of day-to-day life. It involves being aware of and assessing the potential dangers but not letting that stop you from doing what you want to do in your life. Think about the risks that you take daily. This could be something as simple as crossing the road or switching on a light. You know that there is a risk in both, but you assess the situation. For example, you look at the traffic lights and wait for them to turn red so the cars have stopped and you can cross, and you manage the risk, as you know that drivers have a legal duty to stop at the lights and must wait for you to cross. You therefore take the risk.

Individuals who have care and support needs also have the same rights as everyone else to take risks so that they can live their lives how they want to. Supporting individuals to take the risks they choose is therefore a key part of a person-centred approach as it can make a positive difference to individuals' lives. We have discussed how person-centred approaches are all part of giving individuals the rights to choose and allowing them their independence so that they are in control. Risk-taking is part of this as individuals should be given the choice to decide which risks they take. However, you should be there to:

- inform them about the risks
- support them in the risk assessment by explaining what the risks involve and how they can be managed, how they can stay safe and the measures that you can all put in place to ensure that the risks do not pose a threat or harm them
- encourage individuals who do not want to take risks to do so, so that they can live more independently and grow in confidence
- stop individuals from taking risks if the risks pose a danger to them.

Risk taking has many potential benefits, as Figure 8.2 shows.

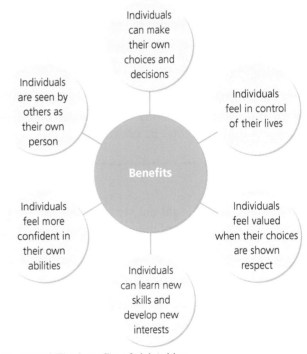

Figure 8.2 The benefits of risk taking

Understanding the risks and handling risks positively

Risk taking by individuals who have care and support needs is not always seen as something positive. Sometimes adult care services and professionals perceive risk taking to have negative consequences such as:

- putting the individual at risk of danger, harm or abuse (the individual may get lost or targeted) because they are seen as vulnerable
- enabling unwise decisions (the individual may have a seizure when they are cooking and burn themselves or cause a fire)
- conflict with their **duty of care**, the individuals' rights to take risks may be in conflict with services and professionals' duty of care. This can have serious consequences for the services provided and the careers of the professionals involved.

The key is not to avoid risk taking but to find ways of handling these risks positively. When risk taking is part of a person-centred approach you can reduce the potential negative consequences of risk taking. For example:

- if an individual with dementia wants to go out shopping without staff, perhaps you could suggest that the individual uses a taxi to get to and from the shops or that they identify someone who they may like to go shopping with that is not staff, such as a family member or friend.
- if an individual with **epilepsy** wants to cook their meals independently, perhaps you could suggest that someone be present at meal

times while the individual does so or that the individual avoids using the cooker but instead uses the oven or the microwave to cook their meals. If there is a pattern to when their seizures occur perhaps you could suggest that they avoid these times for cooking meals.

The examples above show how the individuals want to live independently, even taking part in small activities, such as going shopping on their own (or with someone of their choosing) or cooking a meal. Risk taking, therefore, when part of a person-centred approach, can help individuals to achieve their goals in life, allow them to see what they are capable of achieving and live the way that they want to – a right that we all have and cherish.

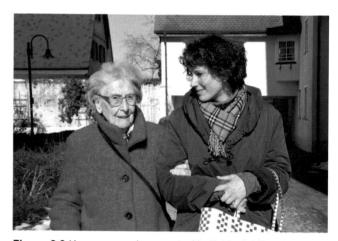

Figure 8.3 How can you be a part of individuals' lives?

Key terms

Duty of care is the legal duty to ensure the safety and well-being of individuals who have care and support needs. You will learn more about how this concept relates to your job role in the care setting where you work in Unit 205, Duty of care.

Epilepsy is a condition that affects the brain and causes repeated seizures or fits.

Evidence opportunity

1.3, 5.2 Risk-taking and person-centred approaches

Find out more about the 'risk-decision' policy and practice in the care setting where you work. You may find it useful to speak with your manager about this. Create a summary of the key points that ensure best practice in your care setting when supporting individuals to take risks. Why is this important and central to high-quality person-centred care? You could include some specific examples, although you must bear in mind confidentiality.

AC 1.4 Explain how using an individual's care plan contributes to working in a person-centred way

A care plan is the document where day-to-day requirements and **preferences** for **care** and support are detailed and may also sometimes be known by other names, such as a support plan or individual plan. Care plans can be developed and updated by the individual receiving the care, along with the help of others who know the individual well, such as family and friends. You or the manager will then look at the care plan, assess and agree to it. As well as looking at the overall plan, it may be that the manager needs to approve any budget with regard to the plan.

What is included in a care plan?

A care plan will include personal details of the individual, such as their name, date of birth, address, likes, dislikes, interests, the individual's care and support needs, the names and contact details of those involved in the provision of care and support.

As well as these details, the care plan will also focus on more specific details of the individual's agreed

Key term

Preferences refer to an individual's wishes. These may be based on an individual's beliefs, values and culture.

goals and what the individual wants to achieve, how they would like to be helped to achieve those goals, what the care worker or setting can do to help them to achieve the goals and by when. However, as you have learned, a key part of person-centred care is to encourage the individual to do as much as possible themselves, so a very important part of the care plan will be to identify the areas that the individual is able to manage by themselves – and then work out where the individual requires some help. By being focused on the individual, the care can be based on what he or she wants and tailored to match their needs. This is why the care plan is so important when it comes to delivering person-centred care. Essentially, the care plan should be informed by what the individual wants from their care and then how you can provide that care and support.

Figure 8.4 on page 282 is an extract from an individual's care plan to give you an example of what one might look like. It is important to remember that, as care plans are personal and unique to the individual, no two care plans will be the same. Just imagine if someone were creating a plan for your development at work. What would happen if you were told that you would be given no choice in your role?

How does a care plan contribute to person-centred care?

Using an individual's care plan contributes to working in a person-centred way.

- **It promotes the individual's rights**. The individuals you care for are fully involved or lead how their care and support needs are met. They may not only write the plan, but may also have a copy of what has been agreed in their care plan. They can also maintain control over their personal information.

- **It supports individuality**. The care and support you provide meet an individual's unique needs and preferences. The plan is drawn up in a format that the individual understands and may even use photographs or video.

- **It enables the individual to live independently**. By focusing on their strengths, abilities and wishes, a care plan can enable an individual to have the quality of life they desire and allows them to achieve as much as they can for themselves.

Sophie's care plan
All about me
My name is Sophie Donning. I am 26 years young and up until a year ago I lived with my mum, dad, younger brother and two dogs. My family and friends are very important to me and I enjoy spending time with them and enjoy visiting them at weekends and going away on holiday.
My family and friends know me very well and are the people who are the closest to me. They say that I am fun to be around and admire my patience and kindness, especially towards my younger brother who, like me, also has a physical disability. I enjoy helping people and always try to keep busy.
How to support me
When I need support, I will let you know; I am very good at asking for help when I need it. Some things I can do for myself. These include getting washed, dressed, doing the laundry and cleaning my flat.
There are other things that I need you to support me with. This is because I use a wheelchair and sometimes I may feel a bit low in myself and might feel unable or not confident enough to do these things on my own. These things usually involve going out shopping, attending appointments – especially those at the hospital and going to new areas or places I've never been to before.
Please remember not to assume I will always need your support when I go out. Sometimes if I'm having a good day I won't need your help. Always ask me, just to make sure.

Figure 8.4 Example of a care plan

Reflect on it

1.1, 1.2, 1.4 Person-centred values and care plans

Reflect on your previous learning at the beginning of this unit around the meaning of person-centred values and how to embed these in your working practices.

What person-centred values are you promoting when using an individual's care plan for the provision of their care and support?

Evidence opportunity

1.4 Care plans and person-centred care

Identify an individual's care plan that you have used in your day-to-day work practice – you may find it useful to refer to this while you are completing this activity.

Remember that this holds personal information that does not belong to you, so make sure that you have the individual's and your manager's permission to access it and that you do so in private. You must also pay strict attention to confidentiality.

With your manager, discuss the reasons why you used it in your working practice and how it helped you deliver person-centred care according to the needs of the individual. Then, provide two examples of how you used it. Include in your discussion that, by doing so, it had a positive influence on the individual and the quality of care and support you provided. Write up notes to evidence your discussion. This discussion might be observed by your assessor or could be a witness testimony account.

LO1 Knowledge, skills, behaviours
Knowledge: what are person-centred approaches in care and support?
Do you know the meaning of person-centred values and why it is important to work in ways that embed person-centred values?
Do you know why supporting individuals to take risks is important? Why is this part of a person-centred approach?
How can an individual's care plan contribute to working in person-centred ways?
Did you know that you have just shown your understanding of what person-centred working involves?

→

LO2 Be able to work in a person-centred way

Getting started

Make a list of all the people who are important in your life and who know you well. For each person write down one aspect that they know about you. For example, this could be something about your background, family, likes, interests. Why are these aspects of your life important to you?

Now think about an individual who has care or support needs and who you know. Write down what you know about this individual. How well do you think you know this individual? Why? Is there anything else you'd like to know about them? How could you find out?

AC 2.1 Find out the history, preferences, wishes and needs of the individual

As we have discussed, the needs of the individuals that you care for should be at the centre of all the care and support you provide. In order to make sure this happens, first you will need to find out as much as you can about the individual for whom you will be caring. You must not only understand what they would like from their care, but also find out as much as possible about their history to enable you to understand them as a person, which will in turn allow you to meet their needs and allow them to live their life as they want to.

There are different ways you can build up a picture of who the individual is and what makes them the person they are. In order to find out more about the individuals you care for, you will need to explore different ways to find out this information. The best way is to speak to the individual and ask them. You will learn more from speaking to them than you will from other sources. It may be that you can also

speak to their family, carers or advocates and they may also be able to help you build up a better picture of who the individual is. Other professionals, such as GPs may also be able to help you understand their medical history, but this will not necessarily help you understand the person as a whole.

Finding out about an individual's history

By speaking to individuals about their history, you will be able to understand more about the experiences that have informed the person they are. You can do this by asking them about their childhood and family background. This is very important especially when you work with older people. It is important to remember that all individuals have a history and they may even be eager to share it with you. You could ask if they would like to show you any photographs or tell you any memories. By doing this, you are valuing the person you care for as an individual, one for whom you should have a genuine interest. Other people involved in their lives who know the individual well, such as their family, friends and advocates may also be a useful source of information.

Think how you feel when someone asks you for your opinion, or how you are feeling, what your likes and dislikes are or to talk a little about your own history. Do you feel that the person asking cares about you and your opinion? Do you feel that they are interested in who you are as an individual? Similarly, asking people about their history will not only allow you to provide better care but will also allow the individual to feel respected and valued and not simply feel like another older person that requires care.

The individual's preferences

These may be based on the individual's beliefs, values and culture. You can find out about an individual's beliefs by asking the individual what they view as important. For example, these may be religious values and will impact the support needs that they have, such as nutrition and personal care. You can find out about an individual's values by discussing this with the individual. These may include not eating meat, washing with running water and only being assisted with their personal hygiene by a person of the same gender. You can find out more about an individual's culture by asking them (and others who know them well) questions about their culture and the associated practices they follow and how. This might affect how they communicate with others, what they eat and what they wear.

Reflect on it

2.1 Finding out about a person

Reflect on someone who you do not know very well. This may be a neighbour or a colleague from work. Imagine you would like to find out more about their beliefs, their values and their culture.

As you do not know them very well, you may find this a little difficult. How could you make this easier? Think about how you approach them, what you are going to say, the reasons why you are asking them personal information.

The individual's wishes

You can find out about an individual's wishes by asking the individual what their hopes and dreams are for the present and the future. Others who know the individual well may also be helpful when drawing up a picture of what the individual's wishes are.

The individual's needs

You can find out about an individual's needs by asking the individual what care and support needs they have and what they require to meet these. These might include asking them what their needs are with regards to nutrition and what activities they would like to participate in so that they can live as actively as possible. You will need to identify the gaps between where they are independent and able and where support is required. Others who know the individual well may also be a useful source of information about the needs they have.

It is only by finding out about the individuals that you can truly provide person-centred care. Remember to discuss all aspects of their life that make up the person they are so that you build up a holistic and overall more rounded impression of the person they are.

Find out about their health so that you can understand what their health and medical needs are. How long have they been suffering from an illness? How does it affect them and make them feel? How can you support them in both dealing with the illness and the effects of it? Perhaps the illness has meant that they cannot do as much as they used to, how can you support the individual to cope? Has this changed them as a person?

Find out about their social interactions. How does their family and social life affect who they are? Are there people that they have difficult relationships with? How can this affect who they are as a person and their support needs? If they are in a care setting, do they find it difficult to be away from their family?

Find out about their religious and cultural backgrounds, if they have any religious and cultural needs and what these are. How will this affect their interactions with others? How will this affect their nutritional needs and personal care needs? Are there any activities and practices that they will not participate in and is there any food and drink that they will not consume? How do they prefer to wash? How do they prefer to dress? Do they prefer to have a care worker of a particular gender? Will they need somewhere quiet to reflect and pray?

Find out about their educational and employment background. Have they been previously employed or unemployed for a period of time? How does this make up the person they are? What is their quality of life and how has their job or social class had an effect on this? Do they have a poor diet and lifestyle, perhaps as a result of lack of employment and access to money? How about their educational background? Do their literacy and numeracy levels affect their day-to-day life and life in the setting? Do you need to adjust your communications with them because they are unable to read and understand information?

Collating all this information takes time and may have to be built up over days, weeks and even months. It may involve not only discussions with individuals and others who are involved in their lives but it may also involve reviewing previous care plans the individuals may have had (letters about the care and support they have received, reports, other records, such as communication records and risk assessments, photographs and images of different activities they have participated in and goals they have achieved).

Some of this information may have already been collated by your manager upon the arrival of the individual at the care setting where you work or by other staff who have worked closely with the individual – do not forget to ask them and involve them too.

AC 2.2 Apply person-centred values in day-to-day work taking into account the history, preferences, wishes and needs of the individual

Working in a person-centred way is not only about finding out about an individual's history, beliefs, values, culture, wishes and needs but it also involves taking these into account in your day-to-day work and putting into practice the person-centred values you learned about earlier on in this unit. This is a good time for you to recap your previous knowledge learned about person-centred values for care and support in AC 1.1. Before doing so, how many do you know already? Can you name them?

Now look back at AC 2.1 and think of all the considerations we discussed, such as, an individual's health, family background and religious needs.

Table 8.2 on page 286 provides some examples of how you can apply person-centred values when carrying out your day-to-day work tasks in the care setting where you work. The 'Reflect on it' activity that follows provides you with an opportunity to think about some of your own examples.

Evidence opportunity

2.1 Finding out about the individual

Develop a written plan for the different methods you can use to find out about an individual who accesses the care and support provided in the care setting where you work.

Once you have agreed these with your manager put them into practice. Did you find out anything you didn't know about the individual? How did you find the process? If you did this again would you use the same methods? Explain why. Write down your responses to all of these questions. Remember that you cannot include the care plan or personal details about individuals in your portfolio.

Table 8.2 Examples of how to apply person-centred values

Day-to-day work task	Examples of how to apply person-centred values
Supporting an individual with their personal hygiene	Ask the individual what support they require with their personal hygiene.
	Provide the individual with the opportunity to choose whether they would like a bath or shower and whether they would like their hair washed.
	Show respect for an individual's culture and beliefs by asking them if there is a personal hygiene routine they prefer to follow, such as using running water when washing.
Supporting an individual with preparing a meal	Find out the individual's requirements for eating and drinking. For example, if there are some foods they are unable to eat (due to their beliefs) or their likes and dislikes for food and drink (personal preference).
	For example, they may prefer to eat only vegetarian, vegan, halal or kosher food.
	Find out whether the individual has any allergies or food intolerances. For example, a nut allergy, or perhaps they are gluten intolerant. This is something you will need to check with medical professionals caring for them and others that know them.
	Promote an individual's independence by enabling them to do as much for themselves as they are able to when preparing a meal.
	Ask the individual where they would prefer to eat. Do they prefer to eat in the kitchen, lounge or their own room? You should respect their choice.
Supporting an individual with attending a GP appointment	Ask the individual how they would prefer to travel to their GP appointment. Is this by taxi or bus for example?
	Ask the individual what support they require from you. For example, do they want you:
	• to travel with them only
	• attend the appointment with them
	• speak up for them? Promote an individual's right to make their own informed choices by ensuring the individual understands the information that has been communicated to them by their GP.
Supporting an individual with activities	Ask the individual what activities they would like to do and what support they would like. For example, this may be daily activities, such as cooking and shopping or recreational activities, such as gardening and going to the gym.
	Find out whether there are any activities the individual would like to do but hasn't tried yet like participating in a new activity, such as bowling or learning a new skill like sewing or painting.
	Promote an individual's independence by encouraging them to lead the activity – give only as much support as required and ensure that you do this by going at the individual's own pace.
	Encourage the individual to reflect on their participation in the activity and discuss what they thought worked well. Ask them what they enjoyed, what they didn't like or what they think could be improved.

Reflect on it

2.1, 2.2 Individuals' history

Reflect on why knowing about an individual's history is important when providing care and support. What can an individual's history tell you about the person behind the individual? How can this help you when supporting them with a task, such as taking part in a cooking activity, or when supporting the individual to socialise with others? How would you show the individual that you are taking into account their history?

Applying person-centred values in day-to-day work is a key part of being able to provide high-quality care and support. Working in this way can also have a significant impact on the quality of individuals' lives and can make a positive difference, as Case study 1.1, 1.2 shows.

Case study

1.2, 2.2 Person-centred working in practice

Kian is a **Shared Lives carer** and is married with two children. Stacey has learning disabilities and lives on her own. She is joining Kian and his family this weekend as they are planning a camping trip to take place the following week to which Stacey has also been invited. As Stacey has never been camping before she is keen to find out more about what Kian and his family are planning and she agrees to discuss the trip with Kian and his family over afternoon tea.

Kian begins by showing Stacey photographs of previous camping trips they have done together as a family. Kian asks Stacey to take her time to look through these and then as she does so he asks one of the children to tell Stacey where it was taken and what is happening in the photograph.

Kian has been observing Stacey closely and he can see that she is looking a little upset and so once they have finished looking through the photographs Kian asks Stacey if she can help him with the washing up. Stacey agrees and while the two of them are in the kitchen, Kian asks Stacey what she thinks about camping. Stacey explains that she's feeling very anxious because she has never spent time away from home before.

Kian asks Stacey if she would prefer not to go away at first for a whole weekend – and instead try a day trip to see how she feels. Stacey explains that she would really enjoy that. Kian asks Stacey to have a think about where she would like to go and then perhaps she could visit again one afternoon next week and together they could discuss this again as a family over tea. Stacey agrees and says that she will also try to bring information with her about different places where they could all go together.

Discussion points

1 The person-centred values applied by Kian.
2 Examples of how Kian takes into account Stacey's individual preferences, wishes and needs.
3 The impact of Kian's person-centred approach on Stacey.

Key term

A **Shared Lives carer** is someone who opens up their home and family life to include an adult with support needs so that they can participate and experience community and family life. The individual may stay with them for the weekend, or they may even go on holiday together.

Research it

2.2 Shared Lives Plus

Research Shared Lives Plus, an organisation for Shared Lives carers and schemes. Find out about who they are and what they do. Produce a poster with your findings.

You will find the link below useful:

http://sharedlivesplus.org.uk/about-shared-lives-plus

Research it

2.2 Person-centred thinking tools

Helen Sanderson Associates (www.helensandersonassociates.co.uk) have developed a range of person-centred thinking tools. Research the tools they have developed and think about how they might help you in your care setting.

LO2 Knowledge, skills, behaviours
Knowledge: what is person-centred working?
Do you know what person-centred working means?
Do you know what applying person-centred values in your day-to-day work means?
Did you know that you have just showed your knowledge of the key aspects of working in a person-centred way?
Skills: how can you show that you are able to work in a person-centred way?
Do you know how to find out about an individual's history, needs and preferences?
Do you know how to work in a person-centred way?
Did you know that you have just demonstrated a few of the skills required for using person-centred approaches in care settings?
Behaviours: how can you show the personal qualities you have in your day-to-day working practices?
Do you know how to respect and treat an individual with kindness?
Do you know how to promote an individual's choices and independence?
Did you know that you have just demonstrated a few of the essential behaviours required when using person-centred approaches in care settings?

LO3 Be able to establish consent when providing care or support

AC 3.1 Explain the importance of establishing consent when providing care or support

You will already know that person-centred care involves respecting individuals' choices and decisions. To do so also requires you to provide the individual with sufficient information to be able to understand the choices and decisions they are making. Similarly, before providing individuals with any form of care and support, you must ensure that you have their agreement to do so and that you have provided them with sufficient information about their options, the benefits and consequences of not doing so, to ensure their understanding – this is referred to as 'informed consent'.

Reflect on it

3.1 Consent

Reflect on an occasion when you gave your consent. For example, this may be when you were asked where you wanted to go out or what you wanted to eat. How did this make you feel?

Now imagine how you would feel if you were not asked for your consent?

For example, before you support an individual to move from one position to another, make sure that you have asked the individual:

- the position they want to move to, i.e. to another chair, to their bed?
- when they want to move, i.e. now, after lunch?
- how they want to move, i.e. with support from your arm, on their own?

You must also sure that you have explained to the individual:

- the benefits of moving to another chair, i.e. this will provide more support for their back, and the drawbacks of moving back to their bed, i.e. lying down for long periods may be uncomfortable
- the benefits of moving now, i.e. they will feel more comfortable when eating their lunch, and the drawbacks of moving after lunch, i.e. they may feel uncomfortable when eating
- the benefits of moving with support from your arm, i.e. they will find the move from one position to another easier, and the drawbacks of moving on their own, i.e. they may fall.

It is important to remember that you must ask these questions, have such discussions and obtain consent **before** you carry out the activity. You must have agreement from the individual regardless of whether the task you are about to perform is something that is done daily. It may be that the individual was happy for you to carry out a slightly invasive procedure one day but not on another day. Consent must also be obtained whether it is for something as important as medical treatment or as simple as whether the individual would like the lights in their room turned off.

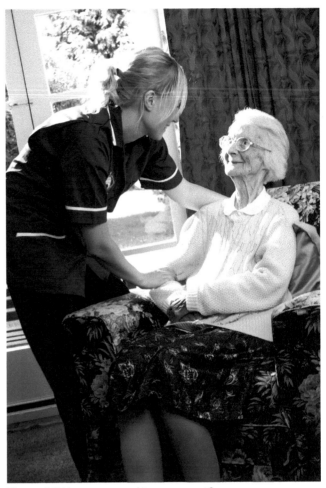

Figure 8.5 Have you sought my consent?

Why is it important to obtain consent?

Obtaining an individual's **consent** when providing care or support is important because:

- it is a legal requirement – to comply with legislation, such as the Mental Capacity Act 2005, the individual must give their consent for the provision of care or support. When an individual is unable to give their consent because they **lack the capacity** to perhaps due to having a condition such as dementia then a representative may decide on their behalf but only if they act in the individual's best interests at all times. It is important to note that lacking capacity to make one decision does not mean an individual lacks capacity to make every decision. The 'best interests' principle in the Mental Capacity Act 2005 means that all decisions made on behalf of an individual who lacks capacity must benefit the individual – this

Research it

3.1 Mental Capacity Act 2005

Research what the Mental Capacity Act 2005 says about the importance of establishing consent when providing care or support and promoting individuals' rights. There is a useful link below:

www.mind.org.uk/media/1834262/mental-capacity-act.pdf

Key terms

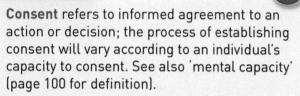

Consent refers to informed agreement to an action or decision; the process of establishing consent will vary according to an individual's capacity to consent. See also 'mental capacity' (page 100 for definition).

This is a key part of person-centred care as it means respecting the individuals we provide care for and ensuring that they remain in control of the care they receive.

Lack of capacity is a term used to refer to when an individual is unable to make a decision for themselves because of a learning disability or a condition such as dementia or a mental health need, or because they are unconscious.

may be in relation to the individual's health, care or support. You can learn more about what to do when consent cannot be established in AC 3.3 on page 292. Obtaining consent also means that the individuals you care for have given their agreement for their care and as a result you and your setting are protected legally.

- it is necessary for working in a person-centred way – obtaining an individual's consent when providing care or support means that you are respecting the individual's right to agree or refuse and promoting their dignity by not assuming that you know what care or support the individual wants or needs or prefers.

Remember it is the individual who knows best. It is the individual or their representative who

Evidence opportunity

3.1 The importance of consent

Develop a case study of an older individual who has care or support needs and who will be having adult care workers providing support in the mornings and evenings with maintaining their personal hygiene. This could be someone you know or it could be a fictitious individual. Then explain from the individual's perspective why it is important that they have given their consent for support from adult care workers.

decides what care or support is needed and/or preferred. The care and medical professions are able to advise on care and medical treatment, but individuals and their representatives must be able to decide what happens to them.

AC 3.2 Establish consent for an activity or action

Establishing consent with an individual for an activity or action can only be successful if you:

- work together with the individual. This ensures their rights are respected and their preferences supported

- are flexible in the methods you use. Some individuals may be able to consent verbally, others in writing.

When establishing consent with an individual for an activity or action in any adult care setting it is important to comply with the following best practice guidance.

Top tips for establishing consent:

- Respect the individual's views about the activity or action, for example you should discuss when it is to be carried out.

- Listen to the individual and find out about their preferences about the activity or action.

- Discuss or explain what carrying out the activity or action will involve, for example you should tell them about the number of staff required to support the activity and the process to be followed.

- Provide the individual with relevant and accurate information; this may also be in response to any questions or concerns the individual may have.

- Support the individual to make their own decisions and respect these. For example discuss with the individual the related benefits, drawbacks and consequences, respect their decisions even if you disagree with them.

- Do not try to persuade the individual into making a decision, even if you think it is in their best interests.

- If the individual lacks capacity, then you should speak to their advocate but make sure that in the first instance, you consult the individual. Also make sure that you support those with language and communication difficulties to communicate their consent, and seek the assistance of translators and communication aids.

Remember that if you are unsure about anything or do not have the knowledge about any of this, then you should refer the individual to someone who does (e.g. a medical professional). This means the individual has access to the most correct and accurate information available. Also remember the things you have learnt about confidentiality when you are communicating information, especially to those other than the individual. You may be dealing with sensitive and private information, so it is important that you are sure the individual is happy for the information to be communicated to others.

Establishing consent is not a process that is completed by adult care workers at the beginning of their shift or once a day, it is an ongoing process that takes place for every activity or action they complete with an individual. This is because an individual's preferences, like yours, may change from one day to another and, like you, respecting individuals' preferences and right to change their mind is a must. For example, just because an individual chose to have a shower yesterday morning does not mean they want to have a shower every morning; the individual may prefer to have a bath instead, or to have a wash at night before going to bed. You will only know if you seek the individual's consent; not doing so will result in you not providing good care and support.

How is consent communicated?

We have already discussed informed consent, where individuals are asked for their consent or agreement based on the information they have received about the benefits, risks and consequences. However, how do individuals give or communicate their consent? You will find that this will vary depending on the types of things for which you are requesting consent. For example, it might be done verbally (*verbal consent*) when you ask an individual whether they are happy to have lunch, or would like to take part in a group activity, and they tell you that it is okay. You may need *written consent*, for example, when individuals are agreeing to serious medical procedures, when an individual agrees for someone to be their advocate or when consent is required around financial matters. However, you will also find that consent is not always communicated. It may often be implied. For example, if you ask an individual who is in bed whether they would like to get up and get dressed, and they sit up in bed and look at their wardrobe, then they are implying that they are ready to do so. It is important that you are aware of these different methods and the situations in which it is important to gain more formal written consent.

Research it

3.2 Health and Social Care Act 2008 (Regulated Activities) Regulations 2014

Research the Health and Social Care Act 2008 (Regulated Activities) Regulations 2014: Regulation 1. What does it state about how consent must be established when providing care or support to an individual?

There is a useful link below:

www.cqc.org.uk/guidance-providers/regulations-enforcement/regulation-11-need-consent

Discuss your findings with a colleague in the care setting where you work. Make notes based on your discussion.

3.2 Obtaining agreement

Reflect on an occasion when you visited an adult care or health setting, for example the dentist, optician, hospital or doctors. How did the care professional obtain your agreement for the treatment being provided to you? How did this make you feel? Why?

Evidence opportunity

3.2, 1.4 Obtaining consent

Identify an individual you provide care or support to in the care setting where you work and that you know well. Using the individual's care plan and your knowledge of the individual's background, needs and preferences, write down which methods you can use to obtain their consent when providing care or support.

Do you use these methods already? If not, why not? What are the benefits of doing so? What could be the consequences of not doing so? Ensure you cover all of this in your written work.

Remember that you cannot include the care plan in your portfolio, and that you cannot include individuals' personal details in your portfolio.

AC 3.3 Explain what steps to take if consent cannot be readily established

As you will have learned in AC 3.1, sometimes it may not be possible to establish consent with an individual. This may be because:

- the individual lacks capacity
- the individual is undecided over whether to give their consent
- it is unclear whether an individual has given their consent

3.1, 3.3 When an individual lacks capacity

Reflect on your previous learning in AC 3.1. What is the meaning of the term 'lacks capacity'? How can this impact on how consent is established with individuals?

- it is unclear whether an individual has understood the information provided to them.

Whatever the reason for not being able to establish consent, remember that you cannot proceed with a task or procedure unless you have obtained consent. If an individual outright refuses consent, you cannot proceed.

If any of the above situations do arise you must do something.

- Try explaining the information to them again. This is so that they understand what the procedure entails, the benefits, risks and consequences.
- Seek advice from for example your manager – it is your duty to not ignore the concerns you have but to report that the individual has not given consent, seek further guidance and discuss your concerns. Settings will have their own policies and procedures in place in case of such situations. Doing so reflects your **competence** for providing good care and support and ensuring that the best outcome for the individual can be reached.
- Consult with the individual's representative – in some cases you may be able to seek further clarification from a person who knows the individual well; this may be the individual's advocate, for example. Discussing this with someone else may help. You must always check before doing so with your manager as this information is personal to the individual and is therefore protected data.
- Record your findings – in relation to the actions you took to establish consent with an individual and the actions you took when you

Key term

Professional Councils are organisations that regulate professions, such as adult social care workers who work with adults in residential care homes, in day centres and who provide care in someone's home. They can provide advice and support around working with individuals who lack capacity to make decisions.

were unable to establish consent with the individual. Include what happened, what the individual said/expressed, the guidance you were given, by whom and when.

If, after trying all these options consent can still not be established with an individual then it may be that you are unable to do anything. However, this will depend on a number of things, such as the individual's capacity, and whether refusal means their health will be in danger. Advice may need to be sought by your manager from external agencies, such as the Courts, who can provide legal clarification, and **Professional Councils** who can provide additional support.

Evidence opportunity

3.3 Steps to take when consent cannot be established

Think about an occasion when you or someone you work with found it difficult to establish consent with an individual. What happened and why was it difficult?

Produce a step-by-step diagram that shows the steps you or your work colleague could take if this situation arose again. Remember to explain the reasons why each step is necessary.

Case study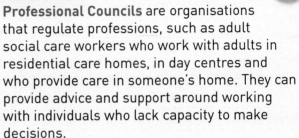

3.1, 3.2, 3.3 The Cheshire West case

Mr P, a 39-year-old man with cerebral palsy and Down's syndrome, lacked the capacity to make decisions about his own care. He was living at home with his mother but when his health deteriorated, Cheshire West and Chester Council placed him in the care of the local authority. Mr P's mother successfully argued that her son's care should be regularly reviewed to ensure that he was not being deprived of his liberty, because once placed in care he was under constant supervision and was not free to leave. The outcome of the case was that he would have regular independent

care reviews to ensure that the care provided was appropriate and met his needs.

Discussion points

1 'A gilded cage is still a cage.' What does this phrase mean? Reflect on how this is relevant to individuals who lack the capacity to make decisions.
2 How can independent care reviews mean that individuals who lack capacity have their human rights upheld?
3 What do you think of individuals who lack mental capacity being equated to birds trapped in cages?

L03 Knowledge, skills, behaviours
Knowledge: why is establishing consent important when providing care or support?
Do you know what consent means?
Do you know the consequences of not establishing consent and the steps to take if it cannot be established?
Did you know that you have just showed your knowledge of why establishing consent when providing care or support is important and also a legal requirement?
Skills: how can you show that you are able to establish consent with an individual?
Do you know how to choose the methods that best match the individual's needs and preferences to establish consent?
Do you know what to do when you cannot establish consent with an individual?
Did you know that you have just demonstrated a few of the skills required to be a competent adult care worker when establishing consent?
Behaviours: how can you show the personal qualities you have when you are establishing consent?
Do you know how to respect an individual's decisions about their care or support?
Do you know how to show that you are able to listen to an individual's views about their care or support?
Did you know that you have just demonstrated a few of the essential behaviours required to provide high-quality care and support?

LO4 Be able to encourage active participation

Getting started

Think about an occasion when you were tasked with an activity to complete. How did this make you feel? How involved were you in the task? Did anyone else support you with it? If so, how? Now imagine being tasked with the same activity but not being allowed to be fully involved in completing it. How do you think this would make you feel? Why? What do you think are the benefits for individuals who are fully involved in all aspects of their lives?

AC 4.1 Describe how active participation benefits an individual

Active participation is a person-centred way of working that can lead to improved care and support. This is because it recognises:

- an individual's rights – for example, to participate in activities fully, to maintain relationships in everyday life as independently as possible
- an individual's abilities – for example, to be an active partner who is involved in their own care or support rather than a passive recipient who is not involved and on the receiving end of care or support
- an individual's potential – for example, to be in control over their care or support and influence how their care or support needs are met.

Active participation means supporting individuals to live their lives as independently as possible. This does not mean doing things for them but instead helping them to do things for themselves as much as possible. This might mean enabling

Key term

Active participation is a way of working that recognises an individual's right to participate in the activities and relationships of everyday life as independently as possible; the individual is regarded as an active partner in their own care or support, rather than a passive recipient.

them to go out shopping on their own or taking part in a social group.

Being able to do things for ourselves and being active members of our society and community can impact positively on our lives through increased social interactions, the achievement of our own personal goals, and living independently, and it can have numerous positive impacts on our health such as feelings of well-being and increased self-esteem. Just think about how you feel when you have achieved

a goal. Perhaps you ran a 10k race and achieved a finish time that you had aimed for. Perhaps you successfully cooked a dish that you had been trying. Such things can give us feelings of well-being and thus impact positively on our health.

Likewise, there are many benefits of active participation for individuals who have care or support needs. Some of the main ones are included in Figure 8.6. Can you think of any others?

Reflect on it

4.1 The benefits of active participation

Reflect on the benefits of active participation identified in Figure 8.6. Now think about the difference each of these benefits would make to your life.

- What impact could it have if you feel good about making your own decisions?

- How can an increase in confidence benefit you?
- Why is being in control of your life important?
- Why is your unique needs and preferences being taken into account and understood important?

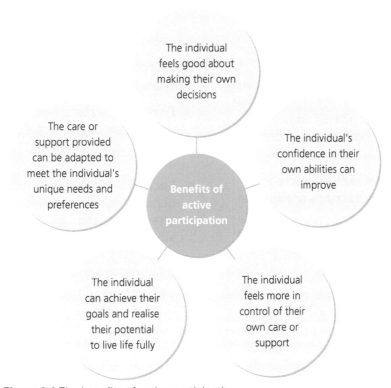

Figure 8.6 The benefits of active participation

Evidence opportunity

4.1 How active participation can benefit an individual

Discuss with your assessor how you would explain to a member of staff who is new to care how active participation benefits an individual.

Include the reasons why, examples of how active participation benefits an individual, and give examples of the benefits for two individuals with whom you have used active participation.

AC 4.2 Identify possible barriers to active participation

As you have learned in AC 4.1 there may be times or occasions when it is difficult to encourage active participation, for example when a new adult care worker lacks the knowledge or skills to know how to do so. There are also many other reasons why.

- **Insufficient time**: when adult care workers are very busy or when they are working in a team where some staff are unwell or away on leave then active participation may be difficult. For example, it may be quicker to make a cup of tea for an individual then support the individual to walk to the kitchen to make a cup of tea for themselves.

- **Lack of training**: it is not only new adult care workers that may lack the knowledge or skills but experienced staff may also become complacent about best practice if they do not actively attend training updates on how to encourage active participation when providing care or support.

It is not always the care worker that acts as a barrier, there may also be **barriers around the individual**:

- **Individuals' understanding**: for active participation to be successful it is crucial that individuals understand how they can be involved and lead on the care or support provided. Sometimes an individual's condition, such as dementia, may make active participation more difficult to achieve if the individual is for example feeling confused about what they are trying to achieve.

- **Individuals' needs**: for active participation to be successful it is crucial that individuals' needs are met. Sometimes an individual's needs, such as their mental health, may mean that their personal confidence in themselves is low and therefore the individual may be reluctant to become actively involved in their own care or support.

- **Individuals' families and carers**: for active participation to be successful it is crucial that families and carers also encourage individuals to be active participants and do not do things for them. This may be difficult given the close relationships they may share with the individual but it is important that care workers also support families and carers in this.

Resources and the environment may also pose barriers to active participation:

- **Physical barriers**, such as a lack of ramps for wheelchair users, may stop individuals from accessing buildings and taking part in social events.

- **Lack of information**: if individuals are unaware of how they can participate, or events they can attend, then they will be unable to partake in such activities.

- **Accessible information**: if information is not available in formats or languages the individual can understand, then this also poses a barrier to participation.

4.2 Barriers to active participation

Develop a profile of an individual who has care or support needs. Write down what their unique needs are and then identify how these may affect the individual when they are involved in their care or support.

Remember to include anything else that may help or hinder this individual's active participation in their own care or support. For example, this may be in relation to the care setting, or to those who work with the individual. How is this a help or hindrance? You may want to think about the role other health professionals might play too.

Remember that you cannot include personal details about individuals in your portfolio.

4.2 Barriers

Reflect on how barriers to active participation can have a negative effect on an individual's wishes and hopes for the future. You could also reflect on how barriers to active participation could affect how individuals think about achieving their goals.

AC 4.3 Demonstrate ways to reduce the barriers and encourage active participation

For this assessment criterion, you will be observed demonstrating both how to reduce the barriers to active participation and how to encourage the active participation of individuals.

You have already taken the first step towards being able to encourage active participation by learning about the different barriers that can exist for individuals who have care and support needs and by raising your awareness of what these are and how they can vary for different individuals and care settings.

You are now therefore ready to take the next step towards encouraging active participation; that is finding out about the different ways and approaches that can be used to reduce these barriers.

Thinking back to the barriers we identified in AC 4.2, there are a number of ways you can reduce these barriers and encourage active participation. For example:

- Where you do not have enough time and think it is quicker to complete the task for the individual, you must remind yourself that it is part of person-centred practice to promote active participation so that the individual is able to do as much for themselves as possible.

- Where you do not have enough training, you should seek out training opportunities and discuss these with your manager.

- Where the individual lacks understanding about how they can involve themselves in activities and do things for themselves, if they suffer from illness, you will need to make sure that you use communication methods to aid their understanding, and you should refer to Unit 203, Communication in care settings.

- Where individuals lack confidence, you should help to build their confidence and self-esteem, which will in turn encourage them to participate.

- Where individuals' families and carers are perhaps doing too much for them, which hinders the individual so that they are unable to do things for themselves, you should discuss this with families and carers so that they are aware of the importance of encouraging active participation and how they can enable the individual in this.

- Where there are physical barriers, you should support the individual in finding out how they can gain access, or request access to places where there may be none. It may be that they require a disabled parking badge or more information about gaining access to buildings; again you should support them in overcoming these physical barriers.

If information is not available, then you will need to support them in accessing this information.

It may be that you can support them with some research on the internet or tell them where they may find more information.

Similarly, if information is unavailable in formats they require, then you should support them in gaining access to information in a form that they can access. It may be that you could request a leaflet in a different language, or ask for one to be translated.

Other ways to reduce barriers and encourage active participation include:

- **Keeping your knowledge and skills about best practice up to date when encouraging active participation** – this enables you as an adult care worker to ensure that your working practices and approaches are effective. Maintaining your knowledge and skills through continuing professional development activities, such as training, reading articles, working with experienced colleagues, can be crucial for encouraging positive ways to encourage individuals' active participation.

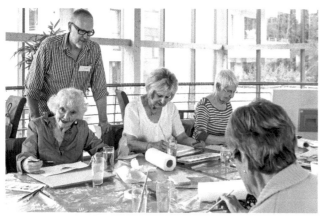

Figure 8.7 How can you make sure I'm fully involved?

- **Spending time getting to know the individual** – this enables you as an adult care worker to build up a good working relationship with the individual that can be crucial for encouraging active participation. You will get to know their needs and preferences which means that you can take these into account when encouraging them to become more involved. For example, if you know that an individual does not like noisy environments then you could make arrangements to discuss their care or support in a quiet area where the individual will feel relaxed and you will not be disturbed. At the same time, the individual will get to know you which means that they will feel valued by you and respected therefore making them more likely to trust you and want to get involved in their own care or support.

- **Accessing sources of information, support and guidance** – this enables you as an adult care worker to increase the opportunities an individual has made available to them to actively participate. Your manager can be one such source of information and guidance. For example, your manager can ensure that you are aware of different ways of supporting individuals' choices about their care or support as well as your responsibilities for doing so. The individual's representative, such as their advocate or a family member, can also act as good support for ensuring the individual understands the information you are providing, including their options. In addition, involving others can ensure that the individual's rights and preferences are being supported and continue to be the main focus of all care or support provided.

Reflect on it

4.3 CPD

Reflect on your understanding of the term 'continuing professional development'. What is best practice when encouraging active participation? How is this useful to your own working practice and how does it benefit the individuals you provide care or support to?

You will find it useful to refer to Unit 207, Personal development in care settings.

Research it

4.3 Best practice

Research some examples of best practice when providing care or support to individuals. Useful sources of information for carrying out your research could include the care setting where you work, care settings you know about in your local area, newspapers, television and the internet.

Produce an information handout with your findings.

Evidence opportunity

4.3 Reducing barriers and encouraging active participation

Review Evidence opportunity 4.2 where you developed a profile of an individual who has care or support needs that included details of their unique needs and the barriers that may affect this individual with actively participating in their own care or support.

Now put together an information handout that highlights possible ways for reducing the barriers that this individual may face. This information could be used to update the individual's care plan.

LO4 Knowledge, skills, behaviours
Knowledge: what is active participation?
Do you know what it means when an individual is an active participant in their own care or support?
Do you know why active participation is important and what barriers can hinder active participation?
Did you know that you have just answered questions about the meaning and benefits of active participation?
Skills: how can you show that you can encourage active participation?
Do you know how to identify possible barriers to active participation?
Do you know the ways to reduce these barriers and encourage active participation?
Did you know that you have just answered two questions about a few of the skills you need when encouraging individuals to be active participants?
Behaviours: how can you show the personal qualities you have when encouraging active participation?
Do you know how to be respectful of individuals' personal decisions and choices?
Do you know how to show that you are able to be patient when encouraging an individual to be actively involved?
Did you know that you have just answered two questions about a few of the essential behaviours that are expected of all adult care workers when encouraging the active participation of individuals?

LO5 Be able to support the individual's right to make choices

Getting started

Think about what it feels like to make your own choices in life. What about how it feels to be independent and in control of your life? Now think about the individuals you work with. Do you know how to respect every individual you work with as a unique person? Do you know how to support every individual you work with to be involved in and make their own choices about day-to-day aspects of their lives? How do you encourage the individuals you work with to be actively involved in their lives?

AC 5.1 Support an individual to make informed choices

For this assessment criterion, you will be observed demonstrating how to support an individual to make informed choices.

Supporting individuals' rights is crucial to working in a person-centred way because it involves supporting individuals to make choices that they:

- understand
- have been fully involved in
- are in control of.

In other words, person-centred practice involves supporting individuals' rights to make *informed* choices.

Regardless of whether you work with individuals in a setting or in their home, a key part of your role will be to support individuals to make choices. This might be about daily tasks such as their personal care routines, or 'bigger' matters such as their care plan, finances, and where they live. Whatever the choice is about, you will need to make sure that:

- the choices they are making are informed ones. This means making sure that you give them all the information they need in order to make their choices, in a clear and accessible way, one where the individual is able to understand what is being communicated

- individuals are aware of the different options available and that these are clearly communicated to them

- you help them to overcome barriers in order to make those choices. If, for example, they experience communication difficulties, you must make sure that this does not stop them from making their own choices. It may be that where individuals lack capacity, you will need to support their family and advocates to make those choices

- if individuals are already aware of the different choices available to them, you should listen to them and support them to make their choices, at the same time telling them about any alternatives they may not have mentioned.

Dos and don'ts for supporting individuals to make informed choices	
Do	Find out how an individual makes their own choices – to ensure that you are providing support to individuals in ways that have been agreed and that match their strengths, abilities and preferences.
Do	Ensure all information presented to individuals is understood – to ensure that individuals can then use this information to consider and choose from different options that are available to them.
Do	Ensure individuals and/or their representatives are involved – to ensure that individuals and their representatives put forward the individual's views, ideas and preferences.
Do	Keep records of all options available and agreed upon – to ensure that these can be shared with everyone involved and referred to when required.
Don't	Make decisions for individuals – this does not support an individual's rights to make their own choices.
Don't	Present information in a misleading way – this does not enable individuals to make informed choices.
Don't	Ignore individuals and others who know them well – this does not enable you to take into account their personal views, ideas and preferences.
Don't	Only agree options verbally – it does not enable information to be shared accurately and reviewed with all those involved if clear records are not kept.

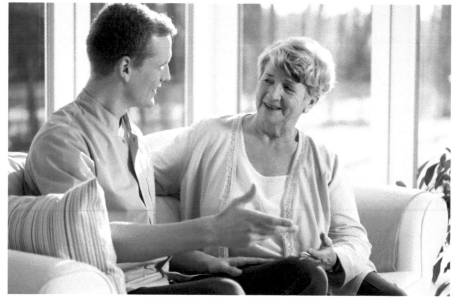

Figure 8.8 Supporting an individual to speak up

Research it

5.1 Informed choices and best practice

Research best practice when supporting individuals to make informed choices. You can conduct your research either in the care setting where you work or in another care setting that you know about.

You could also speak to adult care workers and ask them about the practices they follow when supporting individuals to make informed choices. You could ask them questions, such as: 'What type of care setting do you work in?'; 'What care or support needs do the individuals you work with have?'; 'What ways do you find work best when supporting individuals to make informed choices?'

Reflect on it

5.1 Capacity to make informed choices

Imagine you had an accident, were experiencing temporary confusion and needed support to make informed choices in relation to day-to-day living. How would you feel if you didn't get the support you needed? What impact may this have on how you live your life?

Evidence opportunity

5.1 Supporting individuals to make informed choices

Identify an activity that you can support an individual who has care or support needs with. For example, it could be with putting their shoes on, brushing their teeth, making a shopping list, deciding on how to spend the evening. Think about how you would support the individual with this activity. Ensure you show how you support the individual to make their own informed choices. Alternatively, your assessor might observe you supporting the individual directly or you could get a witness testimony from your manager.

AC 5.2 Use agreed risk assessment processes to support the right to make choices

For this assessment criterion, you will be observed demonstrating how to use agreed risk assessment processes to support individuals' rights to make choices.

Taking risks is part of making choices in everyday life for all of us; not doing so would act as a barrier to us achieving what we want to do. Similarly, when adult care workers support individuals' right to make choices about activities they want to do this too may involve individuals taking risks. This doesn't mean that individuals will be placed in danger or be harmed or abused or persuaded to not take risks but rather that they will be supported to understand what the risks are and how these can be managed.

Explaining the risks and ensuring individuals are aware of the consequences that their choices could have helps to protect both you as a care worker and the individual. Risk might include injury or harm being caused to the individual as a result of their choice. By explaining the risks, the individual is protected because even if they decide to proceed with their decision, they can take measures to make it a safer one, for example, and you as a care worker are protected because you have fulfilled your responsibility by explaining the risks, and also by helping the individual to manage and reduce those risks.

Assessing what the risks are and their impact is crucial when supporting individuals' right to make choices because it involves a careful balance between supporting the rights of individuals to make their own choices while maintaining their safety. A thorough risk assessment is not only a useful tool to use for this but it is also a legal requirement for maintaining individuals' safety while they do the activities that they enjoy.

Level 2 Diploma in Care

Research it

5.2 Risk management

Research what the Management of Health and Safety at Work Regulations 1999 say about managing risks and risk assessment.

You will find the link below useful:

www.legislation.gov.uk/uksi/1999/3242/contents/made

Produce an information leaflet with your findings.

Key terms

Risk assessment is used in work settings for identifying hazards, assessing the level of risk and putting in place processes for reducing the risk identified. In this unit, risk assessment and management are used to support individuals to make informed choices, so that they are aware of the risks involved. It is not to stop people from making their own choices, but to help them to manage and reduce the risks involved.

Hazards are dangers with the potential to cause harm, for example a spillage on the floor or a broken wheelchair.

Risk is the likelihood of hazards causing harm, for example slipping over on the spillage on the floor, an individual falling out of a broken wheelchair.

Risk assessment processes involve the five key steps listed below.

1 Identify the **hazards** of an area, such as a kitchen – or a work task, such as assisting an individual to move from one position to another.

2 Identify those who may be harmed by the hazards (individuals, you or your colleagues or visitors).

3 Evaluate the **risk** by deciding whether it is a high, medium or low risk. Then evaluate how the risks can be controlled or reduced.

4 Record the risk assessment to ensure there is a written record of the risks identified and the methods that have been agreed to control or reduce them, so that this can be referenced by all those involved.

Evidence opportunity

5.2 Risk assessment processes and choice

Develop a risk assessment for an activity that you enjoy doing. Remember to go through each of the five steps listed above.

Discuss your risk assessment with your assessor. Be prepared to show them the risk assessment process you carried out and the reasons why.

5 Review and update the risk assessment to ensure any changes to the level of risk or hazards identified in an area – or work task – are recorded and updated. This means that the risk assessment is an accurate record that can be referenced and used by all those involved.

You can learn more about how to manage risks safely in the care setting where you work in Unit 210, Health, safety and well-being in care settings.

Positive risk taking

Positive risk taking in relation to person-centred care involves weighing up the benefits and drawbacks to the individual of taking the risk. The greater the potential benefits to the individual, the more important it is to try and find a way of managing the risk safely while being able to support the individual to take the risk.

The following reflective exemplar provides you with an opportunity to explore in more detail how adult care workers in care settings use risk assessments as part of working in a person-centred way.

302

Reflective exemplar	
Introduction	I work as a personal assistant providing support to Sean who is 36 years old and uses a wheelchair to mobilise. Sean has panic attacks when he leaves his house and so my role is to support him to manage his panic attacks so that he can visit his local shops independently. I visit him on a weekly basis.
What happened?	This morning I supported Sean to prepare a route that he could use to go to his local shops, which are approximately ten minutes away from his house. While looking together on the internet, on Google maps, at the roads we could walk down together Sean began to get very concerned that he may get into difficulties and not be able to return home safely.
	We discussed Sean's concerns together over a cup of tea. Sean began by saying that he may fall out of his wheelchair when travelling over the uneven pavements; we agreed that with me by his side supporting him and with his lap belt done up this was a low risk. Sean then added that he was afraid that he may have his money stolen again like the last time he went out on his own. I explained to Sean that I would be with him and so this again was a low risk. Finally, Sean had concerns over whether he was able enough to do his own shopping; again, I explained that he had already prepared a shopping list and that with my support he would manage fine.
	After much discussion, Sean apologised to me but said that he wasn't ready to leave the house yet and said that he might try again next week when I visited him.
What worked well?	I think identifying the potential hazards that Sean had concerns over was a good first step towards carrying out a risk assessment and reassuring Sean that he could overcome his fears of leaving the house.
What did not go as well?	I think having identified the hazards and partly evaluated the level of risk we should have discussed together what could be put in place to control or reduce the level of risk identified. This is part of the risk assessment process but also I think would have reassured Sean more fully over the concerns he had; he would have felt safer. He may have refused to go out because he may have thought I didn't take his concerns seriously.
What could I do to improve?	I think I'm going to review my previous learning around the five key steps involved in the risk assessment process and see if I can arrange to attend an update on using risk assessment.
Links to unit assessment criteria	ACs 1.3, 5.2

AC 5.3 Explain why a worker's personal views should not influence an individual's choices

Working in a person-centred way, as you know, involves supporting individuals to make their own choices and decisions. You can only do this successfully if you do not let your own views interfere or influence individuals because this may make individuals:

- make choices that they think will please you rather than make choices that are suitable for them
- make the wrong choices and decisions
- not feel in control of their care or support.

Reflect on it

5.3 Your views

Reflect on how you would feel if you found out that an individual made an important decision about their life because they thought that doing so was what you wanted rather than what they actually wanted.

What can you do to ensure that you do not let your views influence an individual's decision-making and choices?

It is important, firstly, that you do not make choices for the individual, nor let your own personal views influence their choices. Even if you

are asked what you would do, it is better not to say what you would do – even if you feel the choice the individual is making is not one you would make. Instead, you should be **committed** to supporting individuals to make their own choices by giving them the information they need, informing them of their options, and the risks involved.

Ensuring that your views do not interfere or influence individuals' choices is also important because doing so means that you can:

- show that you are supportive and respectful of individuals' rights (i.e. regarding choice, dignity, independence and delivering care or support with **compassion** – showing kindness and consideration)

- show that you are complying with your legal and organisational responsibilities as an adult care worker (i.e. providing care or support to individuals with courage (see page 276) using a person-centred way of working for safe and effective care)

- show that you are enabling individuals to have control and choice in their lives (this is a crucial aspect of person-centred care).

AC 5.4 Describe how to support an individual to question or challenge decisions concerning them that are made by others

Making your own choices in everyday life may also involve coming into conflict with others who may disagree with the decisions you make, or who you may want to question or challenge. For example, in relation to starting a new career or going to university or learning to drive. Doing so requires effective support from others who you trust and know you well, such as family and friends.

Similarly, individuals who have care or support needs may disagree with decisions made about them by others, such as by their GP, social worker or family member, and it is their right to be able to question or challenge any decisions made about them. Individuals may find this difficult to do because of:

- **their needs** – a learning difficulty may mean that the individual finds it difficult to communicate their views to others
- **their relationships** – an individual may feel they are being unkind if they disagree with a decision made by their older parent or anxious if they disagree with a decision made by the adult care worker providing them with care or support in case they withdraw the care or support they are providing
- **their support network** – an individual may feel isolated or not have anyone that they feel they can turn to when they want to question or challenge decisions about them made by others; they also may hold the view that 'others', such as adult care professionals, know best.

Individuals may also lack the confidence to challenge any decisions about them, or may feel that they do not have the knowledge or expertise to challenge such decisions. Supporting individuals to build their self-esteem is all part of providing person-centred care and being a good adult care worker.

It is important that you are aware of the barriers that may prevent or deter individuals from questioning or challenging decisions made about them so that you can support them effectively. Here are some ideas for how you can do so:

- **Encourage good communication** – for example, you should enable the individual to feel relaxed and trust you so that they can feel free to share their concerns. You can also encourage the individual to ask questions and share their views with you. You will need to be patient and be prepared to listen carefully and give individuals the time they need. You will also need to ensure that they have all the information they need so they are aware how they can challenge any decisions made about them.
- **Seek guidance** – for example, speaking to your manager or supervisor can be useful as they can provide additional support to both you and the individual.

6Cs C

Communication

How can you build a positive working relationship with the individuals you provide care or support to? This is crucial for ensuring that they feel relaxed, can trust you and share with you how they are feeling. This is important when you are supporting individuals to challenge any decisions made about them, especially if they feel reluctant to do so.

Research it

5.4 Support groups

Research the support groups that are available in your local area for supporting individuals with mental health needs to speak up for themselves. You will find your knowledge of the local area as well as the internet useful sources of information.

Provide a written account of your findings.

- **Support the individual to ask for a second opinion** – you can do this by supporting the individual to request a second opinion themselves or by you asking for a second opinion and speaking on the individual's behalf.
- **Support the individual to access support** – for example from other people who have been in similar situations so that they can support one another.
- **Support the individual to make a complaint** – support the individual to access the complaints procedure, understand it and then use it. It may be that the individual has made a complaint or challenged a decision in the past and this has not been dealt with well. This could deter the individual from challenging decisions and so it is important to reassure them that support is available and that their complaint will be dealt with respectfully.

Evidence opportunity

5.4 Supporting individuals to question or challenge decisions

Find the complaints procedure for the care setting where you work.

Describe how you can use this to support an individual with care or support needs to question or challenge a decision made about them.

LO5 Knowledge, skills, behaviours
Knowledge: why is it important to support individuals to make their own choices?
Do you know what making an informed choice means?
Do you know why it is important to support individuals' rights to make choices?
Do you know why it is important that your own views do not influence an individual's choices?
Do you know how you can support individuals to challenge any decisions made about them?
Did you know that you have just answered questions about individuals' rights?
Skills: how can you show that you are supporting an individual's right to make choices?
Do you know how you can support individuals to make informed choices?
Do you know how to carry out a risk assessment?
Did you know that you have just answered two questions about a few of the skills you need in relation to supporting individuals to make informed choices?
Behaviours: how can you show the personal qualities you have when supporting individuals' right to make choices?
Do you know how to build individuals' confidence when supporting individuals to challenge decisions made about them?
Do you know how to show kindness and respect when supporting individuals to consider decisions made about them?
Did you know that you have just answered two questions about a few of the essential behaviours that are expected of all adult care workers when supporting individuals' rights to make choices?

LO6 Be able to support the individual's well-being

Getting started

How would you describe yourself? What are your positives? For example, it may be your personality or your kind nature or your sense of humour. How would others describe you? What do they say are your positives? Do you agree with what others say about you? Why? How can what others say about you impact on how good you feel about yourself? Can you think of an example when this happened? As well as what others say about you what other things affect how you feel about yourself? For example, how can your physical health affect how you feel emotionally? How can your emotional health affect your physical health? For example, if you feel unwell does this make you feel more positive or negative? Why?

AC 6.1 Explain how an individual's identity and self-esteem are linked with well-being

Identity

Your individual identity is personal to you and includes the different aspects that make you unique. This can include your gender, your background, your values, your personality, your qualities, your wishes, your views.

We build up our own personal identity through our experiences in life, through both childhood and adulthood. The types of experiences we have will affect what we think about ourselves. For example, if as children we experienced making friends at school as something enjoyable, this will in turn mean that we will feel good about ourselves when meeting new people and making new friends. Making new friends will mean that we will have others to share our lives and experiences with; this in turn will make us feel more confident about ourselves and means we will have a positive view about ourselves, that we are liked by others, that we are needed by others and are part of others' lives. Our friends will reflect back to us who we are and it is through others, such as our friends, that we develop high self-esteem.

Self-esteem

Your self-esteem is what you think and feel about yourself, i.e. this will very much depend on how you value yourself as well as how others close to you think and feel about you too. When others hold you in high regard and praise you then it is likely that you will feel the same about yourself too. When others devalue you however, you are not likely to feel very positive about yourself or your abilities.

Well-being

Your **well-being** refers to your health and whether you feel in good health and happy overall in yourself. It refers to:

- **physical well-being**, for example, living a life free from pain or one where your physical health does not affect your quality of life mentally, e.g. your attitude to life
- **emotional well-being**, i.e. how you feel about life
- **social well-being**, for example, the relationships you have
- **cultural well-being**, for example, your sense of belonging to a group that shares your beliefs
- **spiritual well-being,** i.e. your human spirit
- **intellectual well-being**, for example, your thought processes
- **economic well-being**, for example, your finances, or your housing situation.

Our well-being is also dependent on our identity and self-esteem. For example, if an individual lives alone and feels isolated from family and friends, they will feel low in mood and may feel that they are worthless because they are not part of anyone else's life. This in turn may lead to the individual developing depression that could affect their physical health too; their levels of physical activity, for example, may drop if they do not feel able to get out of bed and do what they used to do. This can lead to the onset of medical conditions such as obesity and pneumonia.

By contrast, if an individual lives alone and enjoys their independence while being supported by family, friends, neighbours or an advocate, then they are more likely to retain their emotional and physical health and well-being because they will feel valued and have purpose in their life. Communications and interactions with others will also be stimulating and motivating and will enable individuals to maintain their current well-being.

Reflect on it

6.1 Self-esteem

Reflect on an occasion when someone praised you for something you had done well. How did this make you feel about yourself? How did this make you feel towards this person?

Now reflect on an occasion when someone devalued you. How did this make you feel about yourself? How did this make you feel towards others?

To summarise, your identity, self-esteem and well-being are all interrelated and one can affect the other. For example:

- A strong sense of identity can promote high self-esteem and high self-esteem can in turn make you value yourself and feel good about who you are. A good sense of identity and high self-esteem can in turn promote good well-being because both will impact positively on different aspects of your health. In addition, if you have good mental and physical health for example, this in turn will positively impact on how you feel about yourself (self-esteem) and who you are (identity).

- Not knowing or being unsure about your own identity can lead to low self-esteem which can in turn make you feel unworthy. A lack of identity and low self-esteem can in turn promote ill-being because both will impact negatively on different aspects of your health. For example, you may find it difficult to meet people (social health) which can in turn lead to isolation (mental health). Poor social and mental health will impact negatively on how you feel about yourself (self-esteem) and who you are (identity).

In your role, you will need to think about how the individual's identity and self-esteem affect their well-being.

Key term

Well-being is a concept that refers to different aspects of an individual's good health, such as their physical, mental, emotional, social, cultural, spiritual, intellectual and economic health.

Dos and don'ts for promoting an individual's identity and self-esteem	
Do	Value each individual, their identity and their unique qualities. This will help individuals to feel like a valued member.
Do	Encourage active participation in the setting, an individual's community and areas that they want to take part in. This will increase their self-esteem, allowing them to feel they have real contributions to make.
Do	Find out as much as you can about the individual and their past experiences to have a better understanding of how those experiences may have made them the person they are. Perhaps they have experienced a particularly traumatic or stressful event such as a miscarriage, abuse or bereavement.
Do	Support them or seek specialist support for them to help them to deal with such experiences. This is all part of person-centred care.
Don't	Ignore situations where you are worried that someone else may be the cause of such distress; you should also report this to your manager. Also, don't ignore situations where you are particularly worried about an individual's well-being, especially if they are showing signs of distress. You should report these to your manager as this could lead to more serious situations such as self-harm.
Don't	Highlight an individual's flaws, because that may lower their self-esteem and sense of self-worth.
Don't	Highlight all the things an individual cannot do because of a disability, for example. Instead, discuss all the things they can do, and how they can overcome barriers.

Evidence opportunity

6.1 Identity, self-esteem, well-being

Write down three different aspects of your health that are important to you and your well-being. For each one explain how they affect a) your identity and b) your self-esteem.

1 Then write down and explain how your identity and your self-esteem affect each of the three aspects of your health that are important to your well-being.

2 Discuss your findings with your assessor.

AC 6.2 Describe attitudes and approaches that are likely to promote an individual's well-being

Attitude, approaches and well-being

You are an integral part of an individual's well-being because the way you think, behave and practise in your work role when providing care or support will affect an individual's identity, self-esteem and overall health.

Your attitudes refer to your thoughts and behaviours and as an adult care worker you need to ensure that your attitudes are positive and promote an individual's well-being because doing so will mean that the individual will:

- feel valued
- feel respected
- build a good working relationship with you
- trust you.

Positive attitudes include being:

- kind
- caring
- considerate
- person-centred
- respectful.

As we discussed in AC 6.1, valuing individuals and helping to promote their well-being by increasing their self-esteem are all part of a positive attitude. Positivity can be infectious and if you have a positive attitude towards your work and the individuals you care for, this can impact positively on them, helping them to see the 'up' side and remain positive!

> **Reflect on it**
>
> **6.2** Attitudes
>
> Reflect on the top three attitudes you show when providing care or support to individuals. You could ask your manager and your work colleagues for their views too – did they say you had the same top three attitudes that you thought you had? What have you learned about yourself?
>
> For each attitude reflect on how you think this influenced the individuals you were providing care or support to.

All of this can increase a sense of well-being in the individual, impacting their health and outlook.

Your approaches refer to the way you work and the skills you demonstrate when providing care or support. You need to ensure that you can demonstrate good working approaches that promote an individual's well-being.

Approaches that you as an adult care worker can use to promote individuals' well-being can include the following:

- **Enabling** – by showing your support of individual's choices and decisions and empowering individuals to do as much for themselves as they are able to.
- **Focused** – by working in a person-centred way, the focus is maintained on the individual, their strengths, abilities, wishes and preferences.
- **Positive** – by showing your support of individuals' views and suggestions and using good communication.

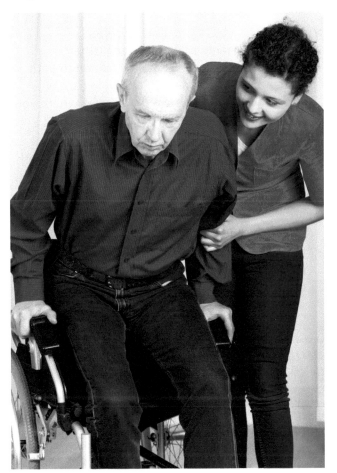

Figure 8.9 Have you got what it takes?

- **Reflective** – by taking time to reflect on achievements and areas for further improvement – this can be in relation to both you and the individuals you provide care or support to; taking time out to review where you are and how to move forward is important.
- **Challenging** – by ensuring individuals are working to their full capacity and provided with opportunities to take risks and further develop.
- **Safe** – by ensuring individuals' safety is maintained while promoting their rights and supporting them to achieve what they want to do.
- **Partnership working** – by encouraging individuals to be 'active partners' in their care or support.

AC 6.3 Support an individual in a way that promotes a sense of identity and self-esteem

For this assessment criterion you will be observed demonstrating how to support an individual in a way that promotes a sense of identity and self-esteem.

Your attitudes and approaches as an adult care worker also include providing support to an individual that promotes their sense of identity and self-esteem. You may find it useful to recap on the meanings of these two concepts that we explored in AC 6.1.

You can support an individual in a way that promotes their sense of identity and self-esteem in the following ways.

- **Spending time getting to know who they are as a person** – their needs, values, preferences. This will show the individual that you are taking a genuine interest in them.
- **Supporting the individual to find out about their history** – their culture, background, beliefs, practices relating to for example nutrition, religion, dress. Doing so means that you will be reflecting back to the individual who they are and why they should feel proud of who they are.
- **Interacting with the individual in a positive way** – by using positive language when speaking, using open body language when interacting, reinforcing good ideas and giving praise. Support the individual to take risks, make mistakes (and learn from them) and promote the individual's rights, i.e. to dignity, privacy, independence.

Evidence opportunity

6.2, 6.3 Promoting well-being, identity and self-esteem

Show how you provide support, with one aspect of their life, to an individual who has care or support needs. For example, this may be in relation to going out, communicating with others or completing household tasks. This can be observed directly by your assessor or through a witness testimony by your manager.

Ensure that you show how you promote the individual's sense of well-being, identity and self-esteem.

It is important, however, to think about the things discussed in Unit 209 on equality and diversity, and remember that when you are promoting identity and trying to find out as much as possible about individuals, that you do not stereotype people based on their race, gender or class, for example. This is counter-productive in promoting identity, and an environment that promotes well-being. Instead, you should learn to see individuals as individuals, ones that may share similar traits, values and beliefs as others, but are unique beings with their own needs.

AC 6.4 Demonstrate ways to contribute to an environment that promotes well-being

For this assessment criterion you will be observed demonstrating different ways of contributing to an environment that promotes well-being.

Supporting individuals' well-being is also dependent on ensuring that the environment around them also promotes their well-being. This includes the following:

- physical environment – rooms in a care setting, layout in a health service, such as a GP surgery, access to the garden, the individual's personal belongings

Reflect on it

6.4 Physical and social environment

Reflect on the differences there are between the physical and social environment. Reflect on the aspects that are important to you in terms of physical and social environments and the reasons why.

- social environment – the atmosphere in a care setting or service, the quality of the working relationships in a service.

How can you ensure that the physical environment promotes an individual's well-being?

- Furniture and furnishings – ensuring furniture and furnishings are clean and attractive can make individuals feel good. Ensuring furniture is maintained and not broken can promote individuals' safety and therefore well-being.
- Personal belongings – ensuring individuals' personal belongings are placed in individuals' rooms and other areas in a care setting will make individuals feel at home and will help to promote a sense of well-being.
- Temperature – ensuring rooms and environments are not too hot or too cold; both have the potential to make individuals feel uncomfortable. Checking with individuals if the temperature is comfortable will make them feel comfortable and promote their well-being.

How can you ensure that the social environment promotes an individual's well-being?

- Items and pictures – ensuring rooms contain items and pictures that are representative of individuals' diverse backgrounds (i.e. in relation to their age, gender and cultures) will ensure that individuals feel a sense of belonging, and therefore can promote well-being.

Research it

6.4 Adapting physical and social environments

Research how the physical and social environment can be adapted to meet the needs of an individual who has dementia. Discuss your findings with a colleague.

You may find the Alzheimer's Society weblink below a useful source of information:

www.alzheimers.org.uk/info/20114/publications_about_caring_for_a_person_with_dementia/957/alzheimers_society_guide_to_the_dementia_care_environment

Evidence opportunity

6.4 Contributing to an environment that promotes well-being

Identify an individual who has care or support needs; this may be an individual with learning or physical difficulties, hearing or sight loss, dementia or a heart condition. Write a case study listing the individual's needs and the different ways that you can contribute to an environment that promotes the individual's well-being.

Remember that you cannot include personal details about individuals in your portfolio.

- Management of a care setting or service – an environment that is managed well and where agreed ways of working are complied with will be less likely to place individuals in danger or at risk of harm or abuse and so will promote feelings of security amongst individuals and in turn a good sense of well-being.

- Atmosphere – an atmosphere that is welcoming and inviting will promote feelings of well-being. A stimulating atmosphere will ensure individuals' needs are met. For example, organising the provision for activities or the availability of adult care workers with special areas of expertise. In turn, this will promote a sense of well-being as the individual will feel valued.

As well as the above, you will need to make sure that the way you work also contributes to an environment that promotes well-being, one where the individual is at the centre. This might mean that your policies and procedures need to be adjusted to place emphasis on finding out about the needs and requirements of individuals that are specific to them, such as cultural or religious needs. Such needs will affect, for example, individuals' dietary requirements, clothing, interactions with different genders, and personal care requirements, and so being understanding and sympathetic to these is crucial. Such considerations will also ensure that you promote the well-being of individuals.

AC 6.5 Recognise and respond to changes in physical and mental health

You will only be able to continue to promote an individual's well-being if you are able to identify any changes that may arise in their physical or mental health and know the actions to take when these arise. Knowing the individuals you provide care or support to well and being observant about changes that happen, however small, are two essential skills that you as an adult care worker will require when promoting an individual's well-being.

It is important to remember that every individual is unique and therefore their experiences of changes to physical and mental health will vary. It is important to recognise any changes that are unusual for the individual. Remember that no two individuals are the same.

Recognising changes to physical health

Changes to physical health include:

- weight – loss of weight, increase in weight
- mobility – becoming frail, mobility lessening or becoming more difficult
- breathing – difficulty with breathing, rapid breathing, shallow breathing
- physical appearance – looking unwell, pale, clammy

- pain – verbally expressing pain in different areas in the body, non-verbally holding or pointing to different areas in the body, for example stomach, arm, back.

Recognising changes to mental health

Changes to mental health include:

- mood changes – mood swings, low in mood, elation
- stress – anxiety and stress levels may increase
- sleep – disturbances in sleep, too much or not at all
- suicide and self-harm – thoughts and/or attempts
- eating – overeating or not eating
- personality changes – becoming obsessive, withdrawn, over-enthusiastic
- hearing and seeing changes – hearing voices, seeing things that aren't there.

Responding to changes in physical and mental health

All changes in individuals' physical and mental health that you notice must be taken seriously and the appropriate action taken. If you are ever in any doubt report any changes you notice to your manager and always record your observations however insignificant you think they may be so that the individual can receive the help they need to restore their well-being. Your manager may then decide to take further action depending on the severity of the physical and mental health changes. They may, for example, administer treatment, book an appointment with the GP,

Reflect on it

6.5 Changes in your physical and mental health

Reflect on any changes you have ever experienced to your physical or mental health. What were they? How did they make you feel? How would you have felt if these were ignored?

contact the Community Psychiatric Nurse, call for an ambulance.

In addition to these actions, you could also respond by doing the following:

- weight – monitor weight loss and increase by keeping records of the individual's weight, the individual's food and fluid intake
- mobility – monitor and observe the difficulties the individual is having, record the tasks that the individual is no longer able to do independently
- breathing – monitor individuals' breathing rates
- physical appearance – observe the individual's physical appearance; ask the individual how they feel
- pain – ask the individual to show you where it hurts or how they feel
- mood changes – monitor whether there is a pattern to when these occur
- stress – monitor when stress and anxiety levels rise and fall, talk to the individual to find out how they are feeling
- sleep – ensure the environment is comfortable for the individual (you will find it useful to recap on your learning for AC 6.4)
- suicide and self-harm – reassure the individual, observe and monitor the individual
- eating – monitor the individual's eating habits
- personality changes – monitor whether there is a pattern to when these occur
- hearing and seeing changes – observe the individual for when these may be occurring, listen to what the individual is saying and expressing, communicating through their facial expressions or body language.

Not responding to changes to physical and mental health is not an option because left untreated one could affect the other and the individual's overall sense of well-being would also be negatively impacted on. It would also be useful to refer to Unit 201, Safeguarding and protection in care settings, AC 2.1 for information on signs and symptoms of abuse.

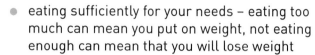

AC 6.6 Explain the importance of good nutrition and hydration

Good nutrition and hydration are crucial for the health and well-being of individuals who have care or support needs. Have you ever had a busy day where you didn't have time to eat or drink properly? Do you remember how this made you feel? Did it make you feel tired, irritable, low in mood? Well, imagine being an individual with care or support needs feeling the same way but being unable to express how you feel.

What does good nutrition look like?

Good nutrition means eating healthily and in a balanced way:

- eating sufficiently for your needs – eating too much can mean you put on weight, not eating enough can mean that you will lose weight
- eating as wide a range of foods as possible so that your body is provided with all the nutrients it needs to work well
- eating lots of fruit and vegetables that are a very good source of vitamins
- eating more fish that contains many vitamins and minerals that are essential for your body
- cutting down on eating salty and fatty foods to avoid putting on weight and conditions such as heart disease
- cutting down on sugary foods to avoid putting on weight, low and high mood swings, tooth decay.

You will need to make sure that you provide the correct level of care and support to meet individuals' nutritional needs. This can mean providing them with eating aids (adapted plates and cutlery) and checking what their dietary requirements are (for example, they may be diabetic, or they may require gluten free, vegetarian, vegan, halal or kosher food). This also means checking whether they have any allergies. You can provide dietary sheets for this.

What does good hydration look like?

Good hydration means drinking healthily and in a balanced way. Consider:

- drinking fluids, such as water and milk – avoiding drinking too many sugary and fizzy drinks that can lead to tooth decay, caffeine-based drinks that can lead to putting on weight and sleep disturbances
- drinking enough and regularly (the UK Government recommends 6–8 glasses every day)
- avoid drinking before meals as this can make you feel bloated and can reduce your appetite.

You will need to make sure that you provide the correct level of care and support to meet individuals' hydration needs. This will mean providing them with drinking aids (for example, adapted cups and straws) and fluid sheets to record the amount and types of fluids they are drinking. Again, you will need to find out which fluids individuals can or cannot drink.

Research it

6.6 Supporting nutrition and hydration

Research the range of aids available to help individuals with care or support needs with their eating and drinking. Produce a poster with your findings.

You will find the link to the 'Living Made Easy' website useful:

www.livingmadeeasy.org.uk/house%20 and%20home/eating-and-drinking-1477/

Why are good nutrition and hydration important?

Good nutrition and hydration are important because:

- they ensure that the individual's body is getting all the nutrients and fluid it needs to work in a healthy way. This can prevent the individual from becoming unwell, developing illnesses, becoming malnourished or dehydrated
- they can improve an individual's health i.e., if they are recovering from an illness or an operation, for example
- they can maintain an individual's weight (at a healthy level)
- good physical health can lead to good mental health (promote an individual's well-being).

Case study 6.5, 6.6 will provide you with further guidance and information about the positive difference that good nutrition and hydration can make to the life of an individual with care or support needs.

Case study

6.5, 6.6 Good nutrition and hydration

Sam works as a care worker providing care and support to older people living in a residential care home. Mavis is a new resident who has up until two weeks ago been living on her own at home. When Mavis arrived at the care home she was very underweight, looked frail and had skin that easily bruised and was very sensitive, almost tissue-like in appearance.

Sam began by finding out about Mavis's favourite foods and drinks, when she liked to eat them and where. Day by day, Sam and Mavis agreed to work together to slowly introduce different foods and drinks to Mavis so that not only was

she eating and drinking foods and drinks she enjoyed but was also being given the opportunity to try new and different foods.

As a result, Mavis is steadily putting on weight, is enjoying meal times again and is finding that she has more energy and is slowly becoming more active again. The other noticeable change in Mavis is that she looks healthier, her skin no longer bruises easily and she feels good in herself.

Discussion points

1 Examples of person-centred ways of working that are used by Sam.
2 The positive effects of good nutrition and hydration on Mavis's well-being.

Evidence opportunity

6.6 Importance of good nutrition and hydration

Develop a profile of an individual who has care or support needs. Provide examples of the different ways you, as an adult care worker, support

the individual with good nutrition and hydration. Explain the importance of doing so. You could also include the negative effects of not doing so.

LO6 Knowledge, skills, behaviours
Knowledge: what is well-being?
Do you know the meaning of identity and self-esteem?
Do you know the links between identity, self-esteem and well-being?
Do you know why good nutrition and hydration are important?
Did you know that you have just answered three questions about what well-being is?
Skills: how can you show that you can support an individual's well-being?
Do you know how to adapt the environment to promote well-being?
Do you know how to recognise and respond to changes in individuals?
Did you know that you have just answered two questions about a few of the skills you have in relation to supporting an individual's well-being?
Behaviours: how can you show the personal qualities you have when supporting individual's well-being?
Do you know the attitudes that promote individuals' well-being?
Do you know the approaches that promote individuals' well-being?
Did you know that you have just answered two questions about a few of the essential behaviours that are expected of all adult care workers when supporting individuals' well-being?

Suggestions for using the activities

This table summarises all the activities in the unit that are relevant to each assessment criterion.

Here, we also suggest other, different methods that you may want to use to present your knowledge and skills by using the activities.

These are just suggestions, and you should refer to the Introduction section at the start of the book, and more importantly the City & Guilds specification, and your assessor, who will be able to provide more guidance on how you can evidence your knowledge and skills.

When you need to be observed during your assessment, this can be done by your assessor, or your manager can provide a witness testimony.

Assessment criteria and accompanying activities	Suggested methods to show your knowledge/skills
LO1 Understand person-centred approaches for care and support	
LO2 Be able to work in a person-centred way	
LO5 Be able to support the individual's right to make choices	
1.1 Research it (page 277)	Provide a written account detailing your findings.
1.1, 1.2, 1.4 Reflect on it (page 282)	Answer the questions in the activity and write a reflective account.
1.1 Evidence opportunity (page 277)	Write down two care and support tasks you carry out on a day-to-day basis in the care setting where you work. For each task, identify two person-centred values that you apply and describe how you do this. Or you could write a personal statement about what person-centred values are and why they are relevant to your job role in the care setting where you work.
1.2 Research it (page 278)	Produce a written account of your findings. Or you could explain what you found out to your assessor.
1.1, 1.2, 1.4 Reflect on it (page 282)	As mentioned above, answer the questions in the activity and write a reflective account.

→

Suggestions for using the activities	
1.1, 1.2 Evidence opportunity (page 279)	Write down how you would explain what person-centred values are to a new member of staff, and think about the things flagged in the activity.
1.2, 2.2 Case study (page 287)	Or you could provide a written account discussing the different ways that you embed person-centred values in your day-to-day working practices. Remember to explain why this is important, as well as the consequences of not doing so.
	The case study will help you to think about working in ways that embed person-centred values.
1.3, 5.2 Evidence opportunity (page 280)	Once you have found out about the 'risk-decision' policy and practice in your care setting, summarise the key points that ensure best practice in your care setting when supporting individuals to take risks. Address the points in the activity.
1.3, 5.2 Reflective exemplar (page 303)	Or you could write a reflective account of an occasion you supported an individual in the care setting where you work to take a risk. Explain how you did this and the benefits of doing so. Explain the reasons why risk-taking is part of a person-centred approach.
	The reflective exemplar will help you think about why risk-taking can be part of a person-centred approach.
1.1, 1.2, 1.4 Reflect on it (page 282)	As mentioned above, answer the questions in the activity and write a reflective account.
1.4 Evidence opportunity (page 282)	Address the points in the activity and write up notes to evidence your discussion. This discussion might be observed by your assessor or could be a witness testimony account.
	You could also write an account of how you have used an individual's care plan in your day-to-day working practices. Explain how this has been part of working in a person-centred way. You could also show your work product evidence of an individual's care plan that you contributed to and helped to develop. Remember that this holds personal information that does not belong to you, so make sure that you have the individual's and your manager's permission to access it and that you do so in private. You must also pay strict attention to confidentiality.
LO2 Be able to work in a person-centred way	
LO1 Understand person-centred approaches for care and support	
2.1 Reflect on it (page 284)	Write a reflective account addressing the points in the activity.
2.1 Evidence opportunity (page 285)	Develop a written plan as instructed in the activity, and answer the questions in the activity.
	You must also make arrangements for your work practices to be observed so that you can show how you use different ways to find out about the history, preferences, wishes and needs of an individual. You could also show work product evidence, or other relevant records or reports, to support your observation.
2.1, 2.2 Reflect on it (page 286)	Write a reflective account addressing the points in the activity.
2.2 Research it (page 287)	Produce a poster with your findings. Or you could provide a written account detailing your findings.
2.2 Research it (page 287)	Write notes detailing your findings.

→

Suggestions for using the activities	
1.2, 2.2 Evidence opportunity (page 288) 1.2, 2.2 Case study (page 287)	Show the diary that you have kept for a week, detailing the different work tasks you have completed with individuals, to your assessor as instructed in the activity. You must make arrangements for your work practices to be observed so that you can show how you apply person-centred values in your day-to-day work practice and how you take into account the history, preferences, wishes and needs of an individual. You could also show work product evidence or other relevant records or reports to support your observation. The case study will help you to think about applying person-centred values in day-to-day working and taking into account the history, preferences, wishes and needs of the individual.
LO3 Be able to establish consent when providing care or support	
LO1 Understand person-centred approaches for care and support	
3.1 Reflect on it (page 289)	Discuss this with a colleague and write a short account detailing your thoughts.
3.1 Research it (page 290)	Discuss your findings with a colleague and write a short account detailing them.
3.1 Evidence opportunity (page 290)	Develop a case study as instructed in the activity. Or you could write a personal statement that explains the importance of establishing consent when providing care or support. You must detail the reasons why it is important and you could also include the consequences of not doing so for you, the individuals you support and the care setting where you work.
3.2 Research it (page 291)	Research the Health and Social Care Act 2008 (Regulated Activities) Regulations 2014: Regulation 1. Discuss your findings with a colleague and make notes based on your discussion.
3.2 Reflect on it (page 292)	Write a reflective account.
3.2, 1.4 Evidence opportunity (page 292)	Provide a written account addressing the points in the activity. You must make arrangements for your work practices to be observed so that you can show how you establish consent for an activity or action.
3.1, 3.3 Reflect on it (page 292)	Write some notes detailing your thoughts.
3.3 Evidence opportunity (page 293) 3.1, 3.2, 3.3 Case study (page 293)	Discuss what steps you must take if you are unable to establish consent with an individual in the care setting where you work. Be prepared to explain why each step is necessary. You could use your work setting's policy/procedures/agreed ways of working for establishing consent as the basis of your discussion. Produce a step-by-step diagram that shows the steps you or your work colleague should take if this situation arose again, and address the points in the activity. The case study will inform your understanding of issues around 'consent' in this learning outcome.

→

Suggestions for using the activities	
LO4 Be able to encourage active participation	
4.1 Reflect on it (page 295)	Write a reflective account addressing the points in the activity.
4.1 Evidence opportunity (page 296)	You could discuss with your assessor how you would explain to a member of staff who is new to care how active participation benefits an individual, as instructed in the activity.
	You could also write a reflective account of your experience of how active participation benefits an individual. Include a range of benefits in your reflection. You could also collect a witness testimony to support your reflective account, and work product evidence such as daily records you have completed or the contributions you have made to an individual's care plan.
4.2 Evidence opportunity (page 297)	Discuss with a colleague the range of possible barriers to encouraging active participation for individuals in the care setting where you work.
	Develop a profile of an individual who has care or support needs. Write down what their unique needs are and address the points in the activity.
4.2 Reflect on it (page 297)	Write a reflective account addressing the points in the activity.
4.3 Reflect on it (page 298)	Write a short account addressing the points in the activity.
4.3 Research it (page 298)	Produce an information handout with your findings.
4.3 Evidence opportunity (page 299)	Produce an information handout as instructed in the activity.
	You must make arrangements for your work practices to be observed so that you can show different ways that you reduce the barriers that can exist for individuals and encourage active participation. You could also collect a witness testimony from your manager to show your skills and support your observation.
LO5 Be able to support the individual's right to make choices	
LO1 Understand person-centred approaches for care and support	
5.1 Research it (page 301)	Produce a written account detailing your findings and address the points in the activity.
5.1 Reflect on it (page 301)	Write a short reflective account.
5.1 Evidence opportunity (page 301)	Complete the activity. Your assessor might observe you supporting the individual directly or you could get a witness testimony from your manager. You must make arrangements for your work practices to be observed so that you can show how to support an individual to make informed choices.
5.2 Research it (page 302)	Produce an information leaflet with your findings. Alternatively you could write notes detailing your findings.
5.2 Evidence opportunity (page 302) 1.3, 5.2 Reflective exemplar (page 303)	Develop a risk assessment for an activity and discuss this with your assessor.
	You must make arrangements for your work practices to be observed so that you can show you can use agreed risk assessment processes to support individuals' rights to make choices. You could also collect a witness testimony from your manager to show your skills and support your observation.
	The reflective exemplar will help you to understand how risk assessment processes can support individuals' rights to make choices.
5.3 Reflect on it (page 303)	Write a short reflective account.

→

Suggestions for using the activities	
5.3 Evidence opportunity (page 304)	Provide a written account detailing the answers to the questions. Or you could write an account explaining the reasons why a worker's personal views should not influence an individual's choices. Include a range of reasons why this is important and also the consequences of not doing so.
5.4 Reflect on it (page 304)	Write a short reflective account.
5.4 Research it (page 305)	Provide a written account of your findings.
5.4 Evidence opportunity (page 306)	Write a reflection or produce a case study that describes how to support an individual to question or challenge decisions concerning them that are made by others.
	Your case study or reflection must include examples of the different methods you can use to support an individual, and must also make clear who made the decisions concerning them.
LO6 Be able to support the individual's well-being	
6.1 Reflect on it (page 307)	Write a reflective account.
6.1 Evidence opportunity (page 308)	Write down three different aspects of your health that are important to you and your wellbeing. For each one, explain how they affect (a) your identity and (b) your self-esteem. Address the points in the activity.
	Or you could write a personal statement about the meanings and links between the following: identity, self-esteem and well-being. Include examples of all three.
6.2 Reflect on it (page 309)	Write a reflective account.
6.2 Research it (page 310)	Produce a written account detailing your findings.
6.2 Evidence opportunity (page 310)	Produce a job profile as instructed in the activity.
	You could also discuss the range of attitudes and approaches that are likely to promote an individual's well-being with a colleague and write up notes detailing your discussion.
6.3 Research it (page 310)	Produce an information handout with your findings.
6.3 Reflect on it (page 310)	Think about the points, discuss with a colleague and write brief notes.
6.2, 6.3 Evidence opportunity (page 311)	Complete the activity. You must make arrangements for your work practices to be observed so that you can show how you support an individual in a way that promotes a sense of identity and self-esteem.
	Remember to think about what you say, how you express it, how you behave. You could also collect a witness testimony from your manager to show your skills and support your observation.
6.4 Reflect on it (page 311)	Write brief notes to document your thoughts.
6.4 Research it (page 312)	Discuss your findings with a colleague and write notes to document your findings.
6.4 Evidence opportunity (page 312)	Write a case study as instructed.
	You must make arrangements for your work practices to be observed so that you can show how to contribute in different ways to an environment that promotes well-being.
	You could also collect a witness testimony from your manager to show your skills and support your observation.

→

Suggestions for using the activities

6.5 Reflect on it (page 313)	Write brief notes to document your thoughts.
6.5 Evidence opportunity (page 314)	Produce a written account.
6.5, 6.6 Case study (page 315)	You must make arrangements for your work practices to be observed so that you can show how you can recognise and respond to changes in individuals' physical and mental health. If an opportunity to do so does not arise naturally, then you could also collect a witness testimony to show your skills on an occasion when it did occur.
	The case study will help you to think about changes in physical and mental health.
6.6 Reflect on it (page 314)	Write a reflective account.
6.6 Research it (page 315)	Produce a poster with your findings.
6.6 Evidence opportunity (page 315)	Develop a profile as instructed in the activity. Or you could write a personal statement or a reflective account that explains the importance of good nutrition and hydration. Remember to explain what good nutrition and hydration mean and the reasons why both are important to individuals' well-being.
6.5, 6.6 Case study (page 315)	The case study will help you to think about the importance of good nutrition and hydration.

Legislation

Relevant Act	It states that:
Data Protection Act 1998	information and data must be processed fairly, lawfully, used only for the purpose it was intended to be used for, be adequate, relevant, accurate and up to date and held for no longer than is necessary. It established how personal information must be recorded, used, stored and shared to ensure the individual's rights are protected and the security of their personal information is maintained.
General Data Protection Regulation (GDPR) 2018	Also see Unit 206 for more information on the GDPR 2018.
Human Rights Act 1998	everyone in the UK is entitled to the same rights and freedoms. This includes individuals who have care and support needs. The Act supports individuals to have the right to take risks and to have their choices and decisions respected.
Management of Health and Safety at Work Regulations 1999	it is a legal requirement for risks in work settings including care settings to be managed safely and for risk assessments to be carried out, documented, reviewed and updated.
Mental Capacity Act 2005	this Act supports person-centred working by supporting individuals' rights to make their own decisions; this includes being provided with the necessary support to do so. The Act also protects the rights of individuals who lack capacity by providing guidance on who can make decisions about them and how to plan ahead for this if it arises in the future.
Care Act 2014	the Act supports individuals' rights to make informed decisions about their care and support and promotes a person-centred approach to care planning where adult care workers can support individuals to develop their care plans.
	It also defines the concept of well-being and how adult care workers can promote individuals' well-being. Also see the Government publications: • Personalised Health and Care 2020, which sets out how technology and data can be used to improve health and the way health and social care services are delivered. • The Adult Social Care Outcomes Framework Handbook of Definitions, which measures how well care and support services achieve the outcomes that are the most important to people.

Legislation	
Relevant Act	**It states that:**
Health and Social Care Act 2008 (Regulated Activities) Regulations 2014	the Act supports the rights of individuals and their representatives to be involved in the planning, provision and review of their care and support.
	Regulation 11 requires that consent is established before any care or treatment is provided to individuals. It also requires the person who obtains the consent from the individual to have the necessary knowledge and understanding of the care and/or treatment that they are asking consent for.
	Regulation 14 requires that individuals' nutrition and hydration needs are assessed, supported and met and that their preferences are also taken into account.

Resources for further reading and research

Books

Baker, C. (2014) *Developing Excellent Care for People Living with Dementia in Care Homes*, University of Bradford Dementia Good Practice Guides, Jessica Kingsley Publishers

Ferreiro Peteiro, M. (2014) *Level 2 Health and Social Care Diploma Evidence Guide*, Hodder Education

Storlie, T.A. (2015) *Person-Centred Communication with Older Adults: The Professional Provider's Guide*, Academic Press

Booklets

Health and Safety Executive (2014) 'Health and Safety in Care Homes', (HSG220 – 2nd edition), Health and Safety Executive (HSE)

Weblinks

www.alzheimers.org.uk Alzheimer's Society – information and guidance about person-centred care and support to individuals who have dementia, including ways to adapt the environment

www.cqc.org.uk Care Quality Commission (CQC) – useful guidance about the requirements for care settings to work in person-centred ways and establish consent

www.gov.uk The UK Government's website for information about current legislation including the Care Act 2014, the Mental Capacity Act 2005, the Management of Health and Safety at Work Regulations 1999

www.hse.gov.uk The Health and Safety Executive's website for information about managing risks in care settings

www.mind.org.uk Mind – resources and information about the Mental Capacity Act 2005, including useful terms

www.nutrition.org.uk British Nutrition Foundation – information, resources and guidance about living healthily, eating and drinking healthily

www.scie.org.uk Social Care Institute for Excellence (SCIE) – resources and information about the Care Act 2014 in relation to the well-being concept

www.skillsforcare.org.uk Skills for Care – resources and information on the Care Act 2014

Health, safety and well-being in care settings (210)

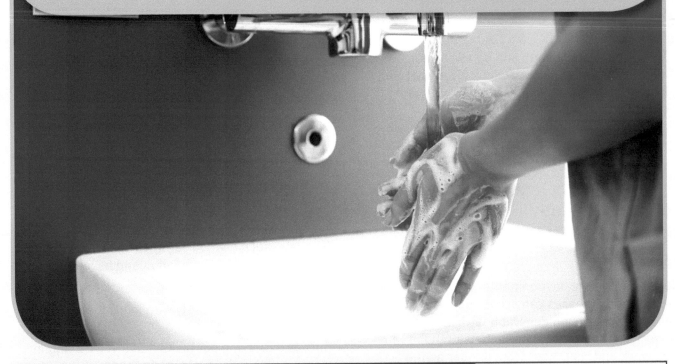

About this unit

Credit value: 4
Guided learning hours: 33

Health, safety and well-being in care settings is everyone's responsibility and promoting it on a day-to-day basis is both interesting and challenging. Health and safety is more than just accident prevention and assessing risks; it involves ensuring care settings are safe environments where individuals feel at home and workers enjoy coming to work.

In this unit you learn about the various aspects that are involved in making sure the environment you work in is a safe one. You will also find out about the various aspects that are involved in making sure that you keep yourself, the individuals you work with and others safe.

Learning outcomes

LO1: Understand your responsibilities and the responsibilities of others, relating to health and safety in the work setting

LO2: Understand the use of risk assessments in relation to health and safety

LO3: Understand procedures for responding to accidents and sudden illness

LO4: Be able to reduce the spread of infection

LO5: Be able to move and handle equipment and objects safely

LO6: Know how to handle hazardous substances and materials

LO7: Understand how to promote fire safety in the work setting

LO8: Be able to implement security measures in the work setting

LO9: Know how to manage stress

LO1 Understand your responsibilities and the responsibilities of others, relating to health and safety in the work setting

AC 1.1 Identify legislation relating to general health and safety in a care work setting

Legislation

Care settings are environments where accidents, injuries and illnesses can occur and so knowing about and practising general **health and safety** at work is important for protecting all those who live, work and visit these from danger as the statistics below show:

- 1.3 million workers were suffering from a work-related illness (new or long standing) in 2015/16
- 0.5 million workers were suffering from work-related **musculoskeletal disorders** (new or longstanding) in 2015/16
- 0.5 million workers were suffering from work-related stress, depression or anxiety (new or longstanding) in 2015/16.

Health and Safety Executive (2016) 'Health and safety at work: Summary statistics for Great Britain 2016'

With many more individuals living in their own homes, you may be providing care to individuals on your own and so it is very important that you are aware of how to maintain your own health and

safety as well as that of individuals and others who may visit their home while you are there.

In care settings, individuals may be more likely to have accidents, sustain injuries and develop illnesses because they may, for example, have:

- difficulties when walking or moving that may result in them slipping and tripping
- vision loss that may result in them having falls
- weak immune systems due to health conditions that may result in them becoming ill.

Adult care workers and others who visit individuals, such as their families and friends, may also be more likely to fall ill and have accidents because:

- they are working closely with individuals who may be unwell
- they are carrying out tasks that involve being in contact with individuals' **body fluids**
- they are carrying out tasks that may be complex, for example using a hoist to move individuals from one position to another
- the environment may generally pose risks and hazards to everyone if it is not maintained.

 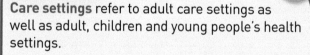

Did you know that the Health and Safety Executive (HSE) is the **regulator** for workers in England, Scotland and Wales and also for individuals in Scotland and Wales and that, in England, from April 2015 the Care Quality Commission (CQC) took over the responsibility for individuals' health and safety for health and social care providers that are registered with them?

Legislation is also in place to ensure that everyone's general health and safety is safeguarded. This includes safeguarding all those who live in, work in and visit care settings.

The main piece of legislation that is relevant to care settings is the Health and Safety at Work Act (HASAWA) 1974; this Act forms the basis of all other current health and safety regulations and guidelines in work settings. The main purpose of health and safety regulations is to amend or supersede current laws.

Table 9.1 provides you with additional information about the key pieces of legislation relating to health and safety.

Research it

1.1 Health and Safety Executive (HSE)

Research some key facts and statistics specifically related to accidents, injuries and illnesses that occur in care settings. The health and social care services page on the Health and Safety Executive's website is a useful source of information:

www.hse.gov.uk/healthservices/index.htm

Provide a written account with your findings.

Key terms

A **regulator** is a body that supervises a particular sector.

Legislation is a process that involves making laws.

Table 9.1 Legislation relating to health and safety

Legislation	
Relevant Act	**What does it say about general health and safety in a care work setting?**
Health and Safety at Work Act (HASAWA) 1974	• It is the basis of all current health and safety legislation and is known as the 'enabling' Act because it enables other health and safety regulations to be made. • It established the Health and Safety Executive (HSE) as the regulator for the health, safety and welfare of people in work settings in the UK. • It aims to protect the health and safety of everyone in a work setting, i.e. in a care setting this includes individuals, adult care workers and those who visit. • It established the key duties and responsibilities of all employers and employees in work settings.
Management of Health and Safety at Work Regulations (MHSWR) 1999	• It requires employers and managers to assess and manage risks by carrying out risk assessments. • It requires work settings to have arrangements in place including appointing competent people to manage general health and safety, for example this may be the manager in a care setting. • It requires work settings to have procedures in place for emergency situations, for example in relation to fire safety. • It requires employers to provide information, training and supervision so that work activities can be carried out safely, for example a training day on health and safety at work.

→

Table 9.1 Legislation relating to health and safety *continued*

Legislation	
Workplace (Health, Safety and Welfare) Regulations 1992	• It requires workplaces to be environments where risks to general health and safety are minimised. • It is concerned with the safety of the working environment, e.g. temperature, lighting, ventilation. • It is concerned with the safety of the building, e.g. windows that can be opened and closed, non-slippery floors. • It is concerned with the safety of facilities, e.g. separate areas for employees to eat and drink, the availability of clean and well-lit toilets supplied with hot and cold water, soap, washbasins and drying facilities. • It is concerned with the safety of housekeeping, e.g. the availability of a clean environment, ensuring spillages are cleaned and removed immediately and that all waste is disposed of safely.
Manual Handling Operations Regulations 1992 (as amended 2002)	• It requires risks associated with moving and handling activities to be eliminated or minimised by employers, e.g. avoiding hazardous activities, such as lifting heavy equipment and using risk assessment for managing moving and handling tasks safely. • It requires employers to provide information, training and supervision about safe moving and handling, e.g. guidelines on moving an individual from one position to another.
Provision and Use of Work Equipment Regulations (PUWER) 1998	• It is concerned with the safety of work equipment used in work settings, e.g. in care settings this may include cleaning equipment. • It requires employees to receive training before using work equipment, i.e. in its use and the safety precautions to take. • It requires work equipment to have visible warning signs, i.e. employees who use work equipment must understand what these mean.
Lifting Operations and Lifting Equipment Regulations (LOLER) 1998	• It is concerned with the safety of lifting equipment used in work settings, e.g. in care settings this may include hoists. • It requires lifting equipment to be maintained and used solely for the purpose it was intended for, i.e. to ensure it is used safely. • It requires that all lifting operations must be planned, supervised and carried out in a safe manner by people who are competent, i.e. the employer must ensure that employees are trained and competent when using lifting equipment such as hoists.
Personal Protective Equipment at Work Regulations 1992	• It is concerned with the provision of personal protective equipment (PPE) to provide protection against infections, e.g. gloves, aprons. • It requires employers to provide PPE free of charge. • It requires PPE to be maintained in good condition so that it is effective. • It requires training to be provided in the use of PPE, i.e. when, why and how to put it on and dispose of it.
Reporting of Injuries, Diseases and Dangerous Occurrences Regulations (RIDDOR) 2013	• It requires employers to report and keep records for three years of work-related accidents that cause death and serious injuries (referred to as reportable injuries), diseases and dangerous occurrences (i.e. incidents with the potential to cause harm). • It requires work settings to have procedures in place for reporting injuries, diseases and incidents. • It requires employers to provide information and training on reporting injuries, diseases and incidents.

→

Table 9.1 Legislation relating to health and safety *continued*

Legislation	
Control of Substances Hazardous to Health (COSHH) 2002	• It requires employers to carry out a risk assessment to prevent or control exposure to hazardous substances, e.g. in care settings substances that may be hazardous to health could include cleaning materials. • It classifies hazardous substances under the following types: very toxic, toxic, harmful corrosive and irritant. • It requires employers to have procedures in place for safe working with hazardous substances, e.g. wearing PPE, carrying out a risk assessment. • It requires employers to provide information, training and supervision so that work activities can be carried out safely, e.g. by monitoring workers' practices to ensure they are safe.
Electricity at Work Regulations 1989	• It is concerned with ensuring that the electricity and the electrical appliances that are used in work settings are safe, i.e. by ensuring they are maintained. • It requires that all electrical equipment installed is safe, i.e. by being tested when it is installed and after installation, by being clearly marked that it has been tested. • It requires employers to provide training to employees in relation to carrying out safety checks on electrical equipment, e.g. how to report faulty equipment, how to carry out tests on electrical equipment.
Regulatory Reform Order (Fire Safety) 2005	• It requires fire risk assessments to be completed by the person responsible for the premises, i.e. in care settings this could be the manager or employer. • It requires fire equipment to be provided and maintained, e.g. fire extinguishers. • It requires fire escape routes and exits to be provided. • It requires employers to provide training to employees in relation to fire safety, i.e. what actions to take if there is a fire.
Health and Safety (First Aid) Regulations 1981	• It requires the provision of first aid to be made available to employees. • It requires employers to have an appointed person in the work setting, i.e. the person/s who will be responsible when an emergency arises. • It requires the provision of first aid facilities, e.g. a first aid box, trained first aiders.
Food Safety Act 1990	• Good personal hygiene is maintained when working with food so that it is safe to eat. • It requires that records are kept of where food is from so that it can be traced if needed. • It requires that any food that is unsafe is removed and an incident report completed.
Food Hygiene (England) Regulations 2006	• Food safety hazards are identified. • It requires that food safety controls are in place, maintained and reviewed. • Environments where food is prepared or cooked are kept clean and in good condition.
Civil Contingencies Act 2004	• Organisations must work together to plan and respond to local and national emergencies. • It establishes how organisations, such as emergency services, local authorities and health bodies can work together and share information. • It requires that risk assessments are undertaken and emergency plans are put in place.
Health and Social Care (Safety and Quality) Act 2015	• Adult social care providers must share information about a person's care with other health and care professionals so that safe and effective care can be provided. • Adult social care organisations should use a consistent **identifier** (the NHS Number, see page 328 for definition) when sharing information about a person's care. • It reduces the risk of harm and abuse by making provision for removing people convicted of certain offences from the registers kept by the regulatory bodies for health and social care professions.

Key terms

An **identifier** is a tool (the NHS Number) used to match people to their health records.

Policies and procedures may include other agreed ways of working as well as formal policies and procedures, for example in relation to how to carry out risk assessments.

Research it

1.2 Policies and procedures

Research what the Health and Safety at Work Act 1974 says about health and safety policies. You will find the link below to the Health and Safety Executive's website a useful source of information:

www.hse.gov.uk/legislation/hswa.htm

Evidence opportunity

1.1 Health and safety legislation

Develop a poster that includes information about the main points that are included in key legislation that relates to health and safety in a care work setting.

Reflect on it

1.2 Your setting's policies and procedures

Reflect on the consequences if you do not understand the health and safety policies and procedures that are in place in the adult care setting where you work.

How could this affect your working practices? What impact could it also have on your colleagues? The individuals you provide care or support to? Those who visit the care setting?

AC 1.2 Outline the main points of the health and safety policies and procedures agreed with the employer

Every adult care setting is required to have in place **policies and procedures** that set out how to put into practice safe working practices and in ways that comply with the health and safety legislation and regulations that you learned about in AC 1.1. Health and safety policies and procedures therefore set out how people's health, safety and well-being will be safeguarded. For example, this may be in relation to how to keep your workplace safe, how to maintain your own safety as well as that of individuals and others you work with or knowing what to do in an emergency, such as a fire at work.

An employer with a workplace that has five or more employees is required to have a health and safety policy in writing that includes:

- a statement that indicates the policy's purpose, i.e. to provide a safe workplace

- who is responsible for the policy and for health and safety activities, i.e. the employer's and employees', and others' responsibilities

- the arrangements in place to achieve the policy's purpose, i.e. the health and safety procedures to follow.

The policy may also include procedures for identifying and reporting health and safety hazards, how to record and report accidents and incidents and the evacuation procedures to follow.

Health and safety policies and procedures are important because they:

- reinforce the importance of health and safety to everyone

- increase everyone's understanding of safe working practices

- reduce the occurrence of injuries, accidents and illnesses.

1.2 H&S policies and procedures agreed with the employer

Read a copy of the health and safety policy that is in place in the care setting where you work. Discuss with your manager or assessor three main points that it explains are important in relation to health and safety. (If you discuss this with your manager, you will need a witness testimony or voice recording to be used as evidence.)

AC 1.3 Outline the main health and safety responsibilities of: self, the employer or manager, others in the work setting

The health and safety policy and procedures in the care setting where you work are essential for ensuring that it is a safe place for you, your colleagues, the individuals you provide care or support to, their families, carers, advocates and any other visitors and contractors. Maintaining health and safety is therefore everyone's responsibility.

Your responsibilities

Under the Health and Safety at Work Act (HASAWA) 1974 you are responsible for the following:

- taking reasonable care of your own and others' health and safety, for example by reporting any hazards that you see, such as a wet floor that may lead to them slipping over. This might also mean ensuring that your clothing and dress does not pose a danger; jewellery can pose hygiene concerns, for example
- taking reasonable care to not put yourself and others at risk, for example by not coming into work when you have the flu as this may lead to you spreading your illness to others, i.e. the individuals you provide care or support to may be frail and so this may lead to their conditions worsening

- co-operating with your employer on all health and safety information, training and procedures to follow, for example by attending health and safety training, by wearing, using and disposing of protective clothing in line with your employer's agreed ways of working
- understanding the meaning of safety signs and following these, for example if a contractor is carrying out some work in an area of the care setting and there is a 'do not enter' sign then you must respect this as not doing so may put you and others in danger
- not misusing first aid facilities, for example not accessing these without authorisation or using the contents of the first aid box for other work activities, such as for crafts
- using the welfare facilities provided, for example using the hand-washing and drying facilities
- using equipment provided and in accordance with instructions and training provided, for example ensuring the hoist is clean and in working order before using it and ensuring it is returned to its storage area after use
- taking reasonable care that you follow safe working practices, for example by complying with all risk assessments in place, by following your employer's agreed ways of working and not carrying out a task that you have not been trained to do
- reporting all accidents, injuries and diseases to your employer, for example by completing the accident book and/or the incident form
- informing your employer if your ability to work is affected. For example, you may be unwell and not be able to assist an individual to move, or you may be taking medication, meaning that you will not be able to operate moving and handling equipment such as a hoist.

You should also remember that in addition to your responsibilities, you have employee rights. These will include receiving health and safety equipment such as PPE to carry out your role, to work in a safe environment, and to be able to report any concerns you may have. Again, these are examples and you can find out more information about your rights from organisations such as the HSE and from your contract of employment as well as directly from your employer or manager.

Your manager or employer's responsibilities

Under the Health and Safety at Work Act (HASAWA) 1974 your manager or employer is responsible for the following:

- providing a workplace that is safe for everyone, for example by ensuring that any hazards, such as a damaged wheelchair or a frayed carpet, are removed and replaced

- ensuring the workplace is free from risks, for example by carrying out risk assessments to identify any risks and taking the necessary actions to reduce them, such as by providing adequate lighting

- providing information, training and supervision around health and safety, for example by making health and safety policies and procedures and training available to employees

- providing safety signs, for example to alert employees that the floor may be slippery as it is being cleaned

- providing adequate first aid facilities, for example a first aid box, a room for first aid

- providing adequate welfare facilities, for example access to clean hand-washing facilities, a separate area where food and drinks can be prepared

- providing protective clothing free of charge, for example aprons and gloves

- providing equipment free of charge, for example a hoist, a bed lift

- assessing risks and taking precautions against risks of injury, for example assessing the risks of moving an individual from one position to another and taking the necessary precautions, such as using lifting equipment

- reporting accidents, injuries, diseases and **dangerous occurrences** to the appropriate authority, for example the reporting of falls, fractures, **hepatitis C** and the failure of equipment while being used, such as a hoist.

Employers have a responsibility to ensure all of the above. In addition, they should ensure that they report any accidents and incidents to the Health and Safety Executive (HSE). They must ensure that machinery and equipment are safe to use, that there are emergency procedures in place, for example in relation to evacuation procedures to follow in the event of a fire. They must also ensure that you do not come across anything that is detrimental to your health including substances or equipment that may pose dangers (electrical equipment for example), and that the environment that you work in is a safe one. These are examples, and your manager/employer will be able to provide a more comprehensive list.

Research it

1.3 Responsibilities

You will find it helpful to refer to the Health and Safety Executive's (HSE) website:

www.hse.gov.uk/workers

This includes links to information on:

- workers' rights and responsibilities
- employer's responsibilities.

Key terms

Others may include team members, other colleagues, those who use or commission their own health or social care services, families, carers and advocates.

Work settings may include one specific location or a range of locations, depending on the context of a particular work role, i.e. a domiciliary carer who may work in individual's own homes and in residential care homes. See Unit 203, pages 3 and 4 for definitions.

Others' responsibilities

Under the Health and Safety at Work Act (HASAWA) 1974, **others** in the **work setting** are responsible for:

- following safe health and safety practices, for example visitors may be required to wash their hands when entering the care setting as part of its infection control procedures, sign a register upon entering and leaving the building, comply with fire emergency procedures
- complying with health and safety procedures, for example not smoking on the care setting's premises, reporting any visible hazards that may pose a danger such as a frayed carpet or a door that will not close
- not misusing anything that is provided in relation to health and safety, for example the first aid box, the fire extinguishers
- maintaining a safe environment, for example not entering a care setting if they are unwell, not behaving in an aggressive way towards the workers in the care setting.

Evidence opportunity

1.3 Health and safety responsibilities

Produce an information leaflet about how health and safety is maintained in the care setting where you work. Remember to include everyone's responsibilities: yours, your manager or employer's and others.

6Cs

Competence

You should feel able and confident to carry out health and safety tasks, such as moving and handling. You can only do so competently if you have received the necessary training, have understood how to carry out the task and are able to do so safely.

AC 1.4 Identify tasks relating to health and safety that should not be carried out without special training

As part of your health and safety responsibilities there are some work tasks that require special training and must not be carried out until your employer has trained you to do so. It is the responsibility of your employer to provide you with the training for these tasks and it is your responsibility to attend this training and only agree to carry them out if you feel **competent** to do so.

As procedures change and evolve, you must ensure that you receive up-to-date training. You cannot simply trust the training you previously received to still be relevant. Instead, your employer should arrange for training to be in line with new procedures, legislation and regulation. Think about the General Data Protection Regulation (GDPR). As the Data Protection Act changed and the GDPR was introduced, employees across various companies and organisations received training sessions informing them of the changes they needed to be aware of.

Figure 9.1 includes examples of some of these tasks.

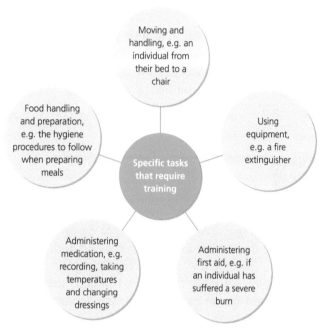

Figure 9.1 Health and safety tasks that should not be carried out without training

Only carrying out health and safety tasks that you are competent in and have been trained to carry out is essential for:

- providing high-quality care or support, i.e. attending training means that you have kept your knowledge and practices up to date and based them on current health and safety legislation and your employer's agreed ways of working
- avoiding putting yourself and others at risk, i.e. ensuring that you only carry out moving and handling when you have been trained to do so will mean that you will use safe practices when moving an individual from one position to another thus reducing the risks to you (i.e. of a back injury) and to the individual (i.e. of a fall).

Remember that this can be dangerous, and so if there are any new procedures you have not received training in you must receive training in these, whether it involves equipment you have used before or not. Remember the legislation relating to the Manual Handling Operations Regulations 1992, Lifting Operations and Lifting Equipment Regulations (LOLER) 1998 and Provision and Use of Work Equipment Regulations (PUWER) 1998 that we looked at in Table 9.1 on page 326.

- carrying out your health and safety responsibilities competently, i.e. complying with the health and safety policy and procedures available in the care setting where you work means that you will be carrying out your job role and responsibilities to the best of your ability.

Tasks that you should not carry out without special training

Tasks that you should not carry out without special training may include those relating to the following.

Use of equipment

Using equipment such as moving and handling equipment requires special training. You must make sure that you receive training in this because not doing so may mean that you use the wrong type of equipment for an individual who wants to be hoisted from their bed to a chair. For example, the wrong size sling may result in you injuring the individual or yourself.

First aid

You must never carry out first aid without having received training first because doing so may mean that you cause the individual unnecessary pain or harm. For example, if an individual has a broken limb it is important that you ensure the individual does not move; doing so will not only cause the individual pain but may also cause additional injuries.

Medication

You have a duty of care towards the individuals you provide care and support for. Administering medication is a highly skilled task because you need to know, for example, how it is administered correctly including any special precautions to take and any observations you may need to

1.4 Tasks that require special training

Discuss with a senior colleague the range of health and safety tasks that you both carry out in the care setting where you work and that require special training. What differences were there between your health and safety responsibilities and those of your senior colleague? Write a self-reflective account of your findings.

carry out. Administering medication without any special training may result in you administering medication to an individual ineffectively; this may have fatal consequences for the individual.

Health care procedures

Health care procedures such as changing used dressings, taking individuals' temperatures and blood pressure requires special training. You must not carry out health care procedures without training because doing so may result in an individual's blood pressure not being obtained or recorded correctly, for example. This may mean that an individual's condition deteriorates without you and others noticing.

Food handling and preparation

Handling and preparing food is also a skilled task and must not be undertaken without special training as doing so may result in you causing individuals to fall ill. For example, providing individuals with food that has not been cooked to the right temperature could result in them being poisoned with harmful bacteria; this may lead to individuals becoming ill and may even lead to fatalities.

AC 1.5 Explain how to access additional support and information relating to health and safety

There may be occasions when you are carrying out your health and safety responsibilities and you are unsure about whether you are carrying out a task correctly or have understood the health and safety procedures in place when carrying out a task. This might include something as simple as the technique to use when washing and drying your hands or how to dispose of your apron and gloves

safely after use. In these situations, it is important that you are able to access further support and information so that you can continue to carry out your health and safety responsibilities effectively.

You have already learned about some useful sources of information, such as, health and safety legislation, the policies and procedures of the care setting where you work. There are many more sources of support and information available to you both within and outside of the care setting where you work.

Sources of support and information

- Your manager can be a valuable source of support and information in terms of providing you with guidance to ensure and information you understand how to comply with the work setting's agreed ways of working. For example, this could be in relation to knowing what to do in the event of a fire in the work setting. You will learn more about fire safety procedures in LO7.

- Your colleagues can also provide you with support particularly in relation to supporting you to follow best practice when carrying out health and safety tasks. They may also provide you with information and show you how to use safe techniques. For example, this could be in relation to carrying out health and safety checks, such as checking that windows are secure and that the smoke alarms are in working order.

- Your **trade union representative** will be able to provide you with support and information if you have any health and safety concerns. For example, in relation to observing unsafe practices in your work setting or not feeling competent to carry out a work tasks that you have been trained to carry out.

- Your **health and safety officer** in the care setting where you work (this may be your manager or another senior member of staff) can provide you with useful and relevant information and training. For example, this could be in relation to changes to health and safety legislation and their impact on your working practices.

- The **Health and Safety Executive (HSE)** provides useful publications about maintaining health and safety in health and social care settings.

Reflect on it

1.5 Additional support

Reflect on an occasion when you or one of your colleagues accessed additional support in relation to health and safety. Why was this necessary? What was the outcome?

Key terms

A **trade union representative** is a member of an organised group of workers who speaks up for the rights and interests of the employees of an organisation, for example in relation to safe working conditions.

A **health and safety officer** is a named person in an organisation that is responsible for overseeing all health and safety matters, for example reviewing health and safety procedures, investigating accidents at work.

The **Health and Safety Executive (HSE)** is the independent regulator in the UK for health and safety in work settings.

The **Care Quality Commission (CQC)** is the independent regulator of all health and social care services in England.

Sector Skills Councils are organisations led by and for specific employment sectors, for example Skills for Care is for the adult social care workforce and Skills for Health is for the healthcare workforce.

- The **Care Quality Commission (CQC)** provides useful information about the health and safety standards that are expected from adult care settings.
- **Sector Skills Councils**, such as Skills for Care and Skills for Health, provide useful information about maintaining good-quality safe working practices and also the standards that are expected from the adult care sector's workforce, i.e. the Care Certificate.
- Additional information sources can include books and journals.

Research it

1.5 Support and information

Research the roles of two organisations that you can access for additional support and information. Write down your findings.

Accessing additional support and information

When you access additional support and information relating to health and safety you need to think about the following.

- What do my work setting's procedures say about accessing support and information in relation to health and safety?
- Which sources are available to me in my work setting? What process must I follow and why? In what situations can I access these?
- Which sources are available to me outside of my work setting? What process must I follow and why? In what situations can I access these?

In most care settings, it would be your manager or health and safety officer who you would approach in the first instance. You can do this formally during supervision with your manager or informally through discussion, for example. This could be a good opportunity to refer to Unit 207, Personal development in care settings, and read about sources of support that are available for personal development where you work.

Evidence opportunity

1.4, 1.5 Accessing additional support and information

Produce a one-page information handout that explains how to access additional support and information about a task that should not be carried out without special training. For example, you may choose a task relating to moving and handling or food handling.

LO1 Knowledge, skills, behaviours
Knowledge: why is health and safety at work important and do you understand responsibilities around this?
Do you know the main points of your employer's policies and procedures when it comes to health and safety?
Do you know what your employers' and others' responsibilities are in relation to health and safety?
Do you know what health and safety tasks you must not carry out without special training?
Do you know how to access additional information about unsafe health and safety practices?
Do you know how to comply with the Health and Safety at Work Act 1974?
Did you know that you have just shown your knowledge of the main legislation relating to general health and safety, and what your responsibilities are in relation to health and safety?
Skills: how can you show that you work in safe ways?
Do you know how to follow the moving and handling procedures in your work setting?
Did you know that you have just shown your understanding of safe working practices in the adult social care sector?
Behaviours: how can you show the personal qualities you have for supporting health and safety in your work setting?
Do you know how to show that you care for individuals' and others' health and safety?
Do you know how to show that you are committed to working in safe ways?
Did you know that you have just answered two questions about a few of the essential behaviours that are expected for supporting health and safety in care settings?

LO2 Understand the use of risk assessments in relation to health and safety

Getting started

Think about an occasion when you wanted to do something that someone else thought was not a good idea because it was too high risk. This may be in relation to doing something daring like a bungee jump or a trip to a country you have never been to before.

What happened? Did you do it? If so, how did you convince the other person that you were going to go ahead and do it? How did this make you feel at the time? If you didn't do it, why not? Did the other person persuade you not to? How did this make you feel at the time?

Reflect back on the situation you described above. Looking back, would you do anything different next time?

AC 2.1 Explain why it is important to assess health and safety risks posed by the work setting, situations or particular activities

Taking risks is not easy but this should not prevent you from doing what you want to do. Taking risks is part of everyday life and when risks are taken in a positive manner they can bring about many benefits.

An essential part of the health and safety responsibilities you and all those in the care setting where you work have involves being aware of how hazards and risks can occur.

Hazards

Hazards are dangers that have the potential to cause harm, i.e. they can be items in the work setting or situations or particular activities that may be the cause of accidents, injuries, ill health, deaths or damage.

Work setting

Hazards in the work setting can include the following.

- Wheelchairs, if not stored away securely when not in use, can be trip hazards.
- Walking aids, if not checked to be safe to use, can lead to individuals falling over.
- Broken furniture, if not replaced or fixed, can lead to individuals using it and injuring themselves.

Situations

Situations in the work setting that pose dangers include the following.

- An individual becomes distressed and throws a chair at the window that results in it being broken.
- An adult care worker forgets to wipe a spillage clean on the floor resulting in their colleague slipping over and hurting their back.
- A visitor leaves their bag in the middle of the hallway resulting in an individual tripping over and fracturing their leg.

Particular activities

Activities can also pose dangers. These can include the following.

- An adult care worker who cleans the floor using a detergent and then forgets to return it to be locked away securely after use. This could lead to it being swallowed accidentally by a child visiting an individual at home.
- Supporting an individual with their personal hygiene requires the effective wearing, use and disposal of personal protective equipment, such as an apron and gloves; not doing so can lead to contact with bodily fluids that can spread illness and result in ill health.
- An adult care worker who does not follow an individual's moving and handling guidelines could cause an injury to themselves and the individual they are supporting.

Risks

Risks are the likelihood of harm occurring as a result of a hazard. The risks may be high, medium or low in terms of their likelihood of occurring and their impact on you, the individuals and others you work with. For example:

Research it

2.1 Common hazards

Research the common hazards that are posed by adult care settings. You can base your research on the care setting where you work. You may also find the HSE's information page, 'Sensible risk assessment in care settings', on its website, a useful source of information:

www.hse.gov.uk/healthservices/sensible-risk-assessment-care-settings.htm

Also research some of the regulations that require risks to be assessed. These include the Noise at Work Regulations 1989 and Control of Asbestos at Work Regulations 2002. Some are also mentioned in Table 9.1 on page 325 (Personal Protective Equipment at Work Regulations 1992, and Control of Substances Hazardous to Health Regulations 2002). What other regulations that require risk assessments to be carried out can you find out about? How do these relate to you? Write down some notes on what you find out.

- there may a high risk of a broken chair in the lounge causing an injury to anyone who sits on it if it is not removed immediately
- there may be a medium risk when moving an individual from their bed to their chair with one adult care worker supporting as the individual is a little unsteady on their feet; two adult care workers may be required to avoid any accidents from happening
- there may be a low risk of an individual who prepares their own meal in the evening forgetting to turn off the oven after they have used it.

Assessing health and safety risks

Assessing health and safety risks forms part of the responsibilities that you and your employer have in the care setting where you work. This process is commonly referred to as risk assessment. Risk assessment is a requirement of the Management of Health and Safety at Work Regulations 1999. The risk assessment process involves five steps, as shown in Figure 9.2.

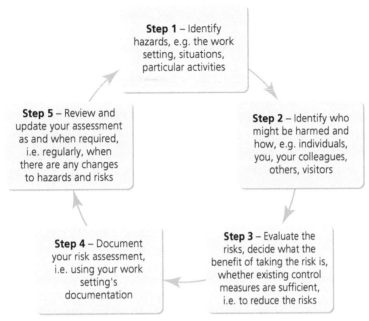

Figure 9.2 Assessing health and safety risks

In addition to the points mentioned in Figure 9.2, when carrying out a risk assessment, remember to question what the purpose of the risk assessment is, who will undertake it, who is at risk, what it is that you should be assessing and when this should be done. You should also consider what the potential benefits of taking the risk are. These are all important considerations to take into account.

Assessing health and safety risks (such as those you learned about that are posed by your work setting, situations or particular activities), is very important because it is part of the provision of good **care**. It shows that you want to make a positive difference to individuals' lives by ensuring their safety at all times. Assessing health and safety risks is also important because it:

- protects the safety of everyone, i.e. to prevent you, your colleagues, the individuals you provide care or support to and others who visit, from being placed in danger, harmed or becoming unwell
- enables potential and actual dangers to be identified as well as their associated risks. This then enables you to decide on the measures that are needed to either eliminate or reduce the risks that could be dangerous, harmful or cause illness
- enables your employer, and you and your colleagues as employees, to comply with the

health and safety legislation that is in place, for example the Health and Safety at Work Act (HASAWA) 1974 and the Management of Health and Safety at Work Regulations (MHSWR) 1999.

Once the risks have been assessed, your setting/employer will need to make sure that they put measures in place to control and reduce these risks. This may include making sure that there are policies in place if a spillage has occurred, or training is given to employees. If you are working in someone's home, then it may be that you can merely advise them about hazards and risks rather than actually make changes to their home.

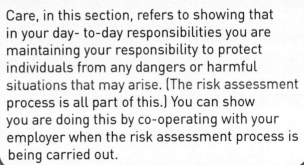

6Cs C

Care

Care, in this section, refers to showing that in your day-to-day responsibilities you are maintaining your responsibility to protect individuals from any dangers or harmful situations that may arise. (The risk assessment process is all part of this.) You can show you are doing this by co-operating with your employer when the risk assessment process is being carried out.

Reflect on it

2.1 Consequences of not assessing risks

Reflect on the consequences if risks in your work setting were not being assessed. How could this impact on your work activities? On the well-being of the individuals you provide care or support to? On working as a team?

Reflect on it

2.2 Reporting risks

Research the procedures that you are expected to follow for reporting health and safety risks that have been identified in the care setting where you work.

Confirm your understanding of these with your manager. Write a short reflective account.

Evidence opportunity

2.1 The importance of assessing health and safety hazards

Identify three health and safety risks that are present in the work tasks you carry out every day and write down explanations of the potential danger they could cause and to whom. Then, for each risk, explain why it is important to assess it using the risk assessment process. State what could happen if you did not follow a risk assessment procedure. What could the outcome and consequences be?

Be prepared to discuss your findings with your assessor.

AC 2.2 Explain how and when to report potential health and safety risks that have been identified

Identifying health and safety hazards and associated risks on their own is not sufficient for protecting the safety of everyone in your work setting. All identified health and safety risks must also be reported so that they can be eliminated or minimised and not continue to pose a danger to those who may be affected by them. It is one of your responsibilities as a care worker to report any unsafe situation or anything that poses a risk.

The health and safety policy in the care setting where you work will include information and guidance about how and when to report potential health and safety risks that you have identified or that others, such as individuals or visitors, have reported to you.

You must report potential health and safety risks as soon as you have identified them or others have told you about them. Not doing so may result in others being put in further danger or harmed. In the first instance, you should report these to your manager. Your manager will then guide you to ensure that the risk poses no further danger or harm and show you how to record the risks you have identified.

Figure 9.3 shows an example of how to report in writing the health and safety risks you have identified; what documents do you use in your work setting?

The Reporting of Injuries, Diseases and Dangerous Occurrences Regulations (RIDDOR) 1995 (amended 2008) mean that you are legally required to report such concerns. You can report any health and safety concerns you have directly to the Health and Safety Executive (HSE). Your manager will need to report these, as well as deaths, to the HSE; your local authority's environmental health department for food hygiene concerns; the Care Quality Commission for failures in individuals' care. These will be recorded and tracked so that if there are regular occurrences of such incidents, they can be acted upon. If it is found that these are occurring on a large scale across the country, it can become an issue for government to deal with.

Risk assessment record Date of risk assessment: 27/01/18					
What is the hazard?	**Who might be harmed and how?**	**What is being done to control this risk?**	**Who needs to take these actions?**	**When do these actions need to be taken?**	**Have these actions been completed?**
The front door of the care home does not lock securely consistently.	J has dementia and may leave the care home with no-one noticing. Staff and individuals could be harmed if an intruder gains access to the home. Individuals' and staff's possessions may be stolen and/or damaged if an intruder gains access to the home.	The contractor has been contacted and will be arriving to repair the door within the next three hours. In the meantime, members of staff are taking it in turns to keep the front door secure by remaining in the hallway at all times.	The manager has phoned the contractor the care home uses. All staff members are to monitor the security of the care home.	Immediately and until the contractor has repaired the front door.	**Yes:** Signed (manager): Date: **No:** Are any further actions needed? If so, by whom? If so, when?

Figure 9.3 Recording the health and safety risks that have been identified

Research it

2.2, 1.1 RIDDOR

Research what the Reporting of Injuries, Diseases and Dangerous Occurrences Regulations (RIDDOR) 2013 says about the reporting and recording of work-related accidents that cause death and serious injuries (referred to as reportable injuries), diseases and dangerous occurrences (i.e. incidents with the potential to cause harm).

You will find the link below to the HSE's information page on their website, RIDDOR – Reporting of Injuries, Diseases and Dangerous Occurrences Regulations 2013, a useful source of information:

www.hse.gov.uk/riddor/

Provide a written account detailing your findings.

Evidence opportunity

2.2 How and when to report potential H&S risks

Discuss with your assessor your reporting of a potential health and safety risk in your work setting. Obtain feedback from your manager about the skills and knowledge you showed in relation to both how and when you reported it. What areas did you do well in? Why? What areas do you need to further improve on? Why?

AC 2.3 Explain how risk assessment can help address dilemmas between rights and health and safety

Risk assessment is, as you know, essential for protecting everyone's safety. However, in adult care settings it can also be a useful process for helping to ensure that individuals' rights to be in control of

2.3 Concerns

Reflect on how you would feel if someone had concerns over your safety in relation to you carrying out an activity that you wanted to do. Would you see this as a positive or negative? Why?

their lives are supported alongside you and your employer's responsibilities to ensure their safety. Supporting an individual's rights against health and safety risks is an all too often dilemma faced by adult care workers because good care and support involves supporting individuals to make their own decisions including taking risks, but it also involves protecting individuals' safety.

Ultimately, measures to protect people's safety may affect or change the way that they live. For example, an elderly person with mobility issues may not want to have a stair lift installed in their home because of the way it will affect the layout of their home, and they have a right over how their home should look. However, this poses a safety issue as climbing and coming down stairs may be dangerous for them. Another example may be if an individual does not wish to stop seeing an abusive family who poses a threat to their safety. In all cases, a risk assessment will be carried out and measures put in place to manage those risks.

Risk assessment can help address dilemmas between individuals' rights and health and safety risks. You can do this by:

- encouraging individuals and adult care workers to talk about the dilemmas and what can be done to address them
- supporting individuals to understand what dangers there are and how these can be balanced against their preferences. Sometimes all you may be able to do is advise them on the best course of action
- making positive decisions with individuals about taking risks.

A risk assessment could be used to address the following examples of dilemmas that may arise in an adult care setting.

- **An individual with a mild learning disability wishes to have a relationship with an individual with a severe learning disability.** You could have a discussion with each individual about their wishes, including what type of relationship, if any, they would like to have and their understanding of what this may involve. For example, you could discuss the benefits as well as the risks of relationships with others. You could explore the rights of both individuals with each of them; both individuals, for example, have a right to have a relationship and to also refuse to be in a relationship. You could all make a decision that balances the safety and rights of both individuals.

- **An individual who is experiencing difficulties with their mobility due to gaining weight wishes to have two desserts rather than one every lunch time.** You could explore the impact this will have on the individual's weight and mobility and on the additional support needed from staff. This will need to be discussed in a **compassionate** way as this is a sensitive issue. You could also discuss the individual's wishes to lose weight and to be more mobile. You could also discuss how this makes them feel. You can then support the individual to make their own decision after balancing the risks to their health and well-being against their preferences.

- **An individual who has recently moved in to a care home wishes to bring with them three large items of furniture and have these placed in their room.** The care home manager is concerned that doing so will mean there will be very little space for the individual and staff to move around in her room which in turn may lead to injuries or falls. You could discuss the dangers of doing so with the individual and also discuss the staff's wishes to ensure the safety of everyone. A decision could be made that balances the safety and rights of both, such as agreeing with the individual for one item of furniture to be placed in her room and for the other two items to be placed in a communal area in the home.

A positive risk assessment process, if done well, can be a very effective way of addressing the dilemmas that may arise between people's rights and their ability to live safely.

Risk assessments in reablement practice

Reablement is an approach that is different to the provision of traditional care at home because it is enables individuals to do things for themselves by supporting them to regain their independence. It is an approach that not only identifies the individual's strengths and areas for development but also finds out from the individual what their hopes are. It is an approach that provides holistic support to individuals so that they can re-learn how to do things for themselves; the process takes place with the individual. For example, an individual may have stopped making their own hot drinks because the last time they did they had a fall. Now they fear that they will have another fall and rely on family members to make drinks. A reablement risk assessment will identify with the individual the benefits of them making their own hot drinks. For example, they can make them as often as they want; it gives them a reason to move around and therefore maintain their mobility; they could also make them for their visitors.

The risk assessment will also consider the individual's overall well-being; for example, an individual's mental and emotional health may also be improved by referring them to their GP for counselling, this may be to help them manage their fear of falling again. Other practical ways of managing the risk of falling can also be discussed with the individual, such as using a kettle tipper to avoid the individual losing their balance when pouring hot water from the kettle, and placing their drink on a walker tray for safety. The individual will be provided with support to use these aids and both you and they will monitor what worked and what didn't. The situation can be assessed again until the individual has reached their goal to make their own drink.

6Cs

C

Compassion

Compassionately discussing a sensitive issue with an individual involves showing that you care about them and how they are feeling. You can show this by being aware of your body language; are you, for example, leaning towards them when speaking to them? The tone of your voice, is it gentle and polite? What you say, are you using kind and thoughtful words?

Evidence opportunity

2.3 Risk assessment and dilemmas

Develop a case study for one or two individuals who have care or support needs. Describe two dilemmas that exist between the individual's rights and your concerns in relation to health and safety. Explain how risk assessment can be used to help address both dilemmas.

LO2 Knowledge, skills, behaviours
Knowledge: why is it important to assess health and safety risks and to use risk assessments?
Do you know what the five stages of the risk assessment process are?
Do you know the consequences of not assessing health and safety risks in your work setting?
Do you know who to go to if you have identified a potential health and safety risk?
Do you know how risk assessment can help address dilemmas between rights and health and safety concerns?
Did you know that you have just shown your knowledge of the risk assessment process?
Skills: how can you show that you are able to report health and safety risks?
Do you know what record to use for reporting a health and safety risk and how to complete it?
Did you know that you have just demonstrated a skill required for reporting health and safety risks effectively?
Behaviours: how can you show the personal qualities you have when balancing an individual's rights with health and safety concerns?
Do you know how to show your sensitivity when an individual's rights conflict with your health and safety concerns?
Do you know how to communicate positively with your manager when reporting potential health and safety risks?
Did you know that you have just demonstrated a few of the essential behaviours required when using risk assessment for managing health and safety risks?

LO3 Understand procedures for responding to accidents and sudden illness

Getting started

Think about an occasion when you or someone you know became unwell or had an accident. Discuss what happened. Why do you think the illness/accident happened? Could anything have been done to prevent it from happening? What treatment was provided? Who provided it? When? Why?

AC 3.1 Describe different types of accidents and sudden illnesses that may occur in your work setting

Accidents and **sudden illnesses** may occur when both hazards and risks have or have not been identified or minimised through the risk assessment process.

Key terms

Accidents are unexpected events that cause damage or injury, for example, a fall.

Sudden illnesses are unexpected medical conditions.

In work settings, accidents and sudden illnesses can happen and can range from being relatively minor to very serious. In adult care settings, there are some types of accidents and sudden illnesses that can occur more frequently than in other work settings because of the work activities that adult care workers carry out on a day-to-day basis. These include supporting individuals with care tasks including eating, drinking, personal care and moving and positioning individuals, as well as supporting individuals who may have conditions that affect their physical and mental health. The statistics below from the Health and Safety Executive (HSE) illustrate the more common types of accidents and illnesses relating to care workers in adult care settings.

The HSE reports that each year for the health and social care sector:

- 5% of workers suffer from an illness they believe to be work-related – of the illnesses reported, 44% are stress, depression or anxiety, 37% are musculoskeletal disorders and 19% are other illnesses
- 2% of workers sustain a work-related injury – of the non-fatal accidents reported by employers in 2015/16, 27% are slips, trips and falls, 25% are lifting and handling and 21% are physical assault.

Health and Safety Executive (2016) 'Statistics for the Health and Social Care sector'

Common types of accidents in adult care settings

- **Slips, trips and falls:** slips, trips and falls may be caused by hazards in the work setting that have not been identified or assessed correctly or because individuals with care or support needs are more susceptible to having accidents if, for example, they have sight loss or difficulties with their mobility. These types of accidents may lead to fractures, back injuries, cuts, bruises and bleeding.
- **Lifting and handling:** lifting and handling in adult care settings may involve both supporting individuals with moving and positioning as well as moving items or equipment, such as hoists, beds, wheelchairs and furniture, for example when cleaning. If you do not follow your agreed ways of working then you may injure your back or cause an individual to fall. You will learn more about safe practices for moving and handling items and equipment in LO5. Equipment may also cause injuries, for example scalds and burns may occur due to electrical equipment; choking may also occur.
- **Physical assault:** physical assault is more commonly experienced by workers in the health and social care sector than by workers in other sectors and can be the cause of **stress** as well as physical injuries. Physical assault may result because of the needs of an individual whose behaviour challenges, and medical conditions or frustration with not having their care or support needs met.

Common types of illnesses in adult care settings

- **Stress, depression and anxiety:** working long shifts, providing support to meet the needs of an individual whose behaviour challenges, such as an individual with mental health needs or dementia on a day-to-day basis, can lead to adult care workers being placed under additional stress. If this is left untreated then it can lead to individuals feeling low in themselves and even to the development of **depression** and **anxiety**.
- **Musculoskeletal disorders:** poor working practices when supporting individuals to move from one position to another, such as, over stretching and lifting, can lead to repetitive strain being placed on the back, arms and legs, which can result in disorders that can cause pain and restrict the body's movements.
- **Other illnesses:** medical conditions, such as, type 2 **diabetes**, **asthma** or **heart disease** can be the cause of sudden illnesses. For example, diabetes may lead to a diabetic coma where the individual loses consciousness, asthma could lead to severe breathing difficulties and heart disease could lead to a heart attack or cardiac arrest. Epilepsy could lead to seizures. Poor working practices, such as lack of good hygiene, may lead to the spread of infections and illnesses such as food poisoning. You will learn more about how to reduce the spread of infections in LO4.

Reflect on it

3.1 HSE statistics

Reflect on the statistics reported by the HSE above. Did any surprise you? Why? Were there any that you were expecting to see? Why?

Research it

3.1 Diabetes

Research the 'BIG 3 signs of diabetes'. Write down your findings.

You will find the link below a useful source of information:

www.diabetes.co.uk/The-big-three-diabetes-signs-and-symptoms.html

Stress is the body's physical and emotional reaction to being under too much pressure.

Depression is a medical condition causing low mood that affects your thoughts and feelings. It can range from mild to severe but usually lasts for a long time and affects your day-to-day living.

Anxiety is a feeling of fear or worry that may be mild or serious and can lead to physical symptoms such as shakiness.

Diabetes is a health condition that occurs when the amount of glucose (sugar) in the blood is too high because the body cannot use it properly.

Asthma is a lung condition that causes breathing difficulties that can range from mild to severe.

Heart disease is a condition that affects your heart and can lead to mild chest pain or a heart attack.

Evidence opportunity

3.1 Accidents and sudden illnesses

Look through your work setting's accident book. How many different types of accidents can you find? What do you think were the causes? Discuss these with your assessor or manager, and record the conversation (if you can) or obtain a witness testimony from them.

Now reflect on the illnesses that you know have been experienced by the individuals and staff in your work setting. How many different types were there? Do you know their causes? Discuss these with your assessor or manager, as above.

AC 3.2 Outline the procedures to be followed if an accident or sudden illness should occur

When an accident or sudden illness occurs in a work setting everyone has a role to play and that includes you! Providing first aid, as you have

learned, is a task that cannot be carried out without special training. Therefore, it is important that if you have not been trained in first aid that you do not provide first aid treatment to a person who has had an accident or sudden illness in your work setting. Doing so may have serious consequences because you may cause the person further pain or discomfort and may make the situation worse. You will also not be complying with your own work setting's agreed ways of working and so you may be disciplined by your employer.

If you work in a residential care home, then it is unlikely you will have to take the lead in a health emergency as you will be working as part of a team; instead you may need to seek assistance from a more senior colleague who is a trained first aider. If, however, you are working on your own as a personal assistant with an individual who lives in their own home then it is likely that as well as seeking help from emergency services you will need to take action yourself. However, you will need to ensure that you have received the relevant training.

Just because you are not a trained first aider does not mean that you cannot play an important role in providing assistance when an accident or sudden illness has occurred by following your work setting's procedures.

Provide assistance and reassurance

You can provide the casualty with support; kind words and reassurance are in high demand when you are in pain. Remember what you have learned about person-centred care and ensure that you listen to the individual and do what you can to respect their privacy. It may be that they do not want others to see them in this way, and so you could find a way to ensure that others do not come near the scene. Of course dealing with the situation first is key.

Call for help

Do this as quickly as you can. This may mean calling 999; for an ambulance or paramedic, or a qualified person in your setting. Again, this will depend on where you work. If this is in someone's home, you will need to call 999; if in a care setting, again the emergency services will be the best point of contact. However, you may also need to alert another staff member who is more qualified to deal with the situation, depending on what the situation is; there may even be a medical professional available. If you are working in a hospital there will be medical professionals around you that you can seek for immediate help.

Provide first aid

The section below covers this, but the important thing to remember is that you should only provide first aid if you have received the proper training and feel confident in carrying this out.

Make the area safe

Make sure the area around the individual is safe, and that there is nothing that has the potential to cause further harm both to the individual or to those who may also be in the area. At the same time, do not attempt to remove anything that may cause further harm until the emergency services arrive. Make sure that others do not come near the scene if this will cause harm. You may even need to put a sign up if there is one nearby.

Assist others

You can provide assistance to the qualified first aider. Make sure you do as the qualified first aider instructs. They will tell you what they need and what to do, and you should do as they say. You may for example need to call for help or an ambulance, or find a blanket to keep the casualty warm. You may need to ensure the area is kept safe as mentioned above, for example by asking other individuals not to approach the casualty so as to protect the casualty's privacy and dignity. Remember that when you are telling others about the situation, whether it is someone on the scene or the emergency/ambulance services, speak clearly, remain calm and answer all the questions they ask you.

Also provide reassurance to others who may be concerned or distressed about what has happened, especially if the incident has been an upsetting one. Inform them of the facts, at the same time as reassuring them. You should also seek support if you have also found the situation

distressing. Again, this will need to be done after the incident but it is important to remember this so that you are able to share your feelings, are supported and can support others.

Report and record

You can report and record the accident or sudden illness. You should ensure that you report it immediately to your manager, a senior member of staff or first aider.

After the incident, you must ensure that all the information is recorded even if it was a minor incident. This is a legal requirement as set out by RIDDOR outlined in Table 9.1. Make sure that you record the incident by completing the accident book or incident form. Record details of the individual, the date, time, place of the accident/sudden illness, their injury/illness, what you witnessed, any information you received, your actions taken in response and the actions taken by others (when you sought help, what time help arrived on the scene, whether you needed any equipment or medication to deal with the situation), the outcome of the incident, your name and signature.

It is important that this is all recorded so that this information can be shared with your manager, if you work in a setting for example, or an inspector. It may even be needed by medical or legal professionals so it is important that you record all of this information.

Reflect

Make sure you take the time to reflect on what has taken place. Could this incident have been prevented? How? How did you deal with the situation? What did you do well? What could you have improved? How would you support others to deal with a similar situation?

Ensure your training and knowledge is up to date

You can keep your knowledge and skills up to date by attending training and reading through your work setting's procedures for what to do in the event of an accident or sudden illness.

Suggest changes and improvements

In light of the accident, illness and procedures followed, is there anything that could be improved to better the procedures, or make the environment safer to prevent further accidents in the setting, home or community? Make sure that you discuss this with your manager for example, or the individual that you care for if you are working in their home. This will lead to improved care and support and a safer environment.

First aid procedures

Although you may not be a qualified first aider it is still useful to have some knowledge of basic first aid when attending an accident or sudden illness. These are stressful situations that you may come across in your work setting and so having an understanding of what to do can help you feel more able to handle them.

You can use **DR's ABC** as a good way of helping you to remember what to do when you come across an accident or sudden illness.

- **D** (Danger): Look around you and check for any risks or signs of danger. Never put yourself in any danger.
- **R** (Response assessment): Assess all casualties. Check whether they are conscious by calling their name, tapping them on their shoulders, observing whether they are breathing normally.
- **S** (Shout for help): Call an ambulance or get someone else to do this for you and ask them to come back and tell you that they have done this.
- **A** (Airway): Check that the casualty's airway is open and not blocked. Check that help is on its way.
- **B** (Breathing): Check whether the casualty is breathing normally. If the casualty is breathing normally place the casualty in the recovery position. If the casualty is not breathing, start CPR only if you have been trained to do so. Check that help is on its way.
- **C** (Circulation): Continue to monitor the casualty and check that help is on its way.

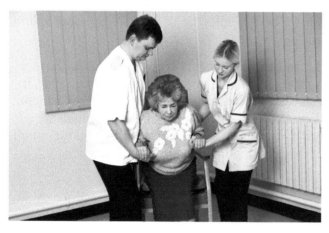

Figure 9.4 What support can you offer?

Research it

3.1, 3.2, 1.5 First aid

Research the basic first aid treatment for two accidents and two sudden illnesses. Write down your findings.

You will find a current first aid book a useful source of information. There should be one available in your work setting. Ask your manager if you can reference it. Your work setting's first aid procedures will also be useful.

Reflect on it

3.2 How you can help

Reflect on an occasion when you witnessed an accident or someone becoming suddenly unwell. How did you feel? What did you do? Why?

Now think about the other ways of helping that you learned about by following your work setting's procedures. Is there any other action you could have taken? Why?

Evidence opportunity

3.2 Procedures to follow if an accident or sudden illness should occur

Identify an accident or sudden illness that may occur in the care setting where you work. Produce a leaflet that outlines the procedures you are expected to follow. Add diagrams and images to support your work.

Research it

3.2 First aid

Research how to treat three conditions that individuals may have with first aid and discuss your findings with a colleague.

St John's Ambulance information page 'First Aid Tips, Information and Advice' is a useful source of information: www.sja.org.uk/sja/first-aid-advice.aspx

It is important that you have an understanding of the different first aid procedures and that you receive training for these before you perform them.

Tables 9.2 and 9.3 outline some useful sources (mainly St John's Ambulance and the NHS) that will explain some of the first aid procedures you will need to know. They are helpful sources of knowledge and information although they will not replace training.

Of course you are not expected to know all of the medical procedures. However, it is useful to be trained in first aid so that you are equipped with the knowledge and skills that you may need until the medical services are at the scene.

You will also find it useful to research and learn more about the first aid procedures for the following:

- **Anaphylaxis (or anaphylactic shock):** www.nhs.uk/conditions/first-aid/#anaphylaxis or www.nhs.uk/conditions/first-aid/#anaphylaxis are useful sources of information.

- **Drowning:** www.sja.org.uk/sja/first-aid-advice/breathing/drowning.aspx or www.nhs.uk/conditions/first-aid/#drowning are useful sources of information.
- **Difficulty breathing:** www.nhs.uk/conditions/shortness-of-breath/ may be a useful source of information.
- **Hot and cold conditions:** www.sja.org.uk/sja/first-aid-advice/hot-and-cold-conditions.aspx is a useful source of information.
- **Loss of consciousness:** www.sja.org.uk/sja/first-aid-advice/loss-of-responsiveness.aspx may be a useful source of information.

The NHS website: www.nhs.uk/conditions/first-aid/#common-accidents-and-emergencies is also a good source of information for the different types of accidents and illnesses we have discussed above.

You will also need to ensure you know how to do the recovery position as you will need this when dealing with various emergencies. Go to: www.sja.org.uk/sja/first-aid-advice/first-aid-techniques/the-recovery-position.aspx to understand the procedure.

The information on these websites will not replace training. You must ensure that you attend all first aid training courses that you are advised to attend. You and your employer are responsible for ensuring you receive the training and guidance that you need.

Table 9.2 Accidents, signs and symptoms and useful sources of information

Type of accident	Signs and symptoms	Useful source of information
Fracture	• Swelling • Oddly positioned limbs • Pain around the fractured area	www.sja.org.uk/sja/first-aid-advice/bones-and-muscles/broken-bones-and-fractures.aspx
Cut	Large or small amounts of blood	Cuts and grazes: www.sja.org.uk/sja/first-aid-advice/bleeding/cuts-and-grazes.aspx

→

Table 9.2 Accidents, signs and symptoms and useful sources of information *continued*

Type of accident	Signs and symptoms	Useful source of information
Bleeding	Large or small amounts of blood	Severe bleeding: www.sja.org.uk/sja/first-aid-advice/bleeding/severe-bleeding.aspx Nose bleeds: www.sja.org.uk/sja/first-aid-advice/bleeding/nose-bleeds.aspx
Burn/scalds caused by heat/flames/hot liquids/chemicals/electrical currents	• Swollen or blistered skin • The person may be in severe pain or shock	www.sja.org.uk/sja/first-aid-advice/hot-and-cold-conditions/burns-and-scalds.aspx
Poisoning caused by chemicals, plants or substances like drugs and alcohol	• The person may be unconscious • The person may be in severe pain • Swollen or blistered skin around the mouth and lips	www.sja.org.uk/sja/first-aid-advice/poisoning.aspx
Electrical injuries caused by high voltages (e.g. railway lines) or low voltages (e.g. electrical appliances such as a kettle or heater)	• The person may have burns • The person may have had a cardiac arrest	www.nhs.uk/conditions/first-aid/#electrocution

Table 9.3 Sudden illnesses, signs and symptoms and useful sources of information

Type of sudden illness	Signs and symptoms	Useful source of information
Cardiac arrest is caused by a heart attack, shock or electric shock	• The person has no pulse • The person is not breathing	Cardiac arrest: www.sja.org.uk/sja/first-aid-advice/heart/cardiac-arrest.aspx Heart attack: www.sja.org.uk/sja/first-aid-advice/heart/heart-attack.aspx
Stroke is caused by blood clots that block the flow of blood to the brain	• The person may have an uneven face • The person may not be able to raise and hold both arms • The person's speech may be confused	www.sja.org.uk/sja/first-aid-advice/illnesses-and-conditions/stroke.aspx
Epileptic seizure is caused by changes in the brain's activity	Involuntary contraction of muscles. This is also referred to as a convulsion or a fit	www.sja.org.uk/sja/first-aid-advice/illnesses-and-conditions/seizures-fits-in-adults.aspx
Choking and difficulty with breathing usually caused by food becoming stuck in the throat	• Coughing, gasping • Difficulty breathing (gasping) • Difficulty speaking	www.sja.org.uk/sja/first-aid-advice/breathing/choking-adults.aspx

→

Table 9.3 Sudden illnesses, signs and symptoms and useful sources of information *continued*

Type of sudden illness	Signs and symptoms	Useful source of information
Shock is caused when blood is not flowing round the body effectively	<ul><li>Cold, clammy and/or pale skin</li><li>Fast pulse</li><li>Fast breathing</li><li>May feel sick</li></ul>	www.sja.org.uk/sja/first-aid-advice/heart/shock.aspx
Loss of consciousness is caused by a faint or a serious illness	Not being responsive, either partial or total unresponsiveness	www.sja.org.uk/sja/first-aid-advice/loss-of-responsiveness/unrespon-sive-and-breathing/adult.aspx This website has information on what to do when dealing with an unresponsive breathing adult. There is more information available on 'responsive and breathing adult' on this website. Or you may want to visit the NHS website.

Some important points to remember:

- Make sure you receive training in first aid and remember the importance of it.
- Only carry out the actions that you have been trained in and are able to do safely without causing the individual harm.
- Do not attempt to treat an individual if you do not have the right training or take any actions that you do not have understanding of as this could harm the individual.
- Make sure you get help as fast as you can and support the individual as best you can.
- Make sure the area around the individual is safe and free of any dangerous objects.
- Support the person who may be dealing with the situation, a medical professional for example.
- Seek the advice of a medical professional first if possible.
- Remember the Data Protection Act (replaced by the new GDPR 2018) when you record the incident and when you record details about the individual.
- The actions you will take will also vary depending on your setting. For example, in a care setting you will be able to seek the advice of colleagues, although they may not be doctors or medical professionals. If you are working in someone's home it may be that you will need to seek help from medical professionals or emergency services in situations where you do not have the expertise and have not received training.

LO3 Knowledge, skills, behaviours
Knowledge: what types of accidents and sudden illnesses can occur in your work setting?
Do you know why some individuals with care or support needs may be more prone to accidents?
Do you know where you can access more information about the different types of sudden illnesses that may occur?
Do you know about the different procedures to follow if an accident or sudden illness should occur?
Did you know that you have just shown your knowledge of the different types of accidents and sudden illnesses you may have to respond to, and the procedures to follow?
Skills: how can you respond to accidents and sudden illnesses effectively?
Do you know what you can and cannot do if an individual has an accident?
Do you know how to report and record accidents and sudden illnesses?
Did you know that you have just demonstrated a few of the skills required for responding to accidents and sudden illnesses?

→

LO4 Be able to reduce the spread of infection

Getting started

Think about an **infection** that you have heard about that was spread in the UK and reported in the media. For example, you may have heard of the spread of **MRSA** or the **norovirus**.

What details do you remember being reported about it? What was the impact of it on, for example, individuals in hospitals or in other adult care settings, such as residential care homes and nursing homes?

AC 4.1 Explain your roles and responsibilities as an employee and those of the employer in the prevention and control of infection

In your work setting both you and your employer have a vital role to play in ensuring that infections are prevented because they can affect everyone. When infections do occur because an individual is unwell, for example, you and your employer are also responsible for ensuring that your actions prevent the spread of these infections onto other individuals, your colleagues and others who may visit the care setting where you work.

Your employer's responsibilities in infection prevention and control

Your employer is required by law to prevent and control infections in the work setting; most of these legal requirements come under the Health and Safety at Work Act (1974) that you learned about earlier on in this unit.

Your employer is responsible for ensuring that you and all employees are safe at work and therefore aware of infection prevention and control. They should be aware of the reasons why this is

Key terms

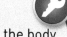

Infection refers to when germs enter the body and cause an individual to become unwell.

MRSA stands for meticillin-resistant *Staphylococcus aureus* and is often referred to as a 'superbug' because it is difficult to treat. It is a bacterium that can cause serious infections.

Norovirus is an infection of the stomach that causes diarrhoea and vomiting.

important and relevant to day-to-day work tasks. Your employer has a responsibility to:

- **provide information:** for example, by displaying information posters such as hand-washing posters above sinks; by providing information leaflets for employees and others who visit; and by keeping relevant records, such as accident and incident records and infection outbreak records.

- **provide education:** for example, by developing infection prevention and control policies and procedures and ensuring these are followed. Your employer needs to ensure that you, as

Research it

4.1 Legislation and responsibilities

Research two Acts that you have learned about in AC 1.1 and that are relevant to infection prevention and control. Write down the key points about what each Act says about your responsibilities and your employer's responsibilities with respect to infection prevention and control.

Reflect on it

4.1 Information available in your setting

Reflect on the infection control posters and information that are available in your work setting. Write down all the ones you know about. Discuss this with your manager; did you find out about any more?

care workers, are aware of what to do if you are informed that an individual in the care setting has the norovirus. They need to provide training on infection prevention and control, provide updates to changes in procedures and legislation and monitor work practices to ensure agreed ways of working are being complied with.

- **provide equipment:** for example, by making available free of charge aprons and gloves for protection against infections (you will learn more about different types of personal protective equipment in AC 4.4). Your employer will need to provide cleaning equipment, such as mops and cleaning agents; provide facilities for the safe disposal of waste, such as used dressings and gloves; provide welfare facilities, such as separate areas for eating and hand washing. If you are working in an individual's home and the individual you are providing care for is also your employer, then the individual will be responsible for providing you with all the necessary equipment you need to carry out your job safely.

Your responsibilities as an employee in infection prevention and control

As an employee, you are responsible for ensuring your work practices are safe and that they protect you, your colleagues and others from infections. As an employee, you have a responsibility to:

- **follow your work setting's agreed ways of working:** for example, by ensuring you read and understand your work setting's infection prevention and control procedures, such as those in relation to food handling and the use and disposal of aprons and gloves. You will also

Evidence opportunity

4.1 Roles and responsibilities

Take it in turns to discuss with your manager, or the most suitable person in your setting, your responsibilities, and theirs, in relation to the prevention and control of infections in your work setting. Produce an information handout with your findings. You will need a witness testimony or recording in order to evidence the discussion.

need to read information updates provided to you by your employer, such as in relation to changes in relevant legislation

- **attend training:** you must ensure that you learn from the training and information provided by your employer about infection prevention and control. You must ensure that you put into your day-to-day working practices the training you have attended

- **record and report:** for example, you must record all infection hazards and risks, such as an overflowing clinical waste bin (see page 358 for definition) that has used dressings or the non-availability of gloves; you must report if you become unwell with an illness such as gastroenteritis, and report all infection hazards and risks immediately.

AC 4.2 Explain the causes and spread of infection in care settings

Infections can make people feel unwell and some are so serious that they can cause people to die.

Table 9.4 The differences between bacteria and viruses

Bacteria	Viruses
Bacteria reproduce in large numbers to cause infections.	Viruses are smaller than bacteria in size and can reproduce in small numbers to cause infections.
Bacteria can multiply outside of the human body.	Viruses can only multiply within the human body.
Bacteria can be treated with antibiotics.	Viruses cannot be treated with antibiotics.
Examples of infections caused by bacteria include: gastroenteritis, tuberculosis, cholera.	Examples of infections caused by viruses include: flu, measles, chicken pox.

Reflect on it

4.2 Infections caused by bacteria and viruses

Reflect on the infections caused by bacteria and viruses named in Table 9.4. Have you or someone you know experienced any of these? What were the symptoms? What treatment was provided?

Research it

4.2 Spread of infection

Research examples of two care settings where the spread of infection was not prevented. Write down what happened and how it affected all those involved in the care setting.

You will find the internet and local newspapers useful sources of information.

What are the causes of infection?

Infections are caused by harmful disease-causing germs referred to as pathogens. Pathogens can be found everywhere, such as inside our bodies and in the air, and they can be spread from person to person. There are many different types of pathogens but the two main types are bacteria and viruses. Bacteria release toxins into our bodies and viruses can damage our bodies' cells which can lead to serious infections. Table 9.4 provides you with some information about each type including the difference between the two.

How can infection spread in care settings?

Care settings are environments where infections can spread easily because:

- **they are places where there are large numbers of people**, some of whom may also be unwell and therefore be carrying an infection, for example an individual who has MRSA, an adult care worker who has gastroenteritis or a visitor with the norovirus. Infections may therefore spread from one person to another in a process called 'cross infection'
- **the work activities that take place are at high risk of carrying infections**, for example,

supporting individuals with care needs involves being in contact with their body fluids. Activities such as assisting individuals with eating, drinking and personal care, handling food, disposing of waste and cleaning areas and equipment can also pose high risks of infection. Infections can also be caused by food that is consumed. Food can become contaminated and infected by bacteria such as *E. coli* and *Salmonella*. This may be due to use of equipment that has not been cleaned properly or bacteria on hands. It may also occur when food is not heated, cooled or cooked properly

- **individuals may be more vulnerable to infections**, for example, older individuals and individuals who are unwell cannot fight off infections as easily as someone who is healthy and well because their bodies' ability to fight off infections has been weakened due to their age or damaged through illness.

Infections can spread in care settings in different ways; such as when you have physical contact with a person who has an infection (e.g. MRSA) or through food that has become contaminated with pathogens (e.g. *Salmonella*), from pathogens present in the air you breathe (e.g. chicken pox) as

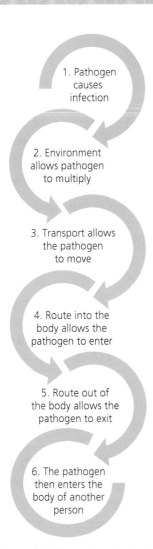

1. Pathogen causes infection

2. Environment allows pathogen to multiply

3. Transport allows the pathogen to move

4. Route into the body allows the pathogen to enter

5. Route out of the body allows the pathogen to exit

6. The pathogen then enters the body of another person

Figure 9.5 The chain of infection

well as through contaminated objects such as bed linen and work surfaces.

Infections spread in care settings through six key stages; these stages are often referred to as the chain of infection and these are identified in Figure 9.5.

This shows that infections can quickly spread from person to person if the conditions are right. For example, the perfect environment for bacteria to grow in is one where there is food and moisture available. This could be in leftover food as well as body fluids, such as urine and faeces. It could be where the temperature is warm and the environment is constant giving the bacteria time to multiply, i.e. in a waste bin that has not been emptied for two days.

Similarly, infections can only spread from person to person if they have transport and a route

through which to enter and exit our bodies, for example, an uncleaned toilet seat or hands that have not been washed (indirect contact) or through coming into contact with an individual's body fluids from coughing or from minor cuts (direct contact).

Preventing spread of infections

In AC 4.3 you will learn about one of the key ways to prevent the spread of infection. However, there are a number of other ways you can prevent the spread of infection. Some of these will be covered in ACs 4.4 and 4.5 but a few things to remember are:

- **Wear protective clothing:** See AC 4.4 for information on personal protective equipment (PPE).

- **Wear gloves:** You will need to ensure you wear gloves when you come into contact with bodily fluids, when you are dealing with broken skin or rashes for example. You will also need to wear them when disposing of waste including soiled bedding or dressings. You will learn more about how to put gloves on in AC 4.4. Where there are serious illnesses or infections like MRSA (see page 350 for definition), you will need to follow your setting's policies and procedures so it is important that you know what these are.

- **Carefully dispose of waste so that you or others do not come into contact with any germs or harmful substances:** You may need to wear gloves and aprons when disposing of waste, and make sure you follow your setting's procedures for doing so. Often there are procedures for disposing of waste in different bags based on whether they are used for dealing with waste that is clinical, soiled or recyclable.

- **Make sure a healthy environment is maintained and equipment is cleaned:** Different individuals and staff may come into contact with equipment (for example, hoists or chairs). Make sure that the setting is working to ensure that equipment is cleaned correctly, and that you are also doing your utmost to do so. Of course, you are not always responsible for this but it is useful to remember this in your practice and look for this in others'. There are also measures placed in the setting to make sure you and others maintain cleanliness, for example through anti-bacterial gel dispensers being placed around the setting so that there are opportunities to clean your hands.

- **Make sure that your health and hygiene does not lead to spread of infection:** See AC 4.5 for more information.

Promoting health and safety in an individual's home

For domiciliary care workers, promoting health and safety in an individual's home is important but there may be other considerations to take into account. For example, in an individual's home you may not have separate waste bins for disposing of household waste (such as paper) and clinical waste (such as used dressings). Effective precautions can still be taken to prevent the spread of infection, for example by ensuring that all waste is placed into a bag and then sealed rather than left open in a black bin bag. There may not be a separate utility area in an individual's home for washing soiled linen; precautions can be taken by ensuring soiled linen is washed separately in the washing machine and on a high setting to destroy any bacteria.

AC 4.3 Demonstrate the recommended method for hand washing in care settings

Preventing the spread of infection can only be done if one or more of the links in the chain of infection you learned about in AC 4.2 are broken; if the chain of infection isn't broken then infections will continue to spread. One of the most effective ways of preventing the spread of infection in care settings is through hand washing.

You must always wash your hands in care settings during your day-to-day work activities because pathogens are likely to be present in the tasks you carry out and can therefore be the cause of infections that can spread.

For example, you must always wash your hands to protect yourself, the individuals and others you work with, as well as the environment, from the spread of germs. You must wash your hands:

- before and after you start work
- before and after contact with individuals who you provide care or support to, i.e. support with eating, drinking, washing
- before putting on and after disposing of gloves
- before preparing and handling food
- before and after eating
- after contact with your own or others' body fluids, or any procedure that means you may come into contact with body fluids
- after going to the toilet
- after coughing or sneezing, or blowing your nose
- after disposing of waste or handling used or soiled linen
- after coming into contact with clinical waste.

The method for hand washing in care settings

The Care Quality Commission recommends that workers in care settings use liquid soap and warm water for washing their hands and that they carry out the following hand-washing techniques for approximately 30 seconds outlined on the NHS's 'Hand hygiene technique for staff' poster (this can be accessed from: www.infectionpreventioncontrol. co.uk/resources/hand-hygiene-technique-for-staff-poster).

Hand-washing technique with soap and water

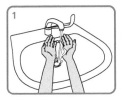

Wet hands
with water

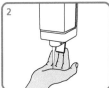

Apply enough soap
to cover all
hand surfaces

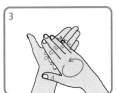

Rub hands palm
to palm

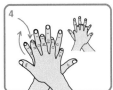

Rub back of each hand
with palm of other hand
with fingers interlaced

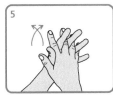

Rub palm to palm with
fingers interlaced

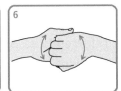

Rub with back of fingers
to opposing palms with
fingers interlocked

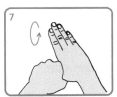

Rub each thumb clasped
in opposite hand using a
rotational movement

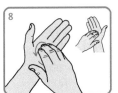

Rub tips of fingers in
opposite palm in a
circular motion

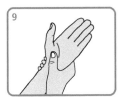

Rub each wrist with
opposite hand

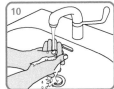

Rinse hands
with water

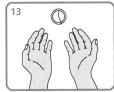

Use elbow to
turn off tap

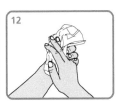

Dry thoroughly with
a single-use towel

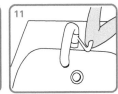

Hand washing should take
15–30 seconds

clean**your**hands
campaign

NHS
*National Patient
Safety Agency*

© Crown copyright 2007 283373 1p 1k Sep07

Adapted from World Health Organization *Guidelines on Hand Hygiene in Health Care*

Figure 9.6 Hand hygiene technique for staff

Research it

4.3 **NHS guidance**

You will also find it useful to refer to the NHS
website for up-to-date guidance on hand hygiene:

www.nhs.uk/Livewell/homehygiene/Pages/
how-to-wash-your-hands-properly.aspx

To summarise:

1&2 Wash your hands under warm running water and apply liquid soap to cover all the hand surfaces.

3 Rub your hands, palm to palm using a circular action.

4 Rub the back of each hand with the palm of the other hand, with fingers interlaced.

5 Rub palm to palm with fingers interlaced.

6 Rub backs of fingers to opposing palms with fingers interlocked.

7 Rub each thumb clasped in opposite hand using a rotational action.

8 Rub tips of fingers in the opposite palm in a circular action.

9 Rub each wrist with the opposite hand.

10 Rinse your hands under warm running water.

11 Use your elbow or a paper towel to turn off the tap.

12 Dry your hands thoroughly with paper towels.

13 Remember that hand washing should take 15-30 seconds.

In addition, it is recommended that staff in care settings also comply with the following hand hygiene practices that are important in the prevention of infections:

- When you provide care to individuals you must roll your sleeves up to the elbows, i.e. this is referred to as Bare Below the Elbows (BBE).
- Jewellery must not be worn i.e. rings, bracelets.
- Finger nails must be kept clean and short.
- Nail extensions, acrylic nails and nail varnish must not be worn.
- Any cuts or abrasions must be covered with a waterproof dressing.

AC 4.4 Demonstrate the use of personal protective equipment (PPE) and when to use it

In care settings, **personal protective equipment (PPE)** refers to the equipment that is worn by adult care workers to protect against the spread of infections. PPE can prevent and control the spread of infections because:

- it protects individuals from infections you may be carrying
- it protects you from infections individuals may be carrying
- it creates a barrier between the infection and you which means that the infection is unable to spread from you to others or vice versa, or from a surface or piece of equipment to you and others; as you have learned, a process known as **cross infection**.

To ensure that you are using PPE appropriately and that it is effective in the spread of infections it is important to:

- read what your work setting's PPE policy states about the different types of PPE you will be using as part of your day-to-day work tasks
- always follow the manufacturer's instructions when using PPE
- always wash your hands before using PPE
- always wash your hands after disposing of PPE.

Table 9.5 describes the two main examples of PPE used in care settings, including the reasons why they are used and examples of when they can be used.

PPE is only an effective tool if you know when to use it and if you know how to put it on and take it off correctly. Table 9.6 provides some guidance on this.

There may be times when PPE is not required. This may, for example, be when you are supporting an individual to get dressed or when supporting an individual living in their own home to prepare a meal.

Key terms

Personal protective equipment (PPE) is equipment that is worn by care workers and is usually disposable to prevent infections from spreading. PPE includes disposable gloves and plastic aprons.

Cross infection is the spread of infection from person to person.

As you have learned earlier on in this unit, the Personal Protective Equipment at Work Regulations 1992 established a set of guidelines for the correct use of PPE in the work setting. You can recap your previous learning from AC 1.1 now.

Table 9.5 Why and when to use PPE

Type of PPE	Why use it	When to use it
Disposable gloves	To provide a barrier for the infections that can be spread through your hands.	For example, when supporting individuals with personal care as you may come into contact with an individual's body fluids, such as vomit, urine and faeces.
		You should wear gloves when dealing with an accident where you may come into contact with an open wound or an individual's body fluids, such as blood and vomit.
		You should also use them when you come into contact with broken skin, rashes or burns for example. When disposing of used or soiled linen or waste, it is also a good idea to wear gloves.
Plastic aprons	To provide a barrier for the infections that can be spread through your clothing.	For example, when handling food as you may come into contact with both cooked and raw foods. You will learn more about food hygiene in practices in LO6.
		You should also wear aprons when carrying out a cleaning task as you may come into contact with a harmful substance. You will learn more about hazardous substances in LO6. You will also need this when coming into contact with bodily fluids.

Table 9.6 How to use PPE

Type of PPE	How to put it on	How to take it off
Disposable gloves	Choose the correct size gloves. If they are too big they may slip off and if they are too small they may tear and let harmful pathogens spread. Wash your hands before putting gloves on so you do not spread harmful pathogens into your gloves.	Remove one glove at a time. Hold the outside of the glove carefully with your opposite gloved hand and, once removed, place it in your gloved hand. Then remove the other glove placing your finger tip on the inside of the top of the glove and remove it without touching the outer surface of the glove. Place them in the **clinical waste bin**. Wash and dry your hands to avoid cross infection (see page 357 for definition), i.e. the infection being passed from the outside of the gloves to your hands and to the surrounding environment.
Plastic aprons	Place the apron over your head and then tie it round your waist to give you maximum protection over any harmful pathogens that may be transported to and from your clothing. Wash your hands before putting plastic aprons on so you do not spread harmful pathogens into your gloves.	Unfasten or break the ties round the waist and then remove the apron by pulling it away from your neck and only touching the inside of the apron while doing so. Roll up the apron and place it in the clinical waste bin. Wash and dry your hands to avoid cross infection from the outside of your apron to your hands and to the environment.

Key term

A **clinical waste bin** is where waste that is contaminated with body fluids (for example used dressings, bandages and disposable gloves) is disposed of as it poses a risk of infection. These are usually located in bathrooms and laundry areas.

Ensure PPE is effective

Disposable gloves and aprons must be changed every time there is contact with a different individual or when there is a change in task, for example supporting the individual with washing and then with eating and drinking. It is also important that you check all PPE; that it is clean and has no tears before wearing it as this may be an opening for a harmful pathogen to enter and cause infection. If you do find any problems with it, do not use it, report this immediately to your manager who will be able to provide you with advice and guidance.

Reflect on it

4.4 Consequences of not using PPE correctly

Reflect on the consequences of not changing your disposable gloves and apron when you have finished supporting an individual to have a shower. What are the consequences for the individual? For you? For others in the care setting where you work? Write a short reflective account detailing your thoughts.

Research it

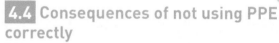

4.4 Your setting's PPE policy

Research what the PPE policy in your work setting says about the different types of PPE you must use as part of your day-to-day work tasks, how to use them, and when and how to report any difficulties you may identify. Discuss with your manager; think about why they are used and when. Write down details of your discussion.

Reflective exemplar	
Introduction	I work as a personal assistant to Joan who requires support with showering, dressing and preparing breakfast. Joan has **cerebral palsy** and finds it difficult to mobilise.
What happened?	This morning I visited Joan as usual and she told me that she wanted to speak with me. I sat down next to her as she explained that she no longer thinks there is any need for me to wear disposable gloves and an apron while I provide care and support to her in the mornings, given that I have been her personal assistant for over a year now and have got to know her very well. Joan added that she would feel a lot more relaxed if I didn't wear these in her home.
	I informed Joan that I was required to follow my work setting's PPE policy and would therefore always have to wear them when providing her with care and support.
	Joan frowned and explained that she didn't feel like getting up this morning and would prefer it if I came back tomorrow. I agreed to come back tomorrow.
What worked well?	The fact that I informed Joan that I have to comply with my work setting's PPE policy.
What did not go as well?	Joan's reaction to the information I gave her, i.e. she does not usually frown.
What could I do to improve?	Perhaps I should have explained the reasons why I must wear PPE to Joan.
	Perhaps I should have referred Joan's request to my manager. The use of PPE could then have been risk assessed with Joan and the work setting to address how to balance her rights with concerns for health and safety.
	I think I need to discuss this situation with my manager and refer back to my work setting's PPE policy in relation to what it says about wearing PPE when an individual asks for it not to be used.
Links to unit assessment criteria	ACs 1.3, 1.5, 2.1, 2.2, 2.3, 4.1, 4.2

Evidence opportunity

4.4 Using personal protective equipment (PPE)

You will be observed for AC 4.4. Practise putting on and disposing of two different types of PPE that you use in your work setting. Ask your assessor for feedback. How did you do? Are there any areas for improvement?

The reflective exemplar provides you with an opportunity to explore in more detail how adult care workers in care settings can seek further support and advice when they are having difficulties complying with their work setting's PPE policy.

Key term

Cerebral palsy is a condition that affects movement and co-ordination, for example, symptoms can include jerky uncontrolled movements, stiff and floppy arms or legs.

AC 4.5 Demonstrate ways to ensure that own health and hygiene do not pose a risk to others at work

Care settings, as you have learned, are perfect environments for the spread of infections. You therefore have an important role to play in the prevention and spread of infections.

Your health

When you are carrying out your work activities, it is crucial that you are in good health to do so. Being in good health means having both physical and mental well-being; you will learn more about

Research it

4.5 Sickness policy

Research your sickness policy in the work setting where you work. Discuss with your manager what types of infections you must report, the reasons why and the procedures for doing so.

how to manage your mental well-being later on in LO10. Mental well-being is crucial for ensuring that you are able to comply with your work setting's infection control procedures.

Physically, it is also important that you are well and able to carry out your work activities; coming into work when you are not well and able can pose a risk to the individuals you work with as well as to your colleagues and other visitors to the care setting. For example:

- If you have the flu it is important you visit your GP and do not return to work until you are well as doing so may mean that you spread your infection onto others.

- If you have gastroenteritis you are most infectious from when your symptoms start until two days after they have passed; it is important therefore to stay off work until your symptoms have stopped for two days.

- If you have a skin rash it is important that you visit your GP and do not return to work until you have been given permission to do so; as this may be passed onto others and therefore can lead to the spread of infections.

Your personal hygiene

Maintaining your personal hygiene to a good standard is not only more pleasant for everyone you come into contact with but it is also an essential part of the control of infection. As you have learned, hand washing and wearing PPE are integral to ensuring that you prevent the spread of infection and are two key aspects involved in maintaining good standards of personal hygiene. Other important aspects of your personal hygiene for controlling the spread of infections include the following.

- **Hair care:** your hair must be regularly washed, brushed and kept clean to prevent infections,

such as head lice. If you have long hair it should be tied back to prevent any unwanted hairs from falling into, for example, food that you are preparing. Your hair may also come into contact with individuals which could lead to the spread of infection and could also be a hazard as it may become caught in equipment or machinery. Likewise, if you wear a head scarf, or head covering, ensure that it is safely tied or in place.

- **Hand and nail care:** your nails must be kept clean and short. Nail varnish and nail extensions must not be worn as these may flake and/or fall off while carrying out your work activities and therefore have the potential to spread any harmful pathogens that they contain. Similarly as you learned about previously, jewellery such as rings and bracelets can also be potential risks of infection as harmful pathogens may become trapped in these. Good hand hygiene, as you have learned, is essential in your role and is also essential when preparing food. See Research it activity 4.5 on page 361 to learn more about the importance of hygiene when preparing food. Remember that food can be a source of infection if hygiene procedures are not followed.

- **Oral care:** you must brush your teeth regularly to avoid infections, such as halitosis, that can cause bad breath.

- **Body care:** you must wash, bathe or shower every day, wear clean clothes and deodorant to ensure that you prevent body odour and the risk of infections to others.

- **Skin care:** your skin must be kept moisturised because with frequent hand washing it is likely to become dry and could therefore flake off during work activities and spread infections. If your skin has open wounds or you have a skin rash then it is important to keep open wounds covered over and to treat all skin rashes to avoid the risk of cross infection.

- **Clothing/uniform:** you must wash the clothes you wear at work and/or uniform regularly so it is kept clean and pathogen free. Wearing an apron will protect the front/outside of your clothes from harmful pathogens. Remember that if you wear your uniform outside of the work setting that you may be at risk of cross infection, for example if visiting the supermarket during your lunch break or travelling home from work on the bus. In these situations, it may be better to change into and out of your uniform at work. In this way you will ensure that your clothing and uniform do not spread infections from person to person and place to place.

Research it

4.5 The importance of food hygiene

Food can be a source of infection if it is not cooked properly or if you do not follow good hygiene practice. You should remember the things that you have learned in this LO as well as this unit when preparing food. Hand hygiene is key; for example, you should remember that if you have a cut, then you should cover this with a bright plaster that can be easily spotted if it does come off while you are preparing food and can be disposed of. It is important that you are aware of how to avoid infection and cross-contamination, how to cook food properly to avoid this from happening, how to ensure that bacteria from food is killed, and the health and safety rules to follow.

You will also need to be aware of best before dates, allergies and special dietary requirements and the rules to follow when preparing food to cater for different requirements.

Below are some useful sources of information that you should read with regard to food safety:

www.gov.uk/food-safety-your-responsibilities/food-hygiene

www.food.gov.uk/business-guidance/food-hygiene-for-your-business

www.food.gov.uk

www.foodsafety.gov

Evidence opportunity

4.5 Your health and hygiene

You will be observed for AC 4.5. Demonstrate to your assessor two or three different ways of ensuring that your health and hygiene do not pose a risk to others in the care setting where you work. Follow up your demonstration with a professional discussion with your assessor.

LO4 Knowledge, skills, behaviours
Knowledge: what roles and responsibilities do you and your employer have in the prevention and control of infection?
Do you know the causes of infections in care settings and how they can spread?
Do you know how to report and record infection hazards and risks?
Do you know the type of information your employer provides in relation to preventing and controlling the spread of infections in the care setting where you work?
Did you know that you have just shown your knowledge of how the responsibility for reducing the spread of infection in care settings is shared between the employer and employees?

➜

LO4 Knowledge, skills, behaviours
Skills: how can your practices reduce the spread of infection in the care setting where you work?
Do you know how to use the recommended method for hand washing after supporting an individual with personal care?
Do you know when and how to dispose of used disposable gloves?
Do you know how to work in ways that do not pose a risk of infection to others?
Did you know that you have just demonstrated some of the skills required for being able to prevent and reduce the spread of infections?
Behaviours: how can you show the personal qualities you have for reducing the spread of infection in care settings?
Do you know how to sensitively tell a colleague about their strong body odour or sensitively critique their personal hygiene?
Do you know how to explain in a kind manner to an individual the reasons why you must wear PPE when assisting them with their care?
Did you know that you have just demonstrated a few of the essential behaviours required when reducing the spread of infections?

LO5 Be able to move and handle equipment and objects safely

Getting started

Think about the different steps involved in moving yourself or items from one position to another. For example, you could think about how you move from sitting in a chair to lying down in bed, how you move when walking from one end of the corridor to the other or how you move a heavy boxed item that has been delivered to your front door upstairs. Think about the different range of movements you perform when carrying out these tasks.

Now imagine you need support with moving or positioning; how would you explain to someone who didn't know you how to support you?

AC 5.1 Identify legislation that relates to moving and handling

Moving and handling in care settings involves providing support to individuals to be able to move from one position to another as well as being able to handle lifting, moving and positioning equipment, such as hoists, slings, bath lifts, standing transfer aids, and other objects, such as wheelchairs and boxes, safely.

Moving and positioning individuals safely is required for ensuring that:

- individuals are being supported to move and position in line with their plan of care and their specific needs

- individuals do not experience pain or distress
- individuals' independence and dignity are promoted
- the agreed ways of working, policies and procedures that are in place in care settings are being complied with.

Policies and procedures

Agreed ways of working for moving and positioning individuals safely are underpinned by specific legislation that relates to moving and handling so that it is carried out safely and accidents can be avoided. Complying with legal requirements will ensure that you protect yourself, individuals and others from injuries and/or accidents. This might prevent back injuries, which can occur if you do not use equipment correctly, or falls which could happen if you do not check that the equipment used is appropriate for the individual.

Moving and handling is required for various activities – it may be that you need to use these procedures for tasks such as moving and lifting boxes, or you may need to move people. It may be that you require special equipment to carry out the moving and handling procedure. You may, for example, require a **sling**. In this case, you can check that the sling being used is appropriate for the individual being hoisted. You will need to check this in relation to the weight, height and shape of the individual as well as whether the individual requires support with their whole body including their head or just with the trunk of their body and whether their condition causes them pain. Remember that slings come in different sizes and shapes and are made out of different materials depending on what the individual requires to be comfortable and maintain their dignity when being hoisted. Individuals with profound and multiple disabilities may require you to use adapted techniques with them such as signs (to involve them during the whole process), adapted equipment and slings.

The following are examples of specific pieces of legislation that relate to moving and handling activities and come under the Health and Safety at Work Act (HASAWA) 1974.

Manual Handling Operations Regulations 1992 (as amended 2002)

These regulations are relevant to moving and handling activities and include lifting, lowering, pushing, pulling and carrying. They require that employers must:

- avoid, as far as is reasonably practicable, any manual handling activity that is hazardous and likely to involve a risk of injury

Key term

Sling refers to the piece of equipment made out of fabric that is placed around the individual's body to enable them to be hoisted.

- carry out a risk assessment of all manual handling activities that cannot be avoided and put control measures in place to reduce the risk of injury*
- provide any equipment necessary for supporting health and safety.

*A manual handling assessment involves five key aspects which can be easily remembered using the TILE (O) acronym:

- **T** – Task (what am I lifting and where am I moving the load to?)
- **I** – Individual (am I capable of lifting the load safely on my own?)
- **L** – Load (how heavy is the load? what shape and size is the load?)
- **E** – Environment (is the load in a small space? Will it be difficult to lift?)
- **O** – Other aspects (do I need to wear PPE?).

As an employee you also have moving and handling responsibilities including:

- maintaining your own safety and those of individuals and others who you work with
- attending moving and handling training provided by your employer
- only carrying out moving and handling activities that you have been trained in
- complying with your work setting's moving and handling procedures and agreed ways of working at all times
- reporting and recording all hazardous moving and handling activities.

Provision and Use of Work Equipment Regulations (PUWER) 1998

These regulations require that all work equipment including moving and handling equipment is used safely. They require that employers must provide moving and handling equipment that is:

- suitable for the intended use
- maintained in a safe condition
- monitored to ensure it is in good working order*
- used only by people who have been trained in its use

- accompanied by suitable health and safety measures, such as emergency stop controls and clearly visible markings
- used in line with the manufacturer's instructions.

*If a risk assessment shows that those handling the equipment are at risk, then employers must make sure that this is checked. Advice can also be sought from the health and safety officer and the manufacturers of the equipment.

Lifting Operations and Lifting Equipment Regulations (LOLER) 1998

These regulations require employers to ensure that lifting equipment used in work settings is safe by requiring that:

- all lifting equipment is used solely for the purpose it was intended for, it must be installed correctly to ensure to reduce any risks
- all lifting equipment is marked with warning and safety signs to show safe working loads
- all lifting equipment is maintained and monitored for safety and records kept (all equipment used must be safe. It must be monitored and examined regularly, not just when defects are reported, to ensure its safety is maintained)
- all lifting equipment that is unsafe is reported and removed from use until it is repaired or replaced and safe to use again
- all lifting activities are planned, supervised and carried out in a safe manner (that it is only by people who have been trained and are able).

Although it is not mentioned as part of LOLER, you should remember that, as an employee, you are responsible for complying with all information, instruction and training you have received from your employer in relation to moving and handling, and to use all equipment you have been trained in safely and in line with the manufacturer's instructions. If you identify that a piece of equipment is faulty then you must report this immediately to your employer and not use it.

AC 5.2 Explain principles for moving and handling equipment and other objects safely

In care settings there is a wide range of moving and handling equipment that is used to meet the diverse needs of the individuals who require support with moving and positioning. This includes:

- **lifting equipment**, such as mobile hoists that lift and lower individuals from, for example, their bed to an armchair and bath hoists that lift and lower individuals into and out of the bath
- **moving and handling equipment**, such as slide sheets that move individuals without lifting them up and down the bed and transfer boards that enable individuals to slide from their wheelchair into an armchair, for example
- **moving and handling aids**, such as hand rails that provide support to individuals going up steps or walking frames that support individuals' weight while walking.

You can use moving and handling equipment safely and move other objects safely by following these good practice rules or principles:

- Follow your work setting's agreed ways of working for moving and handling, for example by only carrying out moving and handling activities that you have been trained for. Not doing so may mean that you or others may get injured.
- Ensure you have read the moving and handling guidelines that are in place for individuals. For example, read through individuals' moving and handling risk assessments before carrying out moving and handling activities or using any moving and handling equipment to ensure the safety and well-being of individuals.
- Complete safety checks before using moving and handling equipment. For example, is it clean? Is it working? Have you noticed any faults? Not doing so may result in a serious failure in the equipment as you are using it which may then cause unnecessary distress to an individual.
- Prepare to move an object safely by completing safety checks, for example, is there enough space in the environment to carry out the move? Is the load too heavy for one person? Not doing so may mean that you will be putting yourself, the individuals and others in danger and at risk of being harmed or injured.
- Report any concerns you have when carrying out health and safety checks. For example, you should report if a piece of equipment is not working and if you witness a colleague using unsafe practices when moving an individual using lifting equipment. Not doing so may mean that unsafe equipment and practices continue in the work setting. Also think about some of the stories you may have read about where individuals have been left in their beds and are unable to move because no assistance has been provided. There have been bans in some organisations on lifting. If you see such practice, it is important to discuss or report this to your manager.
- Always communicate clearly with those involved in moving and handling activities. For example: explain to the individual how you are

---

Research it

5.2 Moving and handling equipment

Research the different types of moving and handling equipment, lifting equipment and moving and handling aids that are used with the individuals in the care setting where you work. Produce a one-page information handout with your findings.

Reflect on it

5.2 Health and safety checks

Reflect on the importance of carrying out health and safety checks before using moving and handling equipment and moving objects in care settings. How can doing so prevent accidents from occurring?

Communication

Good communication when moving and handling is essential for reassuring individuals during moves and for ensuring that you have their permission to carry out the move. Remember the principles of person-centred care that you have learned about. Remember that this is a joint procedure. Good communication enables you to ensure individuals' understanding of how the move will be carried out and it also encourages their active participation, and means that you have considered their rights. Good communication with your colleagues is also essential for ensuring that you work together to enable all moves are carried out smoothly.

5.2 Principles for moving and handling

For each of the principles you learned about in relation to moving and handling equipment, discuss with your assessor their importance for health and safety. Remember to consider how the principles can keep you, individuals and others safe.

AC 5.3 Demonstrate how to move and handle equipment and objects safely

In care settings, moving and handling activities are part of adult care workers' day-to-day work activities. The techniques used involve the use of moving and handling equipment to safely transfer individuals with care or support needs from one position to another as well as following the general principles you learned about in AC 5.2 for moving objects safely.

Expressing the total number of musculoskeletal disorder cases in the Health and Social Care sector as a rate, the HSE statistics show that:

'Annually around 1.7% (per 100,000 workers) workers in the sector were suffering from a musculoskeletal disorder they believed was work-related.

This rate is statistically significantly higher than the rate across all industries (1.3%)'

Health and Safety Executive (2015) 'Health and Safety in the Health and Social Care sector in Great Britain 2014/15' (source: Labour Force Survey)

going to support them with the move, check that the individual is not in any pain and that their dignity is not undermined in any way, encourage the individual to actively participate in the move and check with your colleagues which of you is going to take the lead with carrying out the move. Not communicating with the individual will be disrespectful towards individuals' rights to be actively involved in all care and support activities. Poor **communication** between you and colleagues may result in moves becoming unsafe.

- Use a safe posture when moving objects. For example, keep your legs and feet slightly apart, your knees slightly bent, do not stoop or twist, keep the load as close to your body as possible. Not doing so could result in you injuring your back and at worse this may mean that you may cause your body irreversible damage and result in you experiencing distress.

- Be honest with yourself. For example, if you are unsure about how to follow any of the above principles, seek advice from your manager and discuss these. Not doing so could result in you not complying with best practice and therefore not promoting your health, safety and well-being as well as that of the individuals and colleagues you work alongside.

Using moving and handling equipment safely

Using moving and handling equipment is a skill and to do it safely so that accidents and injuries to yourself, individuals and your colleagues do not happen, you must:

- **be trained in its safe use**: your employer is required to provide you with the training to do so

- **follow your work setting's moving and handling procedures**: you are required to comply with the safe processes your employer has developed for all moving and handling activities that you carry out. For example, this may involve using the type of equipment appropriate for an individual, in line with their height, weight and condition. You may need to use a piece of equipment to move an individual with two staff instead of one

- **check that the equipment is safe to use**: you are required to do this every time you use a piece of moving and handling equipment. For example, you will need to check the battery is fully charged (not doing so may result in it stopping from working during a move), that there is no visible signs of wear and tear and that it has been tested as per legal requirements

- **check that the equipment is clean**: you are required to do this every time you use a piece of moving and handling equipment. Not only will this reduce the risk of cross infection (a concept you learned about in LO4) but it is also showing your respect and consideration for the individuals you are assisting with moving.

Moving objects safely

From time to time adult care workers may need to move objects in care settings from one position to another. For example, boxes of PPE may be delivered to the front door and may need to be moved into the first aid room or a delivery of groceries may be made that needs to be moved into the kitchen. Moving objects safely is also a skill and using the techniques below will help you with this.

- **Plan how you are going to carry out the move**: for example, consider whether you will need assistance to do so, where you need to move the object to and ensure you have prepared the route you plan to use.

- **Ensure you are in a stable position before carrying out the move**: for example, your feet should be apart to maintain your balance and you should avoid wearing footwear with no support or tight clothing that make it difficult to move in safely.

- **Ensure you are in a safe position when handling the object**: for example, keep and hold the object close to your body, do not stoop when lifting the object, keep your knees, hips and back slightly bent, keep your shoulders facing in the same direction as the hips, keep your head up and look ahead and then put the object down in a smooth movement by keeping hold of it until it reaches the surface you want it on (i.e. the ground, table) and only then slide the object into its desired position.

Moving and handling legislation does not indicate what is a safe maximum weight limit that can be lifted by a person. Instead, as you have learned in AC 5.1, it places legal duties on employers to risk assess all manual handling activities and situations including the person who will be carrying out the move, such as in terms of their physical strength and whether they have any health condition that may affect them. In other words it is always best to be safe than sorry when moving and handling! If in doubt, ask your manager to ensure your practice remains safe.

Moving and handling in an individual's home

Equipment such as hoists may be difficult to operate in an individual's home where the space is confined, for example there may be a small bathroom where it may be difficult to manoeuvre. Where possible, risk assessments must take into account the size of equipment and the room available – for instance, two people may be more appropriate to support an individual to mobilise than a large piece of equipment. In all cases you must not put yourself, the individual, or your colleagues at risk. If you have any concerns, do not carry out any actions that you deem to be unsafe.

Evidence opportunity

5.3 Move and handle equipment and objects safely

You will be observed in the workplace for AC 5.3 on how to do the following.

In pairs, show how to:

1 safely use a piece of moving and handling equipment safely, for example a hoist or bath lift
2 safely move an object, for example a box of first aid supplies or stationery.

Case study

5.2, 5.3 Using moving and handling equipment

Jan, a care worker in a residential care home, is assisting May who is 84 years old with having a bath this morning. As it has been a very busy morning, Jan is running a little late and May is not happy that she will be having her bath a little later on than she usually does.

Once Jan agrees with May to assist her to have a bath, Jan carefully reads through May's care plan and moving and handling guidelines. This is to ensure that there have not been any changes to May's care needs and to the moving and handling equipment used to assist her with moving in and out of the bath.

Once Jan has prepared the bathroom and assisted May to prepare herself, Jan supports May to sit in the bath lift. As Jan begins to operate the bath lift so that May can get in the bath, the lift stops working.

Questions

1 How could this situation have been prevented?
2 What equipment checks could have been done?
3 What impact did this situation have on May?

LO5 Knowledge, skills, behaviours
Knowledge: what legal requirements are in place for moving and handling?
Do you know what your employer's responsibility is in relation to moving and handling activities in your work setting?
Do you know what the principles are for moving and handling?
Do you know how moving and handling equipment is maintained in a safe condition?
Do you know why it is important that lifting equipment should only be used for its intended use?
Did you know that you have just shown your knowledge of the three main pieces of moving and handling legislation; the Manual Handling Operations Regulations 1992 (amended 2002), the Provision and Use of Work Equipment Regulations (1999) and the Lifting Operations and Lifting Equipment Regulations (1998)?

→

LO5 Knowledge, skills, behaviours
Skills: how can you show best practice in moving and handling equipment and objects?
Do you know how to plan all moving and handling activities?
Do you know how to position yourself when lifting an object and moving it from one position to another?
Do you know how safe practices can reduce the risk of accidents and injuries?
Did you know that you have just demonstrated some of the skills required for safe moving and handling of equipment and objects?
Behaviours: how can you show the personal qualities you have for moving and handling equipment and objects?
Do you know how to use good communication with an individual during a move?
Do you know how to pay careful attention to your body movements and posture when moving an object?
Did you know that you have just demonstrated a few of the essential behaviours required for the safe use of moving and handling equipment and objects?

LO6 Know how to handle hazardous substances and materials

Getting started

Look around your home and see how many substances and materials you can find that may cause you to become unwell if you come into contact with them. Why are they potentially dangerous? What impact could they have on your health? Why? You could also discuss your findings with a colleague and see if there are any others that you might not have thought about.

AC 6.1 Describe hazardous substances and materials that may be found in the work setting

Care settings are the types of environments where **hazardous substances** and **hazardous materials** can be found and therefore it is very important that you know what these are so that you can carry out your duty to promote your own, individuals' and others' safety in the care setting where you work.

Hazardous substances and materials can come in different forms such as liquids, sprays and powder. In a care setting, care workers are likely to encounter these in everyday products such as cleaning detergents, medication and bodily fluids.

Key terms

Hazardous substances are substances that have the potential to cause harm and illness to others, for example cleaning detergents, medication, acids and bodily fluids such as blood and urine.

Hazardous materials are materials that have the potential to cause harm and illness to others, for example used dressings or PPE that has come into contact with body fluids.

The Control of Substances Hazardous to Health Regulations 2002 (COSHH) that you learned about in AC 1.1 classify hazardous substances into different types depending on the dangers they pose, i.e. toxic, very toxic, corrosive, harmful or irritant.

Research it

6.1 COSHH Regulations 2002 and labels

Research the COSHH Regulations 2002 and find out the meanings of the classifications of different types of hazardous substances. Produce a poster with your findings.

Then do some further research into the different symbols, and find out why they are hazardous and dangerous. You should also find out what the abbreviations for these are. There is more information in AC 6.2.

Evidence opportunity

6.1 Hazardous substances and materials

Find examples of the hazardous substances and materials that there are in your work setting. For each one, write down what type they are and the potential dangers they pose.

Reflect on it

6.1 Protecting individuals

Reflect on the different ways you could protect individuals in your care setting from the dangers of the hazardous substances and materials you identified as being present in the care setting where you work.

AC 6.2 Explain safe practices for storing and using hazardous substances and disposing of hazardous substances and materials

Hazardous substances and materials, such as cleaning fluids, medication, bodily fluids and used dressings, have the potential to cause harm and illness to others when stored, used or disposed of incorrectly. This is why the COSHH Regulations 2002 require your employer to have in place procedures for safely storing, using and disposing of hazardous materials and substances.

Below are some examples of the safe practices to follow.

When storing hazardous substances (such as cleaning fluids and medication) check:

- **where they are being stored:** the temperature and ventilation of the area need to be checked by you and your employer. Some cleaning substances can be highly flammable and therefore must be kept in an area that is cool and well-ventilated
- **how they are being stored:** whether they are being stored in line with the manufacturer's instructions needs to be checked. Hazardous substances need to be stored in their original containers as supplied by the manufacturer, labelled correctly and with their safety lids on and closed. This is so that individuals in care settings do not accidentally mistake them for a drink and swallow them. The COSHH file in your setting will tell you about how to store these substances

Research it

6.2 Safe practices

Go to www.hse.gov.uk/coshh/basics.htm for more information on COSHH. This requires that all employers control hazardous substances.

You should also go to www.healthyworkinglives.com/advice/workplace-hazards/hazardous-substances to find out more information on safe handling, use and storage of hazardous substances in the workplace.

Make notes to detail what you learned.

- **the precautions to take:** you will need to check whether the necessary storage precautions have been taken, for example you will need to ensure cleaning substances and medication have been stored in secure and appropriate areas. This is because doing so could avoid any outbreaks of fires or illnesses. Make sure that you do not change the labels, and also that you do not use the same container for storing another hazardous substance.

When using hazardous substances (such as cleaning fluids and medication) check:

- **the label:** always remember that before you use a hazardous substance, you should check the label for the hazard symbol. You will then need to check the COSHH file to find out about what precautions you need to take and then follow the procedures that have been laid out here by your setting.

- **how to use them:** you need to check whether PPE must be worn. For some hazardous substances, disposable gloves may need to be worn because if they come into contact with your skin they may cause a skin rash or, worse still, burns

- **the techniques to use:** you need to make sure the techniques you use are safe. Some cleaning substances must be diluted before they are used, others must not. Similarly, for medication, this should not be left unattended as doing so may mean that individuals may swallow it or even pass it on to others; this in turn may result in illnesses and even fatalities

- **the precautions to take:** using warning signs to alert others of the dangers when preparing to use a hazardous substance is important so that you are not interrupted while doing so or distracted from the task. In other words, you should alert others beforehand and also alert them just before you are preparing to use the hazardous substance. Remember to report any incorrect labels, containers and lids to your manager, and also if you see anyone else

using these substances incorrectly or in a dangerous way.

When disposing of hazardous substances and materials (such as cleaning fluids, medication, used dressings and PPE with body fluids) check:

- **where to dispose of them:** the location will vary depending on what the waste is. For example, clinical waste that contains body fluids must be disposed of separately to general waste otherwise cross infection may be caused; the bags must be labelled and the labels must say what they contain; sharps must be disposed of separately in a sharps box where they cannot cause an accidental injury, they must be sealed and, like the clinical waste, will be incinerated; leftover cleaning fluids must be disposed of in a separate utility area where they cannot cause any harm. You will need to make sure that you know all the different types of waste and how to dispose of each one safely, including how to label them, especially because you will not be the last person to handle these. Someone else will then have to handle the bags and containers. It is therefore important for their safety as well

- **the techniques to use:** you must know how to dispose of hazardous substances and materials safely. For example, you must wash your hands afterwards; you must wear gloves and aprons that prevent pathogens from transferring from hazardous activities such as handling waste; you should wear a face mask when coming into contact with body fluids or hazardous substances. This will prevent pathogens present in, for example, body fluids from entering into the body through, for example, the eyes or mouth

- **the precautions to take:** you should check whether all necessary precautions for the disposal of hazardous waste have been taken, i.e. so as to avoid accidents, injuries and cross infection.

Your setting should have a COSHH file that should include clear information on hazardous substances. This will include where they are kept, how they are labelled, the effects they have, the maximum exposure you can have to them whilst staying safe, and what to do if there is an emergency involving any one of them.

Safe practice when working in an individual's home

In an individual's home, cleaning materials may be in a 'downstairs' or kitchen cupboard instead of being locked away. Always return any cleaning materials you use to their appropriate location; again if you feel these may pose a risk to either the individual or someone else who visits their home such as a child, then share your concerns with the individual so the appropriate action can be taken.

Research it

6.2 COSHH file

Find out from your manager where the COSHH file is kept in your work setting and the information it contains in relation to storing, using and disposing of hazardous substances and materials. Discuss the key points with your manager.

Does it mention how to store these substances? Does it mention when and in which situations you may need to handle these substances? How about the length of time that people should be exposed to these substances? How about the PPE you must wear when handling these substances?

Good practice when dealing with hazardous substances

The Health and Safety Executive's website includes a list of points to follow for good practice in the control of substances hazardous to health. They have been included here but you should go to their website to research these further:

www.hse.gov.uk/coshh/detail/goodpractice. htm

1 Design and operate processes and activities to minimise emission, release and spread of substances hazardous to health.
2 Take into account all relevant routes of exposure – inhalation, skin and ingestion – when developing control measures.
3 Control exposure by measures that are proportionate to the health risk.

4 Choose the most effective and reliable control options that minimise the escape and spread of substances hazardous to health.
5 Where adequate control of exposure cannot be achieved by other means, provide, in combination with other control measures, suitable personal protective equipment.
6 Check and review regularly all elements of control measures for their continuing effectiveness.
7 Inform and train all employees on the hazards and risks from substances with which they work, and the use of control measures developed to minimise the risks.
8 Ensure that the introduction of measures to control exposure does not increase the overall risk to health and safety.

Disposal of waste

Research the following waste products and find out how each of these needs to be disposed of. This is important as not disposing of these correctly can lead to illness and infections:

- clinical waste such as dressings
- soiled bedding
- soiled clothing
- recyclable equipment and other instruments
- bodily fluids
- syringes, needles, sharps.

You could go to the following webpage to find out more about these:

www.hse.gov.uk/healthservices/healthcare-waste.htm

Reflect on it

6.2 Consequences

Reflect on the consequences of not following safe practices for storing, using and disposing of hazardous substances.

Evidence opportunity

6.2 Safe practices

Produce an information leaflet that explains:

1. Two hazardous substances that are present in your work setting. Explain safe practices for their storage, use and disposal.
2. Two hazardous materials that are present in your work setting. Explain safe practices for their disposal.

LO6 Knowledge, skills, behaviours
Knowledge: what are hazardous substances and materials?
Do you know how hazardous substances are classified?
Do you know the dangers posed by hazardous substances and materials?
Do you know what the safe practices for storing and using hazardous substances are?
Do you know what the safe practices for disposing of hazardous substances and materials are?
Did you know that you have just shown your knowledge of the COSHH Regulations 2002?
Skills: do you know how to handle hazardous substances and materials?
Do you know how to store, use and dispose of hazardous substances and materials safely?
Do you know the checks to carry out when storing hazardous substances and the reasons why?
Do you know how to prepare yourself when using hazardous materials including the PPE to use and why?
Do you know how to dispose of used dressings safely?
Did you know that you have just demonstrated some of the skills required for the safe handling of hazardous substances and materials?
Behaviours: how can you show the personal qualities you have for the safe handling of hazardous substances and materials?
Do you know how to thoroughly read the manufacturers' instructions for hazardous materials?
Do you know how to show your competence when disposing of clinical waste?
Did you know that you have just demonstrated a few of the essential behaviours required for the safe storage, use and disposal of hazardous substances and materials?

LO7 Understand how to promote fire safety in the work setting

Getting started

Read the article about the Cheshunt care home fire that left two dead and 33 people in need of rescue:

www.bbc.co.uk/news/uk-england-39540401

What were your immediate reactions and why?

AC 7.1 Describe practices that prevent fires from starting and spreading

Practices that prevent fires from starting

As a care worker, it is important that you know how to prevent fires from starting as well as the correct actions to take to prevent fires from spreading and causing even more danger and harm.

A fire can only start if it has all three of the following: oxygen (present in the air and can be given off by some chemicals), fuel (any item that can burn, i.e. a solid, liquid or gas) and heat (the cause of the fire such as an unattended cigarette or equipment that has overheated or a trailing electrical wire).

A fire will not start if precautions are taken and safe working practices are followed. These include:

- ensuring that all hazardous materials that may be flammable are stored securely, for example in a locked fireproof cupboard

- ensuring that all hazardous materials that are flammable are kept to a minimum, for example by using non-flammable hazardous materials instead

- ensuring that items that may cause fires are removed and controlled, for example by assessing the risks of individuals smoking and putting in control measures, reporting immediately all defects with electrical equipment

- ensuring that safe working practices are used, and there is regular testing of fire safety equipment such as smoke detectors that can alert you to any fires that may be starting. You will also need to ensure you assess any hazards and risks that any activities, such as cooking, may pose.

Remember that it is good practice to remain vigilant. Be aware of electrical equipment that may cause a fire hazard, and ensure that people do not smoke inside the building or in an unsafe area. Obviously this will vary if you work in the individual's home but it is good practice to ensure that you are aware of fire hazards.

The gov.uk website also offers some guidance on fire safety in the workplace. They suggest a five step fire risk assessment:

1 Identify the fire hazards

2 Identify people at risk

3 Evaluate, remove or reduce the risks

4 Record your findings, prepare an emergency plan and provide training

5 Review and update the fire risk assessment regularly.

You can find out more about these at: www.gov.uk/workplace-fire-safety-your-responsibilities/fire-risk-assessments

Practices that prevent fires from spreading

If a fire does start in your work setting it is very important that you follow your work setting's procedures so that you do not put yourself, individuals or others in danger or at risk. You will also have received training from your employer in fire safety and have practised what to do in the event of a fire.

There are a number of practices that you can follow that can prevent fires from spreading and therefore minimise the danger, harm and damage that fires can cause. You can find out more information about these practices in your work setting's fire safety procedures, for example:

- by ensuring fitted smoke detectors, fire alarms, sprinklers and fire extinguishers are maintained and are in good working order. This is to ensure they work effectively when a fire starts. You can do this by testing them. You should report any defects you or others notice

- by ensuring smoke detectors and sprinklers are not obstructed with items that are piled up underneath them to ensure they work effectively when a fire starts. You can do this by completing health and safety checks on a regular basis

- by ensuring windows and doors are kept closed to keep the fire contained

- by ensuring you know what to do when a fire starts and to be able to keep the fire contained until help arrives, for example by using a fire extinguisher, but only if you have been trained to do so.

Reflect on it

7.1 Your role and responsibilities

Reflect on your role and responsibilities for preventing fires from starting and spreading. If you are unsure about any fire safety aspects, reflect on who and where you can go for information and guidance.

Evidence opportunity

7.1 Practices that prevent fires from starting and spreading

Discuss with your assessor the practices that you use in the care setting where you work that prevent fires from starting and spreading. Do you feel confident in following these practices? If not, what do you need to do? Perhaps you may need further fire safety training or to read through your work setting's fire safety procedures? Write an account to evidence your discussion. You may wish to do some further research before your discussion.

Your employer's responsibilities

Your employer has responsibilities with regards to fire safety. These include:

- appropriate fire safety guidance and training, which you must attend. You must also ensure you keep your knowledge about fire safety practices up to date
- fire safety procedures clearly displayed, and accessible for all those in the setting
- clear fire exit signs, and fire doors
- fire safety equipment, such as correct fire extinguishers, in the setting
- following legislation and regulation with regards to fire safety, including having a fire drill and confirming the actions to take in the event of a fire.

You should know not only what your personal responsibilities in an emergency are but also who else is responsible and what else they are responsible for.

Research it

7.1 Fire extinguishers

It is important that you know that there are different types of fire extinguishers. These are labelled with instructions and will clearly say whether they contain 'water', foam or powder, for example, and they will also include instructions on how to use them. While you do not need to know everything about each type of fire extinguisher, it is important to know which ones are in your setting, understand how to use them and receive training in this.

Go to the following website to read about some of the different types of extinguishers, what they are used for, the dangers around using them, how to use them and how they work:

www.fireservice.co.uk/safety/fire-extinguishers

This is obviously not a substitute for training but it will help you gain an understanding of the different fire extinguishers.

AC 7.2 Describe emergency procedures to be followed in the event of a fire in the work setting

Your work setting's fire safety procedures will detail the emergency procedures you must follow in the event of a fire in the work setting. It is important that you read through and understand what these are so that you do not place yourself or anyone else in danger as these will vary depending on the care setting where you work and your job role.

Most fire safety procedures will include the following points:

1 Raise the fire alarm. Do this as soon as possible.

2 Call the emergency services on 999 or inform someone else to do this immediately.

3 Make sure you ensure the safety of others and that they are moved away from any danger. Your setting will have procedures in place dealing with different people, for example how to safely move people who are not mobile. This might include the use of wheelchairs, and how

to move bed-bound individuals. Make sure you know about the evacuation procedures.

4　If you have received training, you can use the correct fire extinguisher to put out the fire. You must also know where fire safety equipment is kept.

5　Go the assembly point. Workplaces have designated areas, and you must know where yours is. Workplaces have fire drills to ensure that you know where this is and so you know and understand the procedure of what to do in the event of an actual fire.

6　Do not return to the building. You will be told when it is safe to do so.

7　Reflect on your practice. You will need to consider what worked well, what didn't and why, and what you can do to improve.

The 'dos and don'ts' table includes some of the key actions to take that apply to all care settings in the event of a fire.

Evacuation procedures

There may be times when you need to evacuate the building, not because there is a fire but because there is a perhaps a bomb scare or threat of an explosion, for example. In these cases, you will need to follow similar guidance to the above, for example you will need to remain calm, and move people in a safe way. Your setting will have clear guidance on this. AC 7.3 has more information on this. When working in an individual's home you will need to familiarise yourself with the exit to be used in the event that you need to evacuate the individual's home.

Reflect on it

7.2 Fire emergency procedures

Reflect on the importance of being familiar with fire emergency procedures in place in the care setting where you work. How can this help you in promoting fire safety in the event of a fire? How can this reassure the individuals you provide care or support to?

Dos and don'ts when there is a fire emergency	
Do	Immediately alert others that there is a fire (check what to do in your work setting, i.e. it may vary from sounding the alarm to alerting a senior member of staff).
Do	Control and contain the fire (only if you have been trained to do so and it is safe to do so).
Do	Contact the fire brigade (check what to do in your work setting. Some fire alarm systems automatically dial the fire brigade, only allocated members of staff may be able to contact the fire brigade as they have been trained to do so). The fire brigade will require information from the contact person, such as their name, address and details about the fire, for example where it is and how far it has spread, the type of care setting it is and whether anyone is in danger.
Do	Assist with ensuring everyone is in a place of safety either inside or outside of the building. For example, visitors could be supported to leave the building by the nearest fire escape route, individuals who are unable to mobilise can remain in their rooms providing their doors and windows are closed until the fire brigade arrives.
Do	Try and remain calm and wait until the fire brigade informs you that it is safe to re-enter the building.
Do	Walk calmly when exiting. Assemble outside the building in line with your work setting's agreed ways of working.
Don't	Run, as this may cause others to panic and may lead to slips and falls.
Don't	Stop or re-enter the building for any personal items as this could place you in danger. Others may not know that you have returned and may therefore be unaware that you are in the building. Assemble outside the building in line with your work setting's agreed ways of working.
Don't	Panic – remember if you stay calm this will be reassuring for others.

7.2 Your work setting's fire emergency procedures

Research your work setting's fire emergency procedures. Discuss with your manager the steps you are required to take in the event of a fire in the care setting where you work and the reasons why.

Evidence opportunity

7.2 Emergency procedures

Produce a poster to show the actions you must take and not take in the event of a fire in the work setting. Use diagrams and relevant images in your poster.

AC 7.3 Explain the importance of maintaining clear evacuation routes at all times

To be able to safely exit a building where there is a fire, it is very important that your work setting's fire escape routes are kept clear at all times. If they are not kept clear, this may prevent you and others from evacuating the building, which therefore places you and others in danger and/or may result in slips, trips and falls.

Research it

7.3 Fire escape routes in your setting

Research where the fire escape routes are in the care setting where you work. How many fire escape routes are there? Why? You will find your manager a useful source of information.

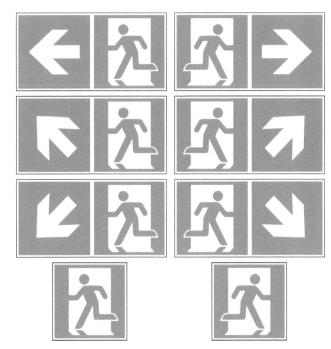

Figure 9.7 Do you know what these fire escape signs mean?

You may work in a variety of different work settings including individuals' homes and residential care homes and so it is very important that you are aware of the escape routes for each setting that you work in because they are the means for ensuring your safety and that of others.

Fire evacuation routes must be:

- clearly signposted, i.e. they must indicate where the fire escape route and exit is
- well-lit so that they can be easily located at night or if there is smoke. Well-lit routes can also help individuals with vision loss to locate these
- fitted with fire safety equipment, for example there must be fireproof doors and fire extinguishers
- suitable as an escape route, i.e. they must not be too narrow and they should be fitted with handrails
- safe to use with no obstructions, such as boxes or mobility appliances, that can make it difficult to escape in an emergency. They must have floor coverings that are not worn or damaged. Wear and tear in floor coverings can cause trips and falls.

Reflect on it

7.3 How can you ensure fire escape routes are safe?

Reflect on how you and others can ensure that fire escape routes are safe to use. You could think about the checks that are carried out.

Evidence opportunity

7.3 Importance of maintaining clear evacuation routes

Produce a one-page information handout about the importance of maintaining clear fire evacuation routes at all times as well as the consequences of not doing so.

LO7 Knowledge, skills, behaviours
Knowledge: what does fire safety involve?
Do you know the causes of fires and what you can do to stop them starting and spreading?
Do you know the emergency procedures to follow in the event of a fire in the work setting?
Do you know why it is important to ensure that fire evacuation routes are clearly signposted?
Did you know that you have just shown your knowledge of fire safety at work?
Skills: how can you show what to do in the event of a fire in your work setting?
Do you know the first action to take when you have discovered a fire in your work setting?
Do you know what your role is in your work setting in the event of a fire?
Did you know that you have just demonstrated a few of the skills required for following your work setting's fire emergency procedures?
Behaviours: how can you show the personal qualities you have for fire safety?
Do you know how to keep calm when others around you are panicking?
Do you know how to be supportive towards others in the event of a fire?
Did you know that you have just demonstrated a few of the essential behaviours required for promoting fire safety at work?

LO8 Be able to implement security measures in the work setting

Getting started

Think about an occasion when you were visiting a building or premises and you were asked to confirm who you were. What were you asked about yourself?

Think about an occasion when you requested information over the telephone in relation to yourself. For example, this may be in relation to blood test results or a doctor's appointment. How did the person on the other end of the telephone check that you were who you said you were? How did this make you feel?

AC 8.1 Use agreed ways of working for checking the identity of anyone requesting access to premises and information

Promoting health and safety at work involves putting into practice **security measures**, such as, checking the **identity** of all visitors. This is because care settings are environments where individuals who have care or support needs live. Due to their conditions or disabilities, they may be more susceptible to not realising the dangers of bogus visitors claiming to be, for example, contractors or adult care workers. Implementing security measures in care settings, therefore, is everyone's responsibility so that we can ensure that all settings are kept safe for you, the individuals you support and others who you work with.

Requesting access to premises

The **agreed ways of working** or the procedures to be followed for checking the identity of anyone requesting access to the premises where you work will vary depending on your work setting and job role. For example, you may be required to refer anyone requesting access to the premises to a senior member of staff or you may be required to check the person's identity yourself. Your work setting's procedures will provide you with guidance on what to do. Whatever the procedures, it is important that you safeguard individuals against unwanted visitors and intruders, and protect individuals' private property and information.

> ### Key terms
>
> **Security measures** are safety measures, which can include checking an individual's identity, and the use of identity and visitor badges.
>
> **Identity** means confirmation of who a person is, for example their name, who they work for, who they are visiting.
>
> **Agreed ways of working** will include policies and procedures where these exist; they may be less formally documented with smaller employers.

Below are some examples of good practice security measures that you can follow.

Before allowing a visitor access to the premises

- **Stop and think:** before you let the visitor enter into the premises, stop and think. Consider whether the visitor is known to you or anyone else, whether the visitor has got an agreed appointment with anyone, whether you can check this information with anyone, such as, with your manager or the person they have an appointment with; if you do check this information with someone else, remember not to let the person enter the premises until you have done so, i.e. politely ask them to wait outside. It is good practice to be vigilant and question anyone that you do not recognise. For example, if you see someone in the setting that you have not seen before, go over to them and ask them if you can help them. If they say they are visiting someone, you could ask them who and why and escort them to where they need to go. Make sure that you stay with them. This is also covered in the section below. You may also need to check the individual's file to see if there are any other reasons you cannot allow visitors. This might be for medical reasons, for example, or to safeguard the individual but you will need to be aware of the reasons.

- **Use security measures fitted to the premises:** these can include a spy hole, a door chain, or the intercom system; you could even look through the window to check the identity of the visitor. Your setting may have electronic entrance systems where identity passes are required for access, or a code is required to enter. You may need to use a key safe to enter into an individual's home. These measures are to help to ensure intruders do not enter the premises.

- **Check the person's proof of identity:** if the visitor gives you an identity card, check that the person looks like the person in the photo and their name matches who they say they are; you could even ring the organisation who they say they are from to further confirm their identity.

If you are unsure about the person's identity do not allow them to enter the premises until you have sought advice from your manager explaining what your concerns are. It may be necessary to call the police.

If the individual you support has said no to receiving the visitor, then you must deny the visitor access in an assertive but polite tone. Remember the principles of person-centred care that you have learned about. If the person is a family member and still requests access, you must remember that the individual you care for is your priority and you must respect their wishes. You could apologise and explain that if the individual changes their mind, then you will give them a call.

After allowing a visitor access to the premises

Once you have confirmed a visitor's identity you can ask them to enter onto the premises. The following 'dos and dont's' table outlines important points to remember when dealing with visitors.

Research it

8.1 **Unwanted visitors**

Research an occasion reported in the media where an individual with care or support needs was targeted by bogus callers. Share the news story with a colleague and discuss what happened and the impact it had. An example of such a news story is available below:

www.bbc.co.uk/news/uk-scotland-south-scotland-34346274

Requesting access to information

The agreed ways of working or the procedures to be followed for checking the identity of anyone requesting access to information where you work will also vary depending on your work setting and job role. For example, you may be required to pass a request for information from an individual's relative onto the manager or you may respond to an email that has been sent by an individual's advocate in relation to their daily activities.

Under the Data Protection Act 1998 (replaced by the GDPR in 2018) you have a responsibility to ensure that you keep safe and secure all personal information you come across about individuals. This may be in relation to their health, care needs or preferences. You will also need to obtain the individual's permission to do so; unless of course it is an emergency or the information is needed to provide care or support to an individual. Doing so will not only ensure that you respect individuals' rights to privacy but will also mean that individuals will learn that they can trust you and feel able to confide in you. You can learn more about the requirements of the Data Protection Act 1998 by reviewing Unit 206, Handle information in care settings. Remember that this was replaced by the GDPR in May 2018 which is also mentioned in the legislation section in that unit.

Dos and don'ts for dealing with visitors	
Do	Ask them to sign in as a visitor with their full name, the company they are from, the date and purpose of their visit.
Do	Ask them to wear a visitor's badge so that others are aware of who they are.
Do	Explain to them that you have let the person they have come to visit know that they have arrived and are expecting them.
Don't	Allow the visitor access to the premises if they have not signed in.
Don't	Allow the visitor access to the premises if they are not wearing their visitor's badge. In some settings, name badges may not be a requirement as this may unsettle individuals but your workplace will have procedures in place with regards to name badges for security purposes. You should check what the policy and procedures are.
Don't	Allow the visitor to walk through the premises unescorted by you.

6Cs

Commitment

This involves being dedicated to good practice and doing your very best to place the individual's needs first and ensure that the way you work has their best interests at heart. This is important for the provision of person-centred care and for establishing good working relationships with individuals. You can show your commitment to following good practice here by ensuring individuals understand why information is disclosed to others and what efforts you and others have made to keep it private and secure.

Below are some examples of good practice security measures that you can follow.

- Check that the person requesting the information has a right to know it: you will need to check with your manager whether you are able to disclose the information requested. If not, then you will need to find out the reasons why so that these can be explained to the person requesting access.
- Check that you have the individual's consent to provide information: if you do have the individual's consent to provide information then you must always check the identity of the person and the purpose of their request. You may have to do this in person or over the telephone or in an email depending on the nature of the enquiry.

If you have to provide information to others without informing the individual, for example when a health emergency occurs, it is good practice to inform the individual afterwards that you did so and the reasons why. In this way you can show your **commitment** to upholding the individual's rights.

AC 8.2 Implement measures to protect own security and the security of others in the work setting

There are a number of measures to protect the security of care workers and others in the care setting. This can include identity checks that you learned about in AC 8.1, such as security passes for access to the setting, a policy of distributing visitor badges, and password and firewall systems to protect digital personal data. Here we discuss some of the measures you can put into place to protect your own security and the security of others in the work setting.

It is important that you know how to put these into practice to protect your own security and the security of others.

- **Maintain everyday security of the premises:** this can include completing daily health and safety checks, such as, checking rooms and

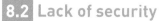
communal areas, checking the doors close securely, the windows are not left open at night, checking visitor badges and ensuring that any security codes for entry to the premises or different rooms are changed regularly to keep them safe.

- **Reflect on your day-to-day practices and those of others:** this can include discussing with your colleagues what security checks have been carried out and reflecting on the security checks that require improvement and the benefits of doing so.

- **Follow your agreed ways of working for lone working:** this includes ensuring others know your whereabouts at all times and signing in and out of the premises.

- **Follow your agreed ways of working for security:** this includes ensuring visitors sign when they arrive and when they leave the premises and keeping any passwords that you may have, such as on key pads on doors, confidential to protect the security of both the premises and all those on the premises.

- **Follow your agreed ways of working for ensuring the security of individuals' personal property and valuables:** this includes recording what items and valuables individuals have with them in the setting, and knowing what to do when things go missing in the setting.

- **Follow your agreed ways of working for security emergencies:** this includes immediately reporting all security emergencies that may arise, such as lost keys for a filing cabinet that contains individuals' personal records, or a broken window or a faulty door latch.

- **Attend training:** this includes accessing training and information provided by your work setting about how to protect your security and the security of others at all times.

Lone working

There are procedures in place for all lone workers to ensure their safety is maintained at all times. Working safely as a lone worker involves always ensuring others know your whereabouts at all times so that they can call for help on your behalf if they become aware that you may be in danger. For example, if you are supporting an individual to go out one evening, ensure you check the individual's risk assessment for anything you need to be aware of. For example, the individual's mental health may have deteriorated and you may need to check if it is still appropriate to support this individual to go out with you on your own. If you do go out with the individual, ensure others know what time you are going out, where you are going and how long you are likely to be. You will need to ensure that others can contact you and that you can contact others so you may need to take a mobile phone with you.

Case study

8.1, 8.2 Implementing security measures at work

Enzo is a care worker in a nursing home for older adults who have a range of different conditions. During the very busy morning shift Enzo hears the front door bell ring. As it is usually the senior care workers' responsibility to answer the front door, he ignores it. Approximately five minutes later the person is still ringing the doorbell. Enzo goes to look for one of the senior care workers on duty; one is on her break and the other is in the middle of the medication round and cannot be disturbed. Enzo walks past the front door and the person standing on the doorstep looks a little familiar and waves excitedly at Enzo to let her in.

Discuss

1 Do you think Enzo should let the person in? Why?

2 What would you do in this situation if it arose in your work setting? Ensure your response is in line with your work setting's agreed ways of working.

AC 8.3 Explain the importance of ensuring that others are aware of your whereabouts

The importance of others being aware of your whereabouts

Ensuring that others are aware of your whereabouts is very important when working in care settings in the event of an emergency, such as a fire, for example. Recap your previous learning for AC 7.2 around the emergency procedures to be followed in the event of a fire, including the reasons why it is important that the fire brigade is aware of everyone's whereabouts.

Ensuring others are aware of your whereabouts is also important in the event of your colleagues requiring your immediate assistance, for example, in the case of an individual having a fall or becoming unwell. For other examples of accidents and sudden illnesses that may occur, recap your previous learning for AC 3.1.

It is also important that others are aware of your whereabouts so that they know you are safe. You may be working with individuals who have a history of violence or you may work with individuals in their homes, and so there are risks that you may face.

How to make others aware

You can make others aware of your whereabouts by:

- signing in and out every time you enter and leave the premises
- letting your colleagues know if you are working after office hours
- informing a named person of your whereabouts if you are not working in the premises. You may need to inform that you will be visiting an individual in their home or meeting with a professional in their office, for example. Make sure that they know details of where you will be and what time you will return.

Accessing immediate help can only be done if others are aware of your whereabouts. Ensuring you comply with your work setting's lone working, staff welfare and health and safety policies and procedures is central to maintaining your own security and that of others.

Precautions to take when outside the setting

You will need to make sure that you have some training in how to protect yourself both in the setting and when working alone. This might include self-defence training in the event of a violent situation. The trainers or your manager will be able to support you with advice and ways to address situations where you feel threatened. You will also need to be aware of other precautions that you can take such as carrying a panic button or personal alarm so that you are able to call for help. There may also be a policy where lone workers are required to call or ring in, and there may even be trackers on mobile phones.

Research it

8.3 Lone working

Research your work setting's procedures for lone working and personal safety while at work. Produce an information leaflet with your findings.

Reflect on it

8.3 Consequences

Reflect on the consequences for you and others if you do not follow your work setting's procedures for maintaining your personal safety while carrying out your day-to-day work activities.

Evidence opportunity

8.3 Informing others of your whereabouts

Make a list of the people you make aware of your whereabouts during your day-to-day work activities. This could include people from your work setting as well as others you know outside of your setting. Write an account of why you should make these people aware of your whereabouts. If you work in an individual's home, who do you make aware of your whereabouts?

L08 Knowledge, skills, behaviours
Knowledge: how can you maintain your own security at work?
Do you know your setting's policies and procedures about checking the identity of visitors?
Do you know why it is important to ensure that others are aware of your whereabouts?
Do you know what your work setting's procedures say about maintaining your personal safety at work and that of others?
Did you know that you have just shown your knowledge of your work setting's agreed ways of working for maintaining your own security?
Skills: how can you show that you put security measures into practice in your work setting?
Do you know how to check the identity of someone who requests personal information about an individual over the telephone and then arrives at the premises requesting to meet with the individual?
Do you know what identity checks you can carry out if someone arrives at your work setting who you do not know?
Did you know that you have just demonstrated a few of the skills required for following your work setting's security measures?
Behaviours: how can you show the personal qualities you have implementing security measures at work?
Do you know how to be assertive if a person you do not recognise wishes to enter your work setting?
Do you know how to be confident when explaining to a person requesting personal information about an individual that you are unable to disclose this?
Did you know that you have just demonstrated a few of the essential behaviours required for implementing security measures at work?

LO9 Know how to manage stress

Getting started

Think about an occasion when you felt stressed.

What made you feel stressed and why? How did you feel physically? How did you feel emotionally? Did you notice any changes in how you were behaving on a day-to-day basis? For example, did you find yourself becoming very tearful but not knowing why or did you feel very negative about yourself? Did you become irritable towards others without meaning to or did you find that you couldn't sleep or concentrate very well?

AC 9.1 Identify common signs and indicators of stress in self and others

Our busy day-to-day lives mean that we frequently experience varying types of pressures, not just at work but also in our personal lives. It is when these pressures begin to build that they can result in us feeling unable to manage with our day-to-day activities. This is often referred to as **stress**. Stress can have positive as well as negative effects, but in this unit the word is used to refer to negative stress.

If stress is not managed in its early stages it can have a significant impact not only on people's health and well-being but also on the workforce in adult care settings. For example, the Health and Safety Executive states that the statistics from the **Labour Force Survey (LFS)** show that:

The total number of cases of work related stress, depression or anxiety in 2015/16 was 488,000 cases, a prevalence rate of 1510 per 100,000 workers.

In 2015/16 stress accounted for 37% of all work related ill health cases and 45% of all working days lost due to ill health.

By occupation, jobs that are common across public service industries (such as healthcare workers teaching professionals, business, media and public service professionals) show higher levels of stress as compared to all jobs.

The main work factors cited by respondents as causing work related stress, depression or anxiety (LFS) were workload pressures, including tight

Key terms

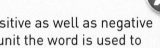

Stress can have positive as well as negative effects, but in this unit the word is used to refer to negative stress.

The **Labour Force Survey (LFS)** is a study of the employment circumstances of the UK population. It is the largest household study in the UK and provides information in relation to employment and unemployment.

deadlines and too much responsibility and a lack of managerial support.

Health and Safety Executive (2017) 'Work-related Stress, Depression or Anxiety Statistics in Great Britain 2016'

The first step to prevent your stress from developing into something more serious involves being aware of the common signs and indicators. Although these vary from person to person and therefore you may not experience all of these, it is still very important that you know about these in the event of you experiencing them in the future and so that you know that you are not the only one that sometimes feels this way. It is also important that you are able to recognise these signs in others so that you can offer them support if they need it.

Signs and indicators of stress

- **Physical signs and indicators**: these can include tenseness, rapid heartbeat, high blood pressure, strokes, dizziness, nausea, diarrhoea or constipation, headaches and migraines. Other physical illnesses include colds, or cold

Research it

9.1 'Fight or flight' response

Research what happens in your body when you are stressed; the body's 'fight or flight' response. You may find the link below useful:

www.psychologistworld.com/stress/fight-or-flight-response

Explain the 'fight or flight' response to a colleague.

Reflect on it

9.1 Effects of stress

Reflect on the impact of the effects of stress on you at work. For example, how might this affect the way you interact with individuals or with others who may visit the care setting where you work?

Evidence opportunity

9.1 Common signs and indicators of stress

Design a poster that identifies the main ways that you think stress affects you and someone else you know. What similarities and differences did you notice? You may want to discuss this with a colleague. You could write an account to evidence the discussion but you may need to omit the name of your colleague.

sores and menstrual issues. These physical symptoms develop because it is how our bodies respond to stress, this is sometimes known as the 'fight or flight' response.

- **Emotional signs and indicators**: these can include low moods, feeling irritable, feeling anxious, an overwhelming sense of being unable to cope, feeling unhappy or angry.
- **Mental signs and indicators**: these can include difficulties with concentration and memory, having racing thoughts and being unable to think logically.
- **Behavioural signs and indicators**: these can include being unable to sleep or sleeping too much, eating more than usual or eating a lot less and withdrawal from situations, particularly those that involve speaking with and socialising with others.

AC 9.2 Identify circumstances and factors that tend to trigger stress in self and others

The second step in preventing your stress from developing into something more serious is recognising that there may be specific circumstances and factors that tend to trigger stress in yourself and others. Again, what causes stress is different for everyone and depends on what is important to you as well as how able you are at dealing with difficult circumstances. This is often referred to as resilience.

Figure 9.8 identifies some examples of circumstances and factors that tend to trigger stress.

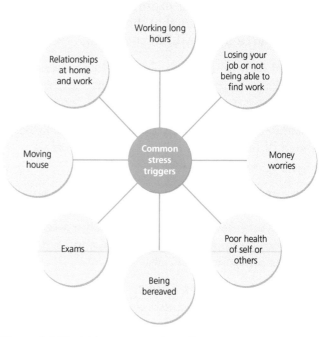

Figure 9.8 What triggers your stress?

Reflect on it

9.2 Reasons for stress

Remember it is important to be aware of the circumstances and factors that trigger stress both at work and outside work.

- Reflect on three reasons for being stressed at home.
- Reflect on three reasons for being stressed at work.
- Reflect on three main reasons for an individual with care or support needs being stressed.

Evidence opportunity

9.2 Circumstances and factors that trigger stress

Choose two stress triggers for yourself and two stress triggers for one of your colleagues. For each one identify the reasons why they make you and your colleague feel stressed. These could include work-related stress triggers, or those outside of work. Write a short piece to evidence this. Again it would be useful to omit your colleague's name in case there are stress triggers that are personal to them.

It is very important to know what triggers stress in yourself and others because in this way you will be able to recognise why you or others are behaving differently. Being supportive and empathetic is a must; not doing so can add more pressure which can leave you and others feeling under even more stress. In addition, understanding the reasons why you are stressed can help you rationalise why you are feeling the way you do so that you can then go about trying to manage it.

AC 9.3 Describe ways to manage stress and how to access sources of support

Once you have identified that you or others are displaying signs of being stressed and can

Key term

Sources of support may include formal and informal support, supervision, appraisal, within and outside the organisation. For more information on this refer to Unit 207, Personal development in care settings.

Reflect on it

9.3 Dealing with stress

Reflect on an occasion when you dealt with stress negatively. Why do you think you did so? How did it make you feel? Is there anything you could you have done positively next time?

identify the triggers for this, then you can begin to look for a way of managing stress. As you know, everyone experiences stress differently and therefore the ways that can be used to manage it are also varied. Remember one size does not fit all – what works for one person may not for another.

Finding ways of managing stress positively means that you will be more likely to avoid the ways that are not beneficial, such as by smoking heavily, 'comfort' eating or drinking excessive amounts of alcohol; all of these are associated with serious health conditions, for example heart attacks and liver cancer.

Positive ways for managing stress can include:

- **Being active**: not only physically but mentally too. For example, by going for a walk in the evening after a long shift at work or doing a crossword. Both activities can help with refocusing your mind and therefore reducing your body's stress levels. You will also feel a lot calmer and able to think clearly again.
- **Staying positive**: thinking about what is going well rather than on what is going wrong will help you feel more in control and able to deal with difficult situations that may arise, such as, the bereavement of someone close to you; you can perhaps think about what that person

would have wanted for you and how you could make them proud by showing them you are in control of your life.

- **Being in contact with others**: agreeing to meet up with friends for a social occasion even when you may be feeling in a low mood can prevent you from becoming isolated from others that can in turn mean that you feel less confident in yourself, for example. Instead, meeting up with others can be a much welcomed distraction and you may find out about circumstances that your friends are experiencing that may be similar, or even worse than yours.

- **Helping others**: doing something for someone else can make you feel good about yourself; a perfect way to boost your self-confidence when you are feeling anxious or withdrawn. You will at the same time meet different people and learn new skills; all examples of ways that can make you feel positive about yourself and your stress less overwhelming.

- **Learning to say 'no'**: this is a useful skill to have that takes some practice! It involves being in control of your stress and being aware of what your limits are.

- **Make time for yourself**: it is very important to take time out to stop and think. Being calm and quiet can help you focus on what is important and put things into perspective.

- **Accessing sources of support for stress**: this involves being honest and **courageous**.

6Cs

C

Courage

Showing courage when accessing sources of support is important so that your stress does not become worse. If it does, it could affect the quality of the care or support you provide to individuals and the relationships you have with your colleagues because you may behave in ways that they are not used to, such as getting upset and becoming irritable very quickly. You can show your courage when managing stress by not being afraid to say 'Help!'

Formal and informal support

Meeting with your manager at work and discussing the triggers for your stress can help with putting together a plan of action, such as, providing you with additional support from a more experienced colleague when working to meet the needs of an individual whose behaviour challenges. Informal support, such as from your colleagues at work, can also be useful in terms of providing useful suggestions for managing stress, for example by socialising or talking through difficult situations that have arisen, like the bereavement of an individual with care needs who you have worked alongside for many years. Workers from outside agencies such as bereavement counsellors can also provide support and understanding at a time when you need it most. You could contact a bereavement counsellor directly yourself or by being referred through your employer or GP.

Supervision

Supervision can help you have some protected time with your manager that focuses solely on how you are managing with your day-to-day responsibilities. Supervision can provide you with an opportunity to share your anxieties as well as what can be done to manage these. This may involve accessing support from outside professionals who can provide training and information on how to develop specific skills and knowledge. Your manager can also help you to identify what circumstances you have managed well and the techniques you have used to do so.

Appraisal

An appraisal provides you with time to reflect and think about what you have learned, what you have achieved and what you would like to achieve next. With the help of your manager, you will able to assess how well you have carried out your day-to-day working tasks and whether any improvements are needed. This is an opportunity to celebrate your achievements; a positive frame of mind is needed for this! It also provides you with time to think about what you would like to achieve next, i.e. it could be a new skill or area of knowledge. Setting yourself targets to achieve makes you feel in control and is an excellent way to build your personal confidence.

Research it

9.3 Procedures for accessing support

Research in your work setting the procedures that you must follow for accessing support for managing your stress.

Evidence opportunity

9.3 Managing stress and accessing support

Discuss with your assessor the support available in your work setting for helping you to manage your personal stress. Did you find out anything you did not know about? You could also provide a written account to evidence your discussion.

LO9 Knowledge, skills, behaviours

Knowledge: how do you know if you and others are stressed?
Do you know two physical signs and two behavioural signs of being stressed?
Do you know two common triggers of stress for you and two common triggers of stress for others?
Do you know the different ways you can manage stress and how to access sources of support?
Did you know that you have just shown your knowledge of identifying signs of stress and the factors that may trigger it, and also the ways to manage stress?
Skills: how can you show that you can access support for your stress?
Do you know what support systems are available in your work setting and how you can access them?
Do you know what to do if you notice one of your colleagues is showing signs of stress?
Did you know that you have just demonstrated a few of the skills required for managing stress?
Behaviours: how can you show the personal qualities you have for managing stress?
Do you know how to remain calm in a stressful situation?
Do you know how to relax after a stressful day?
Did you know that you have just demonstrated a few of the essential behaviours required for managing stress effectively?

Suggestions for using the activities

This table summarises all the activities in the unit that are relevant to each assessment criterion.

Here, we also suggest other, different methods that you may want to use to present your knowledge and skills by using the activities.

These are just suggestions, and you should refer to the Introduction section at the start of the book, and more importantly the City & Guilds specification, and your assessor who will be able to provide more guidance on how you can evidence your knowledge and skills.

Where you are observed during your assessment, this can be done by your assessor, or your manager can provide a witness testimony.

Assessment criteria and accompanying activities	Suggested methods to show your knowledge/skills
LO1 Understand your responsibilities and the responsibilities of others, relating to health and safety in the work setting	
1.1 Reflect on it (page 324)	Write a short reflective account.
1.1 Research it (page 325)	Write down your findings. Or you could produce a handout.

Suggestions for using the activities	
1.1 Evidence opportunity (page 328)	Develop a poster as instructed in the activity or provide a written account.
1.2 Research it (page 328)	Write down your findings.
1.2 Reflect on it (page 328)	Address the questions in the activity. Write a short reflective account.
1.2 Evidence opportunity (page 329)	You can discuss this with your assessor or manager. Remember that your manager will be able to provide a witness testimony. You could also provide a written account or a presentation that details the key points of the health and safety policy and procedures agreed with your employer in your work setting.
1.3 Reflect on it (page 330)	Write a reflective account about your responsibilities with regard to health and safety.
1.3 Research it (page 330) 1.3 Research it (page 331)	Provide a written account detailing information about the training that your employer has planned. Research workers' and employers' responsibilities and provide a written account.
1.3 Evidence opportunity (page 331)	Produce an information leaflet about how health and safety is maintained in the care setting where you work. You could also write a personal statement that outlines the health and safety responsibilities for: you as employee, your employer or manager and others in the care setting where you work. Remember to include examples of the different types of health and safety responsibilities for everyone.
1.4 Reflect on it (page 332)	Write a reflective account answering the questions in the activity.
1.4 Evidence opportunity (page 333)	Address the points in the activity and write a self-reflective account of your findings. You could also discuss the reasons why they must not be carried out unless you have been trained and are competent to do so.
1.5 Reflect on it (page 334)	Write a reflective account. You could also discuss the activity with a colleague and also write about what you learned from them.
1.5 Research it (page 334)	Write down your findings.
1.4, 1.5 Evidence opportunity (page 334)	Produce an information handout as instructed in the activity. Or you could write a personal statement about the procedure you are required to follow in the care setting where you work if you wanted to access additional support and information in relation to health and safety. You will find your work setting's health and safety procedures a useful starting point.
LO2 Understand the use of risk assessments in relation to health and safety	
2.1 Research it (page 336)	Write down notes to detail your findings.
2.1 Reflect on it (page 338)	Write an account reflecting on the consequences of not assessing risks.
2.1 Evidence opportunity (page 338)	Provide a written account addressing the points in the activity. You could also produce a presentation that details the health and safety risks posed by your work setting, situations or activities in your work setting. Include in your presentation, the reasons why it is important to assess these health and safety risks. You will find your manager and your work setting's risk assessment procedures a useful source of information.
2.2 Reflect on it (page 338)	Discuss the procedures that you are expected to follow for reporting health and safety risks that have been identified with your manager. Write a short reflective account.
2.2, 1.1 Research it (page 339)	Provide a written account detailing your findings.

→

Suggestions for using the activities

2.2 Evidence opportunity (page 339)	Discuss with your assessor, your reporting of a potential health and safety risk in your work setting. Obtain feedback from your manager. You could write a personal statement that includes details of the process to follow for reporting health and safety risks that have been identified. Remember to include details of not only how but also when to report health and safety risks and the reasons for this. You will find your manager and your work setting's risk assessment procedures a useful source of information.
2.3 Reflect on it (page 340)	Write a short reflective accounting answering the questions in the activity.
2.3 Evidence opportunity (page 341)	Develop one or two case studies as instructed in the activity. Describe two dilemmas that exist between the individual's rights and your concerns in relation to health and safety. Also write down your explanation about how risk assessment can be used to help address both dilemmas. You will find your manager and your work setting's risk assessment procedures a useful source of information.
LO3 Understand procedures for responding to accidents and sudden illness	
LO1 Understand your responsibilities and the responsibilities of others, relating to health and safety in the work setting	
3.1 Reflect on it (page 343)	Write down some notes to document your thoughts.
3.1 Research it (page 343)	Write down your findings about the big three signs of diabetes.
3.1 Evidence opportunity (page 344)	You can have a discussion with your assessor or manager as instructed in the activity. You could also write down a description of the different types of accidents and sudden illnesses that may occur in your work setting. Remember to also include details about how they can occur.
3.2 Reflect on it (page 346)	You could write a reflective account.
3.1, 3.2, 1.5 Research it (page 346)	Write down your findings about the basic first aid treatment for two accidents and two sudden illnesses.
3.2 Research it (page 347)	You could explain what you have found out from a colleague or write some notes to detail your findings. Useful sources of information have been included in Tables 9.2 and 9.3, so you could pick more than three conditions that you may need to treat with first aid and write about the procedures to be followed if an accident or sudden illness should occur.
3.2 Evidence opportunity (page 346)	Produce a leaflet or provide a written account detailing the outlining the procedures to follow if an accident or illness should occur. Ensure you detail the process you are required to follow within the scope of your job role. You will find your work setting's procedures and your manager a useful source of information.
LO4 Be able to reduce the spread of infection	
4.1 Research it (page 351)	Provide a written account detailing your findings.
4.1 Reflect on it (page 351)	Write about the infection control posters and information that is available in your setting. You could discuss this with your assessor or manager.
4.1 Evidence opportunity (page 351)	Produce an information handout with your findings. If you discuss roles and responsibilities with your manager or the most suitable person in your setting, then you will need a witness testimony or recording to evidence the discussion. You could also produce a presentation that explains your role and responsibilities and those of your employer in relation to infection prevention and control. You will find your work setting's infection control procedures and your manager a useful source of information.

→

Suggestions for using the activities	
4.2 Reflect on it (page 352)	Write a short reflective account.
4.2 Research it (page 352)	Provide a written account.
4.2 Evidence opportunity (page 354)	Provide a written account. You could also produce a handout detailing the main causes of infection and how it can spread in the care setting where you work.
4.3 Research it (page 354)	Develop a poster that includes the key points about what your setting says about how to prevent the spread of infection through effective hand hygiene.
4.3 Research it (page 355)	Write down what you found out about hand hygiene from the NHS website.
4.3 Reflect on it (page 356)	Write a short reflective account.
4.3 Evidence opportunity (page 356)	You will be observed for this assessment criterion so it is important that you make arrangements to be observed here so that you can show that you are able to use the recommended method for hand washing in care settings. Then reflect on the feedback you received.
4.4 Reflect on it (page 358)	Write a short reflective account detailing your thoughts.
4.4 Research it (page 358)	Write down details of your discussion.
4.4 Evidence opportunity (page 359)	You will be observed for this assessment criterion so it is important that you make arrangements for this so that you can show that you are able to use PPE correctly. Then reflect on the feedback you received and answer the questions in the activity.
4.5 Research it (page 360)	Have a discussion with your manager. You could write notes to evidence your discussion.
4.5 Reflect on it (page 361)	Write a short reflective account.
4.5 Research it (page 361)	Make notes detailing findings from your research.
4.5 Evidence opportunity (page 361)	You will be observed for AC 4.5 so it is important that you make arrangements for this so that you can show that your health and hygiene do not pose a risk to others. Follow up your demonstration with a professional discussion with your assessor.
LO5 Be able to move and handle equipment and objects safely	
5.1 Research it (page 364)	Write notes detailing your findings.
5.1 Reflect on it (page 364)	Write a short reflective account. You could also produce a spider diagram of different examples of relevant moving and handling legislation. Ensure the legislation you identify is relevant specifically to moving and handling.
5.1 Evidence opportunity (page 364)	Write down three moving and handling tasks that can be carried out in your work setting, and for each task identify the specific legislation that is in place.
5.2 Research it (page 365)	Produce a handout, or you could write down notes to detail your findings.
5.2 Reflect on it (page 365)	Write a short reflective account.
5.2 Evidence opportunity (page 366) 5.2, 5.3 Case study (page 368)	Have a discussion with your assessor as instructed. Or you could also write an account explaining principles for moving and handling equipment and other objects safely. Ensure you explain how these principles promote safe practices. The case study will help you to understand some of the principles around moving and handling.
5.3 Research it (page 367)	Write down notes to document your findings.
5.3 Reflect on it (page 367)	Write a short reflective account.

→

Suggestions for using the activities	
5.3 Evidence opportunity (page 368) 5.2, 5.3 Case study (page 368)	You will be observed for this AC so it is important you make arrangements for this so that you can show how to move and handle equipment and other objects safely. In addition, if you complete any records in relation to moving and handling you could use these as work product evidence to support your observation. The case study will help you to understand a bit more about moving and handling.
LO6 Know how to handle hazardous substances and materials	
6.1 Research it (page 370)	Produce a written account to detail your findings.
6.1 Evidence opportunity (page 370)	Produce a written account that includes examples of the hazardous substances and materials that are present in your setting. For each one, write down what type they are and the potential dangers they pose. You could also produce a presentation that describes the hazardous substances and materials that are found in your work setting and explain the safe practices to follow with respect to their storage, use and disposal. You will find the COSHH file at work and your manager useful sources of information.
6.1 Reflect on it (page 370)	Write notes to document your thoughts.
6.2 Research it (page 370)	Write notes or produce a handout.
6.2 Research it (page 372)	Have a discussion with your manager. Produce a written account detailing your findings and discussion.
6.2 Research it (page 372)	Make notes to document your findings.
6.2 Reflect on it (page 373)	Write a short reflective account. You could also discuss this with a colleague and this may inform the account you write.
6.2 Evidence opportunity (page 373)	Produce an information leaflet. Or you could provide a written account.
LO7 Understand how to promote fire safety in the work setting	
7.1 Reflect on it (page 375)	You could discuss this with a colleague, and write a reflective account about your roles and responsibilities for preventing fires.
7.1 Evidence opportunity (page 375)	Have a discussion with your assessor as instructed in the activity. Write an account to evidence your discussion.
7.1 Research it (page 375)	Write notes to detail your research.
7.2 Reflect on it (page 376)	Write a reflective account answering the questions in the activity.
7.2 Research it (page 377)	Discuss with your manager the steps that you are required to take in the event of a fire. Make notes to detail your discussion.
7.2 Evidence opportunity (page 377)	Produce a poster or handout. You could also provide a written account detailing the emergency procedures to be followed if there is a fire in your work setting. You will find your work setting's emergency procedures and your manager a useful source of information.
7.3 Research it (page 377)	Have a discussion with your manager. Write notes detailing your discussion.
7.3 Reflect on it (page 378)	You could discuss this with a colleague, and make notes on what you find out.
7.3 Evidence opportunity (page 378)	Produce an information handout or you could write about the importance of maintaining clear evacuation routes at all times. You will find your work setting's emergency procedures and your manager a useful source of information.

→

Suggestions for using the activities

LO8 Be able to implement security measures in the work setting

8.1 Research it (page 380)	Tell a colleague about the news story you have read. Write notes detailing your thoughts.
8.1 Research it (page 381)	Produce a written account detailing your findings.
8.1 Reflect on it (page 381)	Provide a short written account.
8.1 Evidence opportunity (page 381) 8.1, 8.2 Case study (page 383)	You will be observed for AC 8.1 so it is important that you make arrangements for this so that you can show that you are able to check the identity of anyone requesting access to the premises and information. Follow up your demonstration with a professional discussion with your assessor. The case study will help you to understand more about implementing security measures at work.
8.2 Research it (page 382)	Write down notes to document your findings.
8.2 Reflect on it (page 382)	Write a short reflective account.
8.2 Evidence opportunity (page 382) 8.1, 8.2 Case study (page 383)	You will be observed for AC 8.2 so it is important that you make arrangements for this so that you can show that you are able to implement measures to protect your own security and the security of others. Follow up your demonstration with a professional discussion with your assessor. The case study will help you to understand more about implementing security measures at work.
8.3 Research it (page 384)	Produce an information leaflet with your findings.
8.3 Reflect on it (page 384)	Write a reflective account.
8.3 Evidence opportunity (page 384)	Make a list of the people you make aware of your whereabouts during your day-to-day work activities. Write an account of when and why you should make people aware of your whereabouts.

LO9 Know how to manage stress

9.1 Research it (page 386)	Explain the 'fight or flight' response to a colleague and provide a written account detailing this. You could also draw a spider diagram of the common signs and indicators of stress in yourself and others.
9.1 Reflect on it (page 386)	Write a short reflective account.
9.1 Evidence opportunity (page 386)	Design a poster, have a discussion with a colleague and make notes to evidence your discussion but you may need to omit the name of your colleague.
9.2 Reflect on it (page 387)	Write a reflective account.
9.2 Evidence opportunity (page 387)	Write a short account. You may find it helpful to discuss with your manager the circumstances and factors that tend to trigger stress in yourself and others. Remember to include a range of circumstances and factors and ensure these are relevant to both you and others.
9.3 Reflect on it (page 387)	Write a reflective account. You could also more generally write a reflective account on the ways you find most effective for managing your stress. Remember to also describe in your reflection how you access sources of support.
9.3 Research it (page 389)	Write notes to detail your findings.
9.3 Evidence opportunity (page 389)	Have a discussion with your manager and provide a written account to evidence your discussion.

Legislation	
Relevant Act	**It states that:**
Data Protection Act 1998	the right to privacy in relation to personal information must be upheld. Personal information about the individuals and others you may come across, such as individuals' families and your colleagues, must be kept confidential.
General Data Protection Regulation (GDPR) 2018	Also see Unit 206 for more information on the GDPR 2018.
Health and Safety at Work Act (HASAWA) 1974	the health and safety of everyone in a work setting must be protected, i.e. in a care setting this includes individuals, adult care workers and those who visit. It also established the key duties and responsibilities of all employers and employees in work settings.
Management of Health and Safety at Work Regulations (MHSWR) 1999	employers and managers must assess and manage risks by carrying out risk assessments. It requires employers to provide information, training and supervision so that work activities can be carried out safely.
Workplace (Health, Safety and Welfare) Regulations 1992	the working environment must be safe in relation to the building, its facilities and housekeeping and it must be healthy in relation to temperature, lighting and ventilation.
Manual Handling Operations Regulations 1992 (as amended 2002)	risks associated with moving and handling activities must be eliminated or minimised by employers. It also requires employers to provide information, training and supervision about safe moving and handling.
Provision and Use of Work Equipment Regulations (PUWER) 1998	work equipment used in work settings must be safe. It requires employees to receive training before using work equipment and requires work equipment to have visible warning signs.
Lifting Operations and Lifting Equipment Regulations (LOLER) 1998	lifting equipment used in work settings must be safe. It requires lifting equipment to be maintained and used solely for the purpose it was intended for. It also requires that all lifting operations are planned, supervised and carried out in a safe manner.
Personal Protective Equipment at Work Regulations 1992	personal protective equipment (PPE) to provide protection against infections must be provided free of charge by employers. It requires PPE to be maintained in good condition and requires training to be provided in the use of PPE.
Reporting of Injuries, Diseases and Dangerous Occurrences Regulations (RIDDOR) 2013	employers must report and keep records for three years of work-related accidents that cause death and serious injuries (referred to as reportable injuries), diseases and dangerous occurrences (i.e. incidents with the potential to cause harm). It requires work settings to have procedures in place and to provide information and training on reporting injuries, diseases and incidents.
Control of Substances Hazardous to Health (COSHH) 2002	employers must have procedures in place for safe working with hazardous substances and provide information, training and supervision so that work activities can be carried out safely.
Electricity at Work Regulations 1989	electricity and the electrical appliances that are used in work settings must be safe and requires employers to provide training to employees in relation to carrying out safety checks on electrical equipment.
Regulatory Reform Order (Fire Safety) 2005	fire risk assessments must be completed by the person responsible for the premises and requires the provision of fire equipment, fire escape routes and exits, as well as fire safety training.
The Health and Safety (First Aid) Regulations 1981	first aid and first aid facilities including trained first aiders must be provided.

→

Legislation	
Relevant Act	**It states that:**
Food Safety Act 1990	good personal hygiene must be maintained when working with food so that it is safe to eat and requires that records are kept of where food is from so that it can be traced if needed.
Food Hygiene (England) Regulations 2006	food safety hazards must be identified and that food safety controls are put in place, maintained and reviewed so that environments where food is prepared or cooked are safe.
Civil Contingencies Act 2004	organisations, such as emergency services, local authorities and health bodies, must work together to plan and respond to local and national emergencies. It requires that risk assessments are undertaken and emergency plans are put in place.

Resources for further reading and research

Books and booklets

Ferreiro Peteiro, M. (2014) *Level 2 Health and Social Care Diploma Evidence Guide,* Hodder Education

Health and Safety Executive (2016) 'Manual handling – Manual Handling Operations Regulations 1992 – Guidance on Regulations', Health and Safety Executive (HSE)

Health and Safety Executive (2014) 'Health and safety in care homes', (HSG220 – 2nd edition), Health and Safety Executive (HSE)

Health and Safety Executive (2014) 'Risk assessment: A brief guide to controlling risks in the workplace', Health and Safety Executive (HSE)

Health and Safety Executive (2012) 'How the Lifting Operations and Lifting Equipment Regulations apply to health and social care', Health and Safety Executive (HSE)

Health and Safety Executive (2012) 'Manual handling at work. A brief guide', Health and Safety Executive (HSE)

Weblinks

www.asthma.org.uk Asthma UK's website for information and resources about asthma

www.bhf.org.uk The British Heart Foundation's website for information and resources about heart disease

www.cqc.org.uk The Care Quality Commission's website for information and publications about how adult care settings meet the required standards of quality and safety

www.diabetes.org.uk Diabetes UK's website for information and resources about diabetes

www.gov.uk The UK Government's website for information about current legislation including the Health and Safety at Work Act (HASAWA) 1974

www.hse.gov.uk The Health and Safety Executive's website for information and resources about health and safety legislation and regulations including those relevant to care settings

www.skillsforcare.org.uk Skills for Care – resources and information on the Care Certificate, the code of conduct for adult care workers

www.skillsforhealth.org.uk Skills for Health – resources and information on the Care Certificate, the code of conduct for adult care workers

Glossary

Abuse means to mistreat someone, or treat them in a cruel way that causes them pain and hurt and thus violates their human and civil rights. The abuse can be physical, emotional, psychological or sexual. Neglect is also another form of abuse. It is important to be aware of the different types of abuse because you will be working with vulnerable people.

ACAS is an independent organisation that provides impartial and confidential advice to employees for resolving difficulties and conflicts at work.

Accidents are unexpected events that cause damage or injury, for example, a fall.

Accurate refers to ensuring records contain factually correct information.

Active listening is a communication technique that involves understanding and interpreting what is being expressed through verbal and non-verbal communication.

Adult care settings include residential care homes, nursing homes, domiciliary care, day centres, an individual's own home or some clinical healthcare settings.

Adult care workers enable individuals with care and support needs to live independently and safely.

Advocacy services support individuals to speak up when they are unable to; they represent the individual's best interests.

An **advocate** is a person who speaks on behalf of someone who is unable or unwilling to speak for themselves. They represent the views, needs and interests of these individuals and support them to express their views; this might, for example, be for an individual who has an illness or disability. They might put forward a 'case' when reviewing an individual's plan of care, for example.

Agreed ways of working are employers' policies, procedures and working practices. The 'agreed ways of working' may be documented less formally if you are working for smaller employers.

Allegations of abuse are when an individual tells you that they are being abused. Other people may also allege that abuse is happening to individuals.

Alzheimer's Society is the UK's leading dementia support and research charity for people affected by any form of dementia in England, Wales and Northern Ireland.

Anxiety is a feeling of fear or worry that may be mild or serious and can lead to physical symptoms, such as, shakiness.

Aphasia is a condition that affects a person's speech, understanding and use of language. An example of an aspect of this condition may be that they have difficulties putting words together to form sentences.

Asperger's syndrome is a disability that affects how individuals interact with others, i.e. individuals may have difficulty understanding and relating to other people and taking part in day-to-day activities.

The **Association of Directors of Adult Social Services (ADASS)** is a charity whose members are active directors of social care services and whose aim is to promote high standards of social care services.

Asthma is a lung condition that causes breathing difficulties that can range from mild to severe.

Attitude is the way you express what you think or believe through words or your behaviour.

Autism is a condition that affects how people perceive the world around them and interact with others. This can cause difficulties when communicating, interacting and socialising with others.

Autistic spectrum disorder is a lifelong condition that affects how a person perceives the world and interacts with others. For example, they may have difficulties interacting and socialising with others.

Barriers can be anything that prevent or stop you or others from communicating and understanding the communication.

Behaviour is the way in which you act, including towards others.

Beliefs are ideas that are accepted as true and real by the person who holds them. They could be religious, or political. They may also generally be to do with someone's morals or the way they live, for example 'I believe in treating others how I expect to be treated.'

Bodily fluids refer to fluids that circulate around the body or are expelled from the body such as blood, faeces, urine, sputum and vomit.

Boundaries are the limits that you must work within when carrying out your job role.

Braille is a method of written communication used by individuals who are blind. Characters (each letter) represented by patterns of raised dots are felt with the fingertips of the individual.

Brexit is a term that has been used for the United Kingdom leaving the European Union (EU). In 2016, the UK voted in a referendum and decided that they no longer wanted to be a member of the EU. There are a number of 'EU' laws that are in place in the UK. It is uncertain how these laws will be affected when the UK finally leaves the EU, which is likely to be in 2019.

Candour refers to a way of working that involves being open and honest with individuals, your employer and others in the care setting where you work when something has gone wrong. This includes incidents or near misses that may have led to harm.

The **Care Quality Commission (CQC)** is the independent regulator of all health and social care services in England.

Care settings can be residential homes, nursing homes, domiciliary care, day centres, an individual's own home or some clinical healthcare settings. Care settings refer to adult care settings as well as children and young people's health settings. In this qualification, it is adult care settings that are the focus.

Cerebral palsy is a condition that affects movement and co-ordination, for example, symptoms can include jerky uncontrolled movements, stiff and floppy arms or legs.

Chinese New Year, also known as the Spring Festival, is the most important celebration in the Chinese calendar where people share food and celebrate the year ahead together.

Clinical commissioning groups (CCGs) are organisations that are responsible for the provision of NHS services in England.

Clinical healthcare settings are places where healthcare professionals such as nurses, doctors, physiotherapists provide direct medical care to individuals such as in a clinic, pharmacy or in a GP surgery.

A **clinical waste bin** is where waste that is contaminated with body fluids is disposed of as it poses a risk of infection, for example, used dressings, bandages, disposable gloves, aprons. These are usually located in bathrooms and laundry areas.

Communication methods are ways of interacting with others using non-verbal and verbal techniques, and technological aids.

Compassion means delivering care and support with kindness, consideration, dignity and respect.

Compassionate care and support refers to providing care and support with consideration, kindness and while supporting individuals' rights such as privacy, dignity, respect.

Competence means to effectively apply the knowledge, skills and behaviours you have learned.

A **complainant** is the person who makes the complaint.

Complete refers to ensuring records contain full details and all the information that is necessary.

Comply or **complying** means to follow and ensure you are working in line with your employer's agreed ways of working.

Confidentiality means to keep something private. It refers to protecting an individual's personal, sensitive or restricted information and only disclosing it with those who need to know it. This might include information about an individual's diagnosis of a health condition. Confidentiality is important in an adult care setting because it respects an individual's rights to privacy and dignity, it will instil trust between you and others, it promotes an individual's safety and security and it shows compliance with legislation such as the Data Protection Act 1998 (replaced by the GDPR 2018).

Consent means informed agreement to an action or decision; the process of establishing consent will vary according to an individual's assessed capacity to consent. You will need to obtain 'consent' (or agreement or permission) from an individual or their representative if the individual is unable to consent. There are different types of consent and this is covered in Unit 201, AC 3.1 and Unit 211, LO3.

Continuing professional development refers to the process of identifying, documenting and monitoring the knowledge, skills and experience that you learn and apply at work.

Courage means being brave. In a care setting, it can take courage to do the right thing for people and speak up if the individual you support is at risk.

CQC inspectors monitor and check the quality of care settings. They check whether care settings are safe, providing effective care, treating individuals with dignity and respect and meeting individuals' needs.

Cross infection is the spread of infection from person to person.

Culture refers to the particular traditions or customs that describe a group of people who share those certain traditions, customs and values, perhaps from a different country or social group.

A **daily report book** is a record that is completed by adult care workers and includes information on the tasks, care and support provided on a day-to-day basis to individuals.

Dangerous occurrences are incidents that do not cause injury but have the potential to do so.

A **day centre** is a setting that provides leisure, educational, health and well-being activities during the day.

Dementia is a group of symptoms that affect how you think, remember, problem-solve, use language and communicate. These occur when brain cells stop working properly and the brain is damaged by disease.

Depression is a medical condition causing low mood that affects your thoughts and feelings. It can range from mild to severe but usually lasts for a long time and affects your day-to-day living.

Diabetes is a health condition that occurs when the amount of glucose (sugar) in the blood is too high because the body cannot use it properly.

Dignity in a care setting means respecting the views, choices and decisions of individuals and not making assumptions about how individuals want to be treated.

The **Disclosure and Barring Service (DBS)** is a government service that makes background checks for organisations, on people who want to work with children and adults with care or support needs.

Disclosure of abuse is when an individual tells you that abuse has happened, or is happening to them.

Discrimination means treating people unfairly or unlawfully, because they have a disability, or are of a different race, gender or age for example.

Diversity means different types and variation. In an adult care setting you will come across various different people, with different or 'diverse' backgrounds and needs. They may be different, for example, because of where they come from, how they dress, and their age. As a care worker, you will need to recognise, respect and value people's individual differences.

Diwali or Deepavali is the Hindu festival of lights celebrated every year in autumn where people share gifts and pray together.

Domiciliary care is where health and social care workers will provide care and support to individuals who live in their own home but require additional support with household tasks or personal care, for example. This might include assistance with getting dressed, taking medication and preparing meals.

Duties describe all the work and various tasks you are required to carry out as part of your job.

Duty of candour refers to the standards that adult care workers must follow when mistakes are made. This means being open and honest.

Duty of care refers to your responsibility or duty to ensure the safety and well-being of individuals and others while providing care or support.

Dysphasia is a condition that affects how a person understands language and is a less severe form of aphasia. For example, they may have difficulties listening and understanding what another person is saying.

Empathy is the ability to identify with another person's situation and understand how they may be feeling or thinking.

Epilepsy is a condition that affects the brain and causes repeated seizures or fits.

Equality refers to ensuring equal opportunities and rights are provided to everyone irrespective of their differences such as age, ability, race, background or religion. It means treating people fairly and valuing them for who they are. It means not to think of someone as being less important than anyone else.

Female genital mutilation (FGM) refers to a practice where the female genitals are deliberately cut, injured or changed and might be done because of cultural beliefs.

Fluid balance charts are used to record the amount of fluid being taken into and leaving (in the form of urine) a person's body, to monitor their hydration, which is necessary for their wellbeing.

A **formal complaint** is when a complaint may go on file and require an investigation.

Fraud means deliberately misleading a person to commit an unlawful act, for example, pretending to be an individual's relative on the telephone so that you can obtain personal information about the individual.

GDPR refers to the General Data Protection Regulation. This is a set of data protection laws that protects individuals' personal information. This superseded (or replaced) the Data Protection Act 1998 in May 2018.

Harm is caused as a result of abuse. Someone may have come to harm physically; they may experience distress, pain or injury. They may come to harm emotionally and may be frightened or worried as a result. This may be intentional or accidental. An adult at risk of harm may be an individual with care or support needs who is unable to protect themselves. This may include individuals with learning disabilities, mental health needs and older people. Also see definition of 'abuse'.

Hazards are dangers with the potential to cause harm, for example a spillage on the floor or a broken wheelchair.

Hazardous materials are materials that have the potential to cause harm and illness to others, for example, used dressings or PPE that has come into contact with body fluids.

Hazardous substances are substances that have the potential to cause harm and illness to others, for example, cleaning detergents, medication, acids and bodily fluids such as blood and urine.

Health and safety could be in relation to the safety of yourself, your colleagues or the people you support.

Health and safety checklists are used to record safety checks that are made in the environment such as ensuring fire alarms are working, windows locked securely and the first aid box is complete.

The **Health and Safety Executive (HSE)** is the independent regulator in the UK for health and safety in work settings.

A **health and safety officer** is a named person in an organisation that is responsible for overseeing all health and safety matters, for example reviewing health and safety procedures, investigating accidents at work.

Health and well-being boards are health and social care organisations that work together to improve the health and well-being of the people living in the local area they are responsible for.

Hearing impairment refers to hearing loss that may occur in one or both ears. This can be partial (some loss of hearing) or complete loss of hearing.

Heart disease is a condition that affects your heart and that can lead to mild chest pain or a heart attack.

Hepatitis is the term used to describe inflammation of the liver; hepatitis C is caused by the hepatitis C virus. This is usually spread through blood-to-blood contact with an infected person.

Honour-based violence refers to domestic violence committed in the name of 'honour'.

An **identifier** is a tool (the NHS Number) used to match people to their health records.

'In confidence' in a care setting, means to trust that the information will only be passed on to others who need to know.

Inclusion means being included or involved, for example being part of a wider group, or a group of friends. In an adult care setting, this means involving people in their care or the services they use so that they are treated fairly and not excluded. It means ensuring that all individuals are able to be included or partake in everyday life regardless of any differences. This can create a sense of belonging.

Individual refers to someone requiring care or support; it will usually mean the person or people you support.

Induction means an introduction to a new organisation or setting, or a new system of working.

Infection refers to when germs enter the body and cause an individual to become unwell.

An **informal complaint** might be someone highlighting a fault. This may be communicated verbally and may be resolved without requiring an investigation.

Interpreters are professionals who convert spoken/oral or sign language communication from one language to another.

A **job description** is a document that describes the purpose, duties and responsibilities to be carried out as part of your job.

The **Joseph Rowntree Foundation** is an independent organisation that encourages communities in the UK to work together to improve the lives of everyone.

A **key worker** is a person who works closely with the individual to understand their needs, wishes and preferences and who is specifically tasked with working closely with the individual.

The **Labour Force Survey (LFS)** is a study of the employment circumstances of the UK population. It is the largest household study in the UK and provides information in relation to employment and unemployment.

Lack of capacity is a term used to refer to when an individual is unable to make a decision for themselves because of a learning disability or a condition, such as, dementia or a mental health need or because they are unconscious.

Learning disabilities can be defined as a reduced ability to think and make decisions together with difficulties coping with everyday activities – which affect a person for their whole life. A person with a learning disability may experience problems with budgeting, shopping and planning a train journey.

Legible refers to ensuring records are written in a way that they can be easily read and understood.

Legislation is a process that involves making laws.

LGBTQ stands for lesbian, gay, bisexual, transgender, queer, and is used to emphasise the diversity of sexualities and gender identities.

Local systems may include employers' safeguarding policies and procedures as well as multi-agency protection arrangements for your local area, for example, a Safeguarding Adults Board.

Makaton is a method of communication using signs and symbols that is used by individuals who have learning disabilities.

Marie Curie is a charity that provides care and support for individuals and their families living with any terminal illness.

Mental capacity refers to an individual's ability to make their own decisions.

A **mentor** refers to a person in your work setting who has more experience than you and can provide you with guidance and advice in relation to your job role and responsibilities. This person, however, is there to offer advice more informally than your manager. If there is an issue, for example, that you are not sure how to address with your manager, you could talk to your mentor first.

Moving and handling charts are used to record the methods and equipment to be used with an individual for safely moving them from one position to another.

Moving and handling equipment includes hoists, bath lifts and slide sheets.

MRSA stands for meticillin-resistant *Staphylococcus aureus* and is often referred to as a 'superbug' because it is difficult to treat. It is a bacterium that can cause serious infections.

Musculoskeletal disorders refer to injuries, damage or disorders of the joints or other tissues in the upper and lower limbs or the back.

National Occupational Standards ensure that adult care workers provide good care and support and that best practice is followed.

Near misses refer to incidents that have the potential to cause harm such as a delay to administering an individual's medication or a hoist battery that runs out just before an individual is about to be moved from one position to another. It may be that the individual is not actually harmed, but they could have been, and so it is a 'near miss'.

'Need to know' means that you should only give away information that is absolutely necessary in order to protect an individual's privacy and ensure their safety.

Neglect means failing to care for someone so that their needs are not met.

Negotiation means reaching an agreement through discussion.

Norovirus is an infection of the stomach that causes diarrhoea and vomiting.

Nursing homes are homes that provide the same services as residential care homes but have registered nurses for individuals who have health needs.

Objective means to be fair, and not influenced by your own feelings or beliefs.

Ombudsman is a free independent service that investigates complaints against an organisation.

Open or **openness** means being truthful and approachable.

Open questions usually begin with 'What?', 'Why?' or 'How?' in order to encourage the expression of opinions and feelings. This is different to 'closed questions' which normally start with 'Who?' or 'Where?' and encourage short, factual answers.

Others may include team members, other colleagues, those who use or commission their own health or social care services, other professionals, families, carers and advocates.

An **outpatient mental health clinic** is a service that provides mental health treatments in the community rather than in a hospital setting.

Paraphrasing is a way of repeating what has been said or heard using different words.

Participation means to take part, or be involved. This refers to a way of working that supports individuals' rights to be involved in communications.

Personal assistants work directly for one individual with care and support needs, usually within the individual's own home.

A **personal development plan (PDP)** may have a different name but will record information such as agreed objectives for development, proposed activities to meet objectives, timescales for review.

Personal information refers to information that is personal to the individual such as their name, date of birth, weight, care needs.

Personal protective equipment (PPE) is equipment that is worn by care workers and is usually disposable to prevent infections from spreading, for example, disposable gloves, plastic aprons.

Person-centred practice refers to a way of working that takes into account the individual's whole person and focuses on an individual's specific needs, abilities, preferences and wishes. You may also wish to refer to Unit 211 on person-centred approaches.

A **physical disability** is a condition that affects and limits the way an individual moves and their ability to perform physical activities. Physical disabilities include being blind or in a wheelchair.

Physiotherapists are professionals who help people affected by injury, illness or disability through exercise, manual therapy.

Pitch means the quality of a vocal sound made by a person in communication e.g. low or high.

Policies and procedures may include other agreed ways of working as well as formal policies and procedures, for example in relation to how to carry out risk assessments.

Preferences refer to an individual's choices and wishes. These may be based on an individual's beliefs, values and culture.

Prejudice is a negative opinion that you may have of someone which is not based on experience or interaction.

Processing refers to handling information, i.e. recording, storing and sharing information.

Professional refers to carrying out your job in a skilful and knowledgeable way, showing behaviour that is moral and acceptable for the role that you are in.

Professional Councils are organisations that regulate professions, such as adult social care workers who work with adults in residential care homes, in day centres and who provide care in someone's home. They can provide advice and support around working with individuals who lack capacity to make decisions.

Professionalism means demonstrating or showing the knowledge, skills and behaviours expected in your job and showing that you are able to do this successfully and to a high standard.

Provision of care means providing care and support to individuals in line with their individual needs, wishes and preferences. This might include, providing assistance with household tasks, such as personal care tasks, socialising.

A **regulator** is an independent body that supervises a particular sector. It might inspect, monitor and rate adult social care services in terms of their safety, effectiveness, care and management.

Residential care homes are homes in which individuals live in. Care workers will provide meals and assistance with personal care tasks such as washing, dressing, eating.

Responsibilities describe *how* you are required to carry out your duties at work including the care you must show when you carry these out. They can include legal responsibilities (ones that you are required to fulfil like working to the requirements of the Data Protection Act 1998, replaced by the General Data Protection Regulation 2018) and moral duties and tasks that you are required to do as part of your job role.

Rights are legal entitlements to something, for example, to have the information held about you by an organisation kept secure.

Risk is the likelihood of hazards causing harm, for example slipping over on the spillage on the floor, an individual falling out of a broken wheelchair.

Risk assessment is used in work settings for identifying hazards, assessing the level of risk and putting in place processes for reducing or controlling the risks identified.

RNIB stands for the Royal National Institute of Blind People. This is a UK charity that provides information, advice, practical and emotional support to people affected by sight loss.

Safeguarding Adults Boards (SAB) safeguard adults with care or support needs by overseeing local adult safeguarding systems and ensuring all organisations work in partnership.

Schizophrenia is a long-term mental illness that affects how people think, feel and behave. They may see and hear things that others do not and/or hold strong beliefs that others do not have.

Sector Skills Councils are organisations led by and for specific employment sectors, for example Skills for Care is for the adult social care workforce and Skills for Health is for the healthcare workforce.

Services refer to organisations that provide translation, interpreting, speech and language and advocacy.

A **Shared Lives carer** is someone who opens up their home and family life to include an adult with support needs so that they can participate and experience community and family life. The individual may stay with them for the weekend, or they may even go on holiday together.

Signs are outwardly visible to others – you can see them. Signs of abuse can include unexplained or unusual bruises, sores and malnutrition. Signs can also present as changes in behaviour and moods.

Skills for Care is the sector skills council for people working in social work and social care for adults and children in the UK as well as for workers in early years, children and young people's services. It sets standards and develops qualifications for those working in the sector.

A **sling** refers to the piece of equipment made out of fabric that is placed around the individual's body to enable them to be hoisted.

Social workers assess, commission and co-ordinate care services and seek to improve outcomes for individuals, especially those who are more vulnerable. They may work in multi-disciplinary teams and can specialise in areas such as mental ill health, learning disabilities, care for older people or safeguarding.

Sources of support may include formal and informal support, supervision, appraisal, within and outside the organisation.

Speech and language services are providers of specialist communication information and support such as translation, interpreting, advocacy, speech and language services.

Standards may include codes of conduct and practice, regulations and minimum standards.

A **stereotype** is an oversimplified idea of what you think someone or something will be like, based on perhaps their culture or beliefs. For example: all young people are lazy; all older people develop dementia.

Stress is the body's physical and emotional reaction to being under too much pressure.

Sudden illnesses are unexpected medical conditions.

A **supervisor** refers to the person in your work setting that oversees your work and assesses your performance at work; this is usually your manager.

Suspicion of abuse is when you notice signs or are told by someone about signs that make you think or suspect abuse is happening.

Symptoms are experienced by individuals. They are an indication of something, for example feeling upset, angry, scared or alone. Symptoms could be the result of an illness, or abuse.

Technological aids refer to electronic aids that enable a person to communicate and interact.

Tone refers to the sound that you hear, i.e. volume, mood, feeling.

A **trade union representative** is a member of an organised group of workers who speaks up for the rights and interests of the employees of an organisation, for example in relation to safe working conditions.

Translators are professionals who convert written communication from one language to another.

Transparent or **transparency** is making the same information available to everyone.

Up to date refers to ensuring records contain information that reflects current information.

Values are ideas that form the system by which a person lives their life; often a person's beliefs can develop into their values.

A **vetting and barring scheme** ensures that anyone who is not fit or appropriate to work with adults and children does not do so.

Victimised means to single out someone, or pick on them. Here, it means when an individual is treated less fairly when they support or speak up for an individual with a protected characteristic.

Vocabulary means the words that are known and used by a person.

Well-being may include aspects that are social, emotional, cultural, spiritual, intellectual, economic, physical or mental. It can include how a person thinks and feels about themselves with regards to these aspects. More generally, it can also mean being healthy, comfortable, happy and in a positive state.

A **whistle-blower** is a worker who reports incorrect, unsafe or illegal practices at work.

Whistle-blowing refers to exposing any kind of information or activity that is deemed illegal, unethical or not correct. You may, for example, expose unsafe practice, abuse, harm or a serious fault in your setting. It may be a way of working that is not best practice and is having a negative impact on the individual or others.

Work settings may include one specific location or a range of locations, depending on the context of a particular work role. This might, for example, be an individual's home or a communal setting such as a residential care home.

Index

Note: page numbers in bold refer to key word definitions.